WORKBOOK
WITH DRUG CARDS
AND SKILL SHEETS

PARAMEDIC EMERGENCY CARE

SECOND EDITION

WORKBOOK WITH DRUG CARDS AND SKILL SHEETS

Robert S. Porter

BRADY

PARAMEDIC EMERGENCY CARE

SECOND EDITION

Bryan E. Bledsoe, D.O., EMT-P

Medical Director, Emergency Department
Baylor Medical Center
Waxahachie, Texas
and
Clinical Assistant Professor of Emergency Medicine
University of North Texas/Texas College of Osteopathic Medicine
Fort Worth, Texas

Robert S. Porter, M.A., NREMT-P

Director, Central New York Emergency Medical Service Program
Syracuse, New York

Bruce R. Shade, EMT-P

Commissioner, Cleveland Emergency Medical Services
Cleveland, Ohio

With Contributions From:

Richard A. Cherry, M.Ed., NREMT-P

Director of Paramedic Training
Department of Critical Care and Emergency Medicine
State University of New York Health Science Center
Syracuse, New York

Rod Dennison, EMT-P

Emergency Medical Services Division
Texas Department of Health
Public Health Region 1
Temple, Texas

Dexter W. Hunt, M.Ed., EMT-P

Senior Field Paramedic Preceptor
Ada County Emergency Medical Services
Boise, Idaho

Gary P. Morris, EMT-P

Deputy Fire Chief
Phoenix Fire Department
Phoenix, Arizona

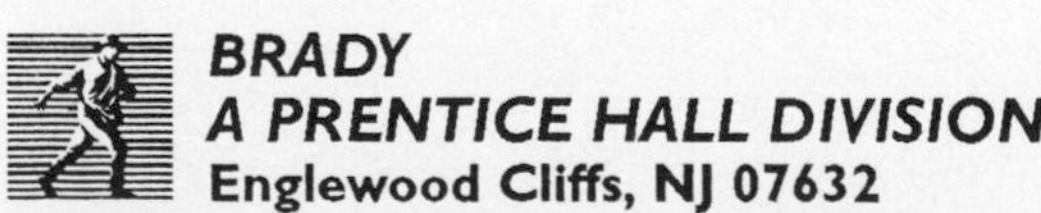

BRADY
A PRENTICE HALL DIVISION
Englewood Cliffs, NJ 07632

Production Editor: *Naomi Nishi*
Acquisitions Editor: *Mark Moscowitz*
Assistant Editor: *Judy Casillo*
Production Coordinator: *Ilene Sanford*

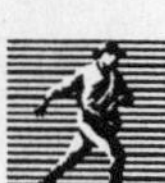
Prentice-Hall, Inc.
A Paramount Communications Company
Englewood Cliffs, New Jersey 07632

Printed in the United States of America

10 9 8 7 6 5 4 3 2

ISBN 0-89303-980-2

Prentice-Hall International (UK) Limited, *London*
Prentice-Hall of Australia Pty. Limited, *Sydney*
Prentice-Hall Canada Inc., *Toronto*
Prentice-Hall Hispanoamericana, S.A., *Mexico*
Prentice-Hall of India Private Limited, *New Delhi*
Prentice-Hall of Japan, Inc., *Tokyo*
Simon & Schuster Asia Pte. Ltd., *Singapore*
Editora Prentice-Hall do Brasil, Ltda., *Rio de Janeiro*

Self-Instructional Workbook

PARAMEDIC EMERGENCY CARE

CONTENTS

DIVISION I

Prehospital Environment

DIVISION 2

Preparatory Information

DIVISION 3

Trauma Emergencies

DIVISION 4
Medical Emergencies

DIVISION 5
Obstetrical and Gynecological Emergencies

DIVISION 6
Psychiatric Emergencies

WORKBOOK ANSWER KEY

National Registry of EMTs

EMERGENCY DRUG CARDS

PATIENT CARE SCENARIOS

Workbook Comment Form

WELCOME
to the
Self-Instructional Workbook
to
PARAMEDIC EMERGENCY CARE

Welcome to the second edition of the Self-Instructional Workbook for Paramedic Emergency Care. We have received many comments about the first edition from both students and instructors and have used them to make the workbook even more helpful and easy to use. Like the first edition, this book can be used either as a stand-alone workbook or with instructor supervision. It addresses the National Standard Curriculum for Paramedic training and meets the content described by the DOT Objectives.

This workbook is designed to help you identify the important principles presented in PARAMEDIC EMERGENCY CARE and direct you to review any material you don't truly understand. The workbook addresses each case study presented in PEC and explains why certain aspects of care are offered. Self-examinations test your reading comprehension and prepare you for the tests within your training course and for state examination.

With this new edition, we're very excited to announce the addition of two new features designed to help you integrate the material in PEC and think on your feet, much as you must do in the field. These are:

Division Reviews

After each unit, a division review now helps you recall and build on your knowledge through scenario-based questions. The scenarios discuss the aspects of care from the preceding chapters and bring all the information learned together.

Patient Scenario Flash Cards

Now, in the back of the workbook, are 40 patient scenario flash cards. Each describes the signs and symptoms of a medical emergency on one side and the field diagnosis and steps of care on the other. Detach the cards and use them to practice your recognition of common medical emergencies. Then practice prescribing the appropriate emergency care steps.

Other features continued with this edition of the workbook include:

Objective Review

Each chapter of the workbook begins with a short review of the focus of each learning objective. Use these objectives and the associated comments to identify what is important to learn during your reading of **PARAMEDIC EMERGENCY CARE**.

Case Study Review

The workbook reviews the case study beginning each chapter of the text. It identifies principles and special considerations of care. It can help you learn about the elements of field care associated with each chapter of the text.

Reading Self-exam

Each chapter contains between 10 and 50 questions which test your comprehension. Take each self-exam carefully and then check your answers against the key in the back of this workbook. If you scored well, just review the questions you missed.

Ambulance Report Form

The workbook enhances the information given by the case study and then asks you to record the appropriate information on an ambulance report form. Check your documentation against the form found in the answer key for completeness and inclusion of the essential points of the run report.

Drug Math Worksheets

The drug math worksheets let you practice working with drug dosages and math required to calculate flow rates and administer field medications. Take the drug math and drip calculation exercises and again check your answers and the math against the key in the back of the book.

Emergency Drug Flash Cards

The workbook contains perforated 3-by-5 inch cards which present the emergency drug name, description, indications, contra-indications, precautions, and dosage/route. Detach the cards and use them in a flash card fashion. Practice until you can give the correct route, dosage, indications, and contraindications for each drug.

ECG Rhythm Strips

Two exercises in the recognition of ECG dysrhythmias are included to assist you in learning how to recognize dysrhythmias that are clinically significant in the care of the patient with cardiovascular problems. Review these dysrhythmia examples until you are comfortable in their recognition.

With these special features and the addition of many new self-exam questions, this revised and expanded workbook aims to smooth your way on the very demanding and rewarding road to becoming a paramedic. Good luck.

Dedication

This effort is dedicated to Russell, my son, whose endless desire for knowledge and naive outlook on life have served as an inspiration to me while authoring this workbook.

Acknowledgments

Special thanks must be given to those whose names do not appear on the cover of this workbook, yet without whom this effort would not have been possible. They are Susan Katz, whose direction of the Brady Publishing line has brought new life into EMS education, and her right- and left-hand person, Natalie Anderson. And thanks are due to Judy Casillo and Tally Morgan, who took the raw manuscript from hen-scratching to a finished product. With the second edition of PARAMEDIC EMERGENCY CARE thanks are extended to Mark Moscowitz, Nancy Brandwein, Lois Berlowitz, and Charly Miller. Charily assured the content accuracy while the others ensured its aesthetic appeal, spelling, and grammar. Thank you.

Patient Care Scenarios

The Patient Care Scenarios found at the end of this workbook have been developed to help you put together the concepts of disease recognition and patient care. Their development was accomplished by James E. Moshinskie, Ph.D., EMT-P. Jim is well respected educator in Texas, and the Director of EMS Education and Assistant Professor of Emergency Medicine for Texas A&M University - College of Medicine, Temple, Texas.

Special Note

PARAMEDIC EMERGENCY CARE and this workbook have been extensively reviewed and edited to make them as accurate and up-to-date as possible. Yet the authors understand that there are constant changes in the knowledge and skills that we call emergency medical service. To that end, we have included a perforated form at the end of the workbook answer key. It is designed to record any comments, concerns, or corrections that you have regarding PARAMEDIC EMERGENCY CARE or this workbook. Please record those comments and mail them to the address found on the form. We are interested in your comments and suggestions. Comments from the first edition have been used in improving this second offering.

I

ROLES AND RESPONSIBILITIES OF THE PARAMEDIC

Review of the Objectives for Chapter I

With each chapter of the workbook we will identify the objectives and the important elements they describe. You should review them and refer to the pages listed if the elements are not clear.

After reading this chapter, you should be able to:

1. Define the role of the EMT-Paramedic.

p. 4

Provide competent medical care
Provide emotional support for the patient
Concentrate on the care and well being of the patient
Provide care to those who may not appreciate the service

2. Define and give examples of professional ethics.

pp. 6 to 9

Ethics are rules or standards of conduct primarily for the benefit of the patient and not laws, but standards for honorable behavior. As a paramedic you are responsible to the patient, society, health professionals, and your profession.

3. Define and give examples of behavior that characterizes the health care professional.

p. 9

Sincerity, compassion, grace, respect for human dignity
Proficient technician
Respectful of patient rights and feelings
Patient well being placed above all except personal safety
Professionalism
- Patient first
- Skills mastery
- Continuing education
- Prepared for response - vehicle, equipment, personally
- Respectful of other health care and public safety personnel

4. List the duties of the EMT-Paramedic in preparation for handling emergency medical responses.

p. 10

Physically fit
Familiar with system policies and procedures, communications, equipment, geography, and support agencies

Personal attributes of self confidence, credibility, inner strength, self control, leadership, and willingness to accept responsibility

5. List the duties of the EMT-Paramedic during an emergency response.

pp. 10 to 11

Drive responsibly
Survey the scene, call for needed assistance, and assure safety
Conduct patient assessment, assign care priorities
Provide basic and advanced emergency medical care in accordance with local protocols
Assess the results of care
Communicate with team members and medical command
Direct transport of the patient to the appropriate medical facility
Maintain rapport with the patient and public safety and hospital personnel

6. List the duties of the EMT-Paramedic after an emergency response.

pp. 11 to 12

Accurately and objectively document all elements of the response
Re-stock the ambulance, assure all equipment is cleaned and operational
Review the call with team members

7. List the post-graduation responsibilities of the EMT-Paramedic.

pp. 12 to 13

Obtain and maintain licensure, certification
Maintain knowledge and skills
Update knowledge and skills
Educate the public - First Aid, CPR, etc.

8. Distinguish between certification, licensure, and reciprocity.

pp. 12 to 13

Certification is recognition that an individual has met a standard of performance
Licensure is the granting of permission to engage in an occupation
Reciprocity is the granting of certification or licensure for comparable certification or licensure by another agency

9. State the benefits and responsibilities of continuing education for the EMT-Paramedic.

p. 13

Maintain initial skills and knowledge
Obtain new skills and knowledge

10. State the major purposes of a national organization.

pp. 13 to 14

Share ideas and concerns
Speak with a unified voice to the issues facing Emergency Medical Service
Continue education (newsletters and conferences)

11. List some national organizations for EMS providers.

p. 13

National Association of Emergency Medical Technicians
National Association of Flight Paramedics
National Association of Search and Rescue
National Council of State EMS Training Coordinators
National Association of State EMS Directors
National Association of EMS Physicians

12. State the major purposes of the National Registry of Emergency Medical Technicians.

p. 14

National testing of EMT-Basic, EMT-Intermediate and EMT-Paramedic
Establishes standards for re-registration
Basis for inter-state reciprocity

13. Describe the major benefits of subscribing to professional journals.

p. 14

Identifies the results of current EMS research
Continuing education
Vehicle for authorship

CASE STUDY REVIEW

As was mentioned within PARAMEDIC EMERGENCY CARE, it is important to review each call you participate in as a paramedic. Similarly, we will review the case study that precedes each chapter. We will address the important points of scene survey, patient assessment, patient management, patient packaging, and transport.

Reread the case study in **PARAMEDIC EMERGENCY CARE** and then read the discussion below.

This is a two-part case study which is designed to examine the changes that have occurred over the past three decades in emergency medical services.

Chapter I Case Study

July 1958:

Communications over thirty years ago were certainly not as efficient as those of today. System entry was a problem, as was the dispatch of the most appropriate ambulance. The vehicle which was dispatched was not as specialized for patient care as those of today. The focus of the 1958 ambulance was speed rather than the ability to house equipment and provide an environment to allow care while en route to the hospital.

Training for personnel was also very different. As identified by the care given, the "Ambulance Drivers" were not concerned with stabilizing injuries or providing any comfort to the patient. Their job was simply rapid transport to a hospital where (presumably) the patient could receive life-saving care.

The Present:

Today the picture is dramatically better. System entry is much improved, as is the response from the personnel. The system is accessed by the 911 telephone system in a large percentage of the country and a trained dispatcher takes the needed information. First responders are quick to arrive, while the paramedic is moving rapidly but safely to the scene. She readies the equipment and places it on the stretcher in preparation for the potentially severe trauma called in by the passer-by and confirmed by the first responders. As the Advanced Life Support ambulance arrives, the first responder communicates the nature and extent of injury for each of the five patients. The authority for patient care is smoothly transferred to the senior paramedic, and personnel are directed to each of the patients.

Specialized prehospital emergency care equipment, not available in 1958, is brought from the unit to the patient's side and she is stabilized quickly. Advanced life support is provided and the most severe patient transported only minutes after the first ambulance arrives. During transport the hospital is alerted to the incoming patients and the nature of the young lady's injuries. As the ambulance backs into the emergency entrance, the trauma team waits to take the patient to the trauma suite.

The paramedic gives a quick update regarding the patient condition and answers a few questions before the doctor and team assume responsibility for the patient. The reports are filed and the IV solutions, trauma tubing, and IV initiation materials are replaced. The ambulance is taken to the base, washed out and inspected before the team is reported as ready for service.

The EMS team sits down over lunch and critiques the call. Jane, the lead paramedic, compliments her assisting EMT for anticipating the equipment she needed. She also is complimentary about the rapid and secure application of the cervical collar and modified short spine board. They talk about better patient calming and reassurance and review the setup for a rapid infusion of fluid for the hypovolemic trauma patient. Later, Jane calls the hospital to find how the patient is doing and asks if the medical command physician felt there was anything the crew could have done better.

Over the past thirty-five years there have been great strides in prehospital care. The equipment is extensive and specially designed for the rigors and unique applications of field service. Training is just as extensive and specially designed. The entire EMS system will continue to evolve as we learn more about trauma and the medical emergency.

GUIDELINES TO BETTER TEST TAKING

Not only is it important to read the text carefully but to also be able to show that you learned from your reading. Here are a few guidelines that may help improve your test-taking performance. (These guidelines may be helpful for both your class tests and those in this workbook.)

1. Relax and be calm during the test.

A test is designed to measure what you have learned. An exam is not designed to intimidate or punish you. Consider it a challenge and just try to do your best. Avoid coffee or other stimulants for a few hours before the exam and be prepared. Reread the text chapters, review the objectives in the workbook and review your class notes.

2. Read the questions carefully.

Read each word of the question and all the answers slowly. Words such as "except" or "not" may change the entire meaning of the question. If you miss them you may answer the question incorrectly even though you know the right answer.

3. Read each answer carefully.

Read each and every answer carefully. While the first answer may be absolutely correct, the rest may also be and the best answer might be "all of the above."

4. Delay questions you don't understand or can't answer.

When a question seems confusing or you don't know the answer, note it on your answer sheet and come back to it later. This will ensure that you have time to complete the test. You will also find that other questions in the test may give you hints to the one you've skipped over. It will also prevent you from being frustrated with an early question and have it affect your performance.

5. Answer all questions.

Even if you do not know the right answer, do not leave the question blank. A blank question is always wrong, while a guess might be correct. If you can eliminate some of the answers, do so. It will increase the chances of a correct guess.

READING COMPREHENSION SELF-EXAM

Each of the chapters within this workbook will include a short self-exam. The questions are designed to test your ability to remember what you read. At the end of the workbook the answers will be given as will the pages where the topic of the question was discussed. If you answer the question incorrectly, review the pages listed.

1. The process by which an organization grants recognition that an individual has met its standards of performance is called ....

   A. licensure.
   B. certification.
   C. an ethic.
   D. reciprocity.
   E. none of the above.

   Answer B

2. The rules or standards governing the conduct of members of a particular group or profession are called ....

   A. ethics.
   B. morals.
   C. licensure.
   D. certification.
   E. registration.

   Answer A

3. The first paramedic training program is generally accepted to have been held in which of the following cities?

   A. Los Angeles
   B. Seattle
   C. Columbus
   D. Miami
   E. Pittsburgh

   Answer D

4. One of the greatest impacts upon the public's feelings toward the Emergency Medical Services system came from the television program "Emergency." Which of the following are aspects of that program's presentation of the paramedics, Gage and Desoto?

   A. clean-cut
   B. responded promptly
   C. remained calm
   D. skillful and compassionate
   E. all of the above

   Answer E

5. The art and science of Emergency Medical Service involves all of the following except ....

   A. sincerity and compassion.
   B. respect for human dignity.
   C. placing patient care before personal safety.
   D. delivery of sophisticated emergency medical care.
   E. none of the above are excluded.

   Answer C

6. As members of the Allied Health Professions, paramedics must recognize a responsibility to ....
   1. their patients.
   2. society.
   3. other health professionals.
   4. themselves.

   Select the proper grouping.

   A. 1, 2
   B. 2, 3, 4
   C. 1, 2, 3
   D. 1, 2, 4
   E. 1, 2, 3, 4

   Answer E

7. Which of the following organizations is responsible for testing EMTs and Paramedics on a national level?

   A. National Association of EMTs
   B. National Registry of EMTs
   C. National Association of Search and Rescue
   D. National Association of EMS Physicians
   E. none of the above

   Answer B

8. Offering of recognition for meeting standards set forth by another agency or state is called ....

   A. licensure.
   B. certification.
   C. reciprocity.
   D. registration.
   E. none of the above.

   Answer C

9. The paramedic, often being the highest trained emergency care professional at the scene, is responsible for the supervision of the members of the emergency medical services team.

   A. True
   B. False

   Answer A

10. The ambulance run-sheet should include which of the following?
    1. accurate and complete documentation
    2. clear and concise opinions
    3. objectively recorded observations

    Select the proper grouping.

    A. 1
    B. 2
    C. 2, 3
    D. 1, 3
    E. 1, 2, 3

    Answer D

11. Upon successful completion of a course of training as an EMT-P most states will ....

A. certify you.
B. license you.
C. register you.
D. recognize you as a paramedic.
E. issue you a permit.

Answer A

12. After a call, the paramedic is responsible for ....
1. re-stocking the ambulance.
2. completing the run-sheet.
3. ensuring that team members are not affected by stress.
4. reviewing the call with team members.

Select the proper grouping.

A. 1, 2
B. 2, 3
C. 2, 3, 4
D. 1, 3, 4
E. 1, 2, 3, 4

Answer E

13. Continuing education is intended to ....

A. maintain a paramedic's initial knowledge.
B. address didactic knowledge only.
C. broaden a paramedic's knowledge.
D. A and C.
E. none of the above.

Answer D

14. Professional journals provide the paramedic with ....

A. an opportunity to write and publish articles.
B. a source of continuing education material.
C. information on new procedures for the field.
D. all of the above.
E. none of the above.

Answer D

15. The EMT-Paramedic will most probably spend more time preparing to perform his or her duties (cleaning and re-stocking the ambulance, reading and attending continuing education sessions, documenting the last call, etc.) than responding to emergency medical calls.

A. True
B. False

Answer A

16. List at least three responsibilities of the paramedic in preparation for the Emergency Medical Service response.

Be mentally, physically, emotionally prepared Optional:
Be Aware of protocals & medical Knowledge. Have leadership Qualitys
Be aware of Support Services Be Aware of local geography.

17. List at least 5 responsibilities of the Paramedic during the emergency response.

Size up and secure the scene.

Patient assessment

Communicate with crew members.

asses effects of treatment

Coordinate Patient transport

Optional:

Determin resource needs.

Initiate Basic & Advanced life Support.

assign priorityes of care.

18. Identify at least five attributes of leadership that should be found in the Paramedic.

Self confidence

Assume controll

willing to except responsibility

Creditability

Communication Skills

Optional:

Knowledge of crew members capibiltys

inner Strength

willing to make decisions

19. Describe the expectations the public has of the Emergency Medical Service System because of the television programs "911" or "Code 3."

Clean cut

Remain Calm

responded promptly

Skill full

Solution for everything

Top quality care.

20. Review the case study for this chapter and identify the shortcomings of the 1958 EMS system.

Slow septen entry

no communication system

limited space to work.

no patient care of stablezation

no scene assesment

limited equipment.

2

EMERGENCY MEDICAL SERVICES SYSTEM

Review of the Objectives for Chapter 2

After reading this chapter, you should be able to:

1. Describe the development of the EMS system in the United States.

pp. 20 to 21

Accidental Death and Disability: The Neglected Disease of Modern Society describes the nature and extent of trauma and the poor state of prehospital care in 1965
1966 Highway Safety Act - first federal funding for the EMS system
1973 Emergency Medical Services System Act - development of regional EMS systems
1981 Block Grant - federal funding for the EMS system

2. List and define the components of an EMS system.

pp. 20 to 21

Personnel
Laypersons trained in CPR and first aid
First Responder
Emergency Medical Technician
Paramedic
Dispatcher
Emergency Physician
Emergency Nurse
Specialty Physicians

Equipment
medical care
communications
the ambulance

Resources
Police
Fire Service
Rescue

3. Explain the oversight duties of an EMS administrative agency.

pp. 21 to 22

Oversees state, regional, and local agencies
Develops policies governing system and personnel function
Selects a Medical Director and advisory council
Identifies who may function within the system
Procures funding
Enacts legislation and/or ordinances
Enforces policies, rules, and regulations

4. Discuss the responsibilities of the physician medical director regarding on-line (direct) and off-line (indirect) medical control.

pp. 22 to 24

Delegates authority to practice medicine - prehospital
Patient remains the patient of medical control whether direct or indirect

Direct

direct communication with medical control physician
responsible for patient - delegate care
paramedic / physician interaction

Indirect

training and continuing education
medical protocols (non-interaction)

Triage	**Treatment**
Transport	**Transfer**

medical audit / chart review / quality assurance

5. Describe public involvement in an EMS system, with regard to system access, recognition of an emergency, and initiation of basic life support.

pp. 24 to 25

Knowledge of system entry, be it 9-1-1, single number or multi-number entry
Training in First Aid and CPR
Early defibrillation

6. Describe the components of an effective medical and operational communications system.

pp. 25 to 26

Citizen access
Single control center
Organizational communications capabilities
Medical communications capabilities
Hardware (radios, towers, pages, etc.)
Software (frequencies, protocols, communications plans)

7. Describe the components of Emergency Medical Service dispatching:

pp. 26 to 28

System status management is a dynamic use of resources to best meet the needs of the service area and the ambulance crews
Interrogation guidelines are used to ensure that the appropriate information is gathered from the caller
Response protocols guide the dispatcher in matching the caller's information with the dispatch of the most appropriate unit(s) and personnel for the patient's need
Pre-arrival instructions communicate care instructions to the caller, assisting them to provide patient care
Dispatcher training assures both medical and technical preparation for their role

8. Describe the use of patient transfer protocols for ground and air transport services.

p. 32

Patient transported to the closest appropriate facility
Special services - trauma, burn, pediatric, neuro, etc.
American College of Emergency Physicians ALS equipment list
Licensed vehicles - KKK-A-1822 - type I, II or III
Air medical transport - rotorcraft or fixed wing ($>$120 mi)
Transfer protocols define criteria for selection of a receiving facility

9. Describe the importance of quality evaluation in EMS, and discuss the similarities and differences between Quality Assurance and Quality Improvement programs.

pp. 32 to 33

An EMS system must be designed to meet the needs of the patient with excellence as the only acceptable quality. Quality Assurance and Quality Improvement programs are designed to continuously move the EMS system toward excellence.

Quality Assurance programs continuously monitor and measure the quality of the EMS system or service. They focus on response times and the standard of care.

Quality Improvement programs focus on patient (the customer) perceptions in addition to the items evaluated by the Quality Assurance programs.

10. Discuss the value of research in EMS.

p. 34

Determine which care procedures/equipment benefit the patient
Determine benefit/risk ratio for procedures
Determine cost/benefit of sophisticated EMS interventions

11. Describe the categorization of receiving facilities, and explain how the coordination of resources is attained.

pp. 34 to 35

Inventory to determine ability of facility to respond to the particular emergency
Emergency department - level I, II or III
Support services - burn, trauma, pediatric, perinatal, cardiac, spinal, psychiatric, or poison control centers

12. List the components of mutual aid and mass-casualty planning.

pp. 36

System tested by frequent drills
Pre-established policies which determine action during times of system overload
Plan for and test personnel, vehicles, equipment, supplies, and communications utilization

13. Outline the various designs and financing methods for an EMS system.

p. 36

EMS service type - hospital, fire department, police department, municipal third service, private commercial, private non-profit
Personnel reimbursement - full-time, part-time, volunteer
Funding - tax subsidies, contributions, corporate sponsorship, Medicare, Medicaid, medical and auto insurance, subscription plans, user fees, HMOs, etc.

CASE STUDY REVIEW

Reread the case study in **PARAMEDIC EMERGENCY CARE** and then read the discussion below.

This case study is an overview of the Emergency Medical Services System with a focus on system entry, the contributions trained bystanders can provide, and the tiered response system.

Chapter 2 Case Study

The case study describes the ideal response to the cardiac arrest or other serious emergency. The only missing component is the recognition of cardiac symptoms by the victim which might have drawn the EMS system into response before the actual arrest. The remaining components include citizen CPR and First Aid, and (included within those training programs) an understanding of how to enter the EMS system. The scenario also identifies the four level tiered response: the bystander, the First Responder, the EMT, and the Paramedic. With each level of training is an increasing ability to provide medical care for the patient.

CPR is being done by bystanders. This alone expands the time from cardiac arrest until brain death, and increases the chance that the EMS system can successfully resuscitate the patient. CPR, First Aid training, and knowledge of EMS system entry (911 or other emergency telephone number) can improve the system response. These programs allow earlier system entry and response to an emergency, and increase the ability of the system to help the person in need. The system described utilizes 911 access to the public safety services; police, fire, and Emergency Medical Service. The number is easy to remember and dial, even in the stress of the emergency. Enhanced 911 telephone systems will display the address of the calling phone and provide directions to the residence or business. The system will allow for immediate call back should the line be disconnected, the caller information found to be incomplete, or the call is suspected as a prank.

The dispatcher is not only able to take information and assure that the best response is provided, he may also calm the caller and elicit further information. In some cases the dispatcher may instruct the caller in some First Aid procedures.

First Responders are able to arrive at the patient's side quickly. They have less training than the EMT or Paramedic but are more available. Many systems use fire fighters, police officers or individuals who are solely trained as First Responders. Not only do they have the ability to apply care rapidly, they are often able to identify the seriousness of the medical problem and help summon the appropriate resources to the scene.

The third tier of response is the EMT, or in this case the EMT-Intermediate. The EMT provides a higher level of medical care through more extensive training and the use of equipment designed for field application. A new and promising adjunct to the care of the EMT is the use of the automatic defibrillator. It is a device that senses and interprets the heart's electrical activity. If it finds the heart is in need of defibrillation, it will send a shock through the chest. Such a device, quickly applied to a cardiac arrest patient, can greatly increase survival.

The final stage of the tiered response is delivery of advanced life support by the paramedics. They are the highest level of EMS prehospital care and the agents of medical command authority. They are directed in their actions by protocols or by direct communications with an emergency department physician. They may employ intravenous routes for the administration of fluid and/or drugs, advanced devices to secure the airway, the monitor/defibrillator to monitor the heart rhythm or electrically shock it, and an expanded knowledge of the anatomy and physiology, pathophysiology, assessment, and management of the patient and the medical problem.

Lastly, this case study identifies the emergency department as a component of the EMS system. It is the transition between the prehospital setting and the intensive care units or surgery. It is where the patient is evaluated (triaged) to determine the nature and severity of the problem. It is also where the care which began in the field will continue. It is staffed by a physician who specializes in emergency medicine and is complemented by nurses and ancillary personnel with the same emphasis. For these reasons, it is more correctly referred to as an emergency department than a room.

READING COMPREHENSION SELF-EXAM

1. The system which makes use of several levels of responding emergency medical services personnel - the First Responder, EMT, and Paramedic - is called ....

A. the tiered response system.
B. a multifaceted system.
C. an advanced life support system.
D. a fail-safe system.
E. none of the above.

Answer A

2. **All prehospital medical care provided by the paramedic is considered an extension of the medical director's license.**

A. True
B. False

Answer A

3. **The hospital health professional responsible for sorting patients as they arrive at the emergency department is usually the ....**

A. emergency physician.
B. ward clerk.
C. emergency nurse.
D. trauma surgeon.
E. A or C.

Answer E

4. **Medical command, which is provided by on-line radio contact between the paramedic and the medical control physician, is which type of medical command?**

A. protocol
B. direct
C. indirect
D. intrinsic
E. none of the above

Answer B

5. **When a paramedic is called by the patient (through the dispatcher) to the scene of a medical emergency, the medical control physician has established a physician/patient relationship.**

A. True
B. False

Answer A

6. **The physician who called for paramedics to transport his patient, without accompanying the patient, remains in charge and responsible for the care provided to the patient until the patient is attended by another physician in the emergency department.**

A. True
B. False

Answer B

7. **Indirect medical command is considered to be ....**

A. treatment protocols.
B. training and education.
C. quality assurance.
D. chart review.
E. all of the above.

Answer E

8. **Protocols standardize field procedures. They should not allow the paramedic flexibility to improvise nor adapt to special circumstances.**

A. True
B. False

Answer B

9. The device which may in the future be used by the First Responder or bystander, and may significantly affect cardiac arrest survival is the ....

A. transcutaneous pacemaker.
B. esophageal obturator airway.
C. automatic external defibrillator.
D. pulse oximetry.
E. all of the above.

Answer C

10. The dispatch system which locates ambulances based upon projected call volume to reduce response times is called ....

A. priority dispatching.
B. system status management.
C. interrogation protocols.
D. medical direction.
E. none of the above.

Answer B

11. The dispatch system which interrogates the caller, prioritizes symptoms, selects the appropriate response, and provides the caller with life-saving instruction is called ....

A. priority dispatching.
B. system status management.
C. interrogation protocols.
D. medical direction.
E. none of the above.

Answer A

12. The ideal EMS dispatch system includes which of the following?
1. caller interrogation protocols
2. pre-determined response configurations
3. system status management
4. pre-arrival instructions for caller
5. strong medical control

Select the proper grouping.

A. 1, 2, 3
B. 2, 4, 5
C. 1, 2, 3, 5
D. 1, 3, 4, 5
E. 1, 2, 3, 4, 5

Answer E

13. Quality Assurance and Improvement programs look at ....

A. response times.
B. adherence to protocols.
C. patient survival.
D. customer perceptions.
E. all of the above.

Answer E

14. Many protocols and procedures that paramedics use today have evolved without clinical evidence of their usefulness, safety, or benefit to the patient.

A. True
B. False

Answer A

15. Quality Improvement programs differ from Quality Assurance programs in that Quality Improvement also looks at ....

A. customer satisfaction.
B. dispatch procedures.
C. quality of care.
D. mortality and morbidity.
E. none of the above.

Answer A

16. Place the following elements in order as they would occur in a research project.
1. develop a hypothesis or question to be asked
2. prepare a paper for a magazine
3. collect and analyze data
4. search the literature
Select the proper grouping.

A. 1, 4, 3, 2
B. 2, 3, 1, 4
C. 3, 1, 4, 2
D. 4, 1, 3, 2
E. 1, 2, 3, 4

Answer A

17. Which of the following is an example of hospital categorization?

A. a Burn Center
B. a Trauma Center
C. a Perinatal Center
D. a Cardiac Center
E. all of the above

Answer E

18. EMS system funding can come from ....

A. tax subsidies.
B. Medicare, Medicaid.
C. subscription plans.
D. user fees.
E. all of the above.

Answer E

19. The elements of a mass-casualty plan should include ....
1. closely defined geographical boundaries.
2. a flexible communication system.
3. major dispatch staff changes when the disaster occurs.
4. a central management agency.
Select the proper grouping.

A. 1, 3
B. 1, 4
C. 2, 3
D. 2, 4
E. 1, 2, 3

Answer D

20. EMS systems are designed with the patient as the highest priority. They begin with a strong administrative agency, which structures the system around the patient's needs, and grants the medical director ultimate authority in all issues of patient care.

A. True
B.False

Answer A

21. Identify the purpose of each of the four types of protocols.

Triage:

Guidelines to determining what levels of EMS Response
Guidelines to determining where a particular patient will go.

Treatment:

Guidelines for Patent Care
Direct orders by physician (on-line)
Standing orders (off line)

Transport:

Guidelines to determine mode of transport (air or ground)
level of care determined by nature of Illness or injury
patient conditional, transport time.

Transfer:

guidelines for inter-hospital transports
ensure patient travels to an appropiate facility

22. What skills are associated with each level of Emergency Medical Services certification?

EMT - Basic: (at least 5)

CPR

hemmorage Controll

emergency Childbirth

Communication

Automatic defibrillation

Optional:

Airway management

Stabilization of fractures.

Basic extrication

use of the PASG

EMT - Intermediate: (at least 2)

Skills of the Emt Basic

fluid therapy

Optional:

use EOA or EGTA

other Advanced Skills

EMT - Paramedic: (at least 4)

Skills of Emt Basic

Advanced Patient Assesment

Et tube

Cardiology Stuff.

Optional:

Skills of Emt intermediate

trauma management.

Pharmacology and drug Administration

other medical emergency care.

23. Identify and describe the four elements of the priority dispatch system.

A. Caller Interogation - ask standard questions

B. Prioritization of Symptoms - determines level of response.

C. Appropiate response - type of personal - Number of Vehicals mode of response.

D. Life Saving instructions - first aid techniques while units are responding.

SPECIAL PROJECT

Using your knowledge of basic life support, design a research project that investigates the value of air splints in fracture care.

Hypothesis: Write a hypothesis. (a statement which defines what you are trying to prove or disprove)

air splints are an inexpensive, easy to use, and effective method to Splint longbone fractures.

Literature review: Where would you look for information? (search of the literature: magazines, journals, etc.)

Magazines – Jems – emergency ect.

Journels – Annals of Emergency medicine ect.

Textbooks – Basic level; Paramedic

Study methods: Describe how you would test your hypothesis. (describe what you would do to verify your hypothesis: field study, clinical trial, etc.)

Apply full leg air, Hare traction splint ect.

Six people fill out Survey forms on the procedures,

Conclusion: Describe the results of the research, and how it supports or rejects your hypothesis. (this is only done once the results of the research are known)

air splint is inexpensive and easy to apply. The patents rated it 3rd. for its ability to Immobilze the femur.

3

MEDICAL-LEGAL CONSIDERATIONS OF EMERGENCY CARE

Review of the Objectives for Chapter 3

After reading this chapter, you should be able to:

1. Describe the two general categories of law in the United States.

p. 41

Criminal law addresses crime and punishment and involves legal action against an individual by the state.

Civil law deals with non-criminal matters such as contracts, domestic matters and torts.

2. Define the following terms:

pp. 41 to 47

Tort - a legal action involving noncriminal charges brought by one individual against another. Malpractice is an example of this.

Negligence - to cause harm to another by failing to meet the expected standard of care.

False imprisonment - the intentional and unjustifiable detention of a person against their will.

Abandonment - the termination of a health care provider-patient relationship without either the consent of the patient or the opportunity for the patient to gain the needed services elsewhere.

Duty to act - the obligation to respond to a situation.

Slander - the act of injuring someone's name or character by the use of false or malicious spoken words.

Libel - the act of injuring someone's name or character by the use of false or malicious written words.

3. Discuss the Medical Practices Act and its implications in prehospital care.

p. 41

The Medical Practices Act generally sets the standards for the practice of medicine. It allows certain individuals to function and describes their scope and role. It allows the paramedic to perform under the license of a physician as his agent.

4. Explain what is meant by the term "delegation of authority."

p. 41

The delegation of authority refers to the physician-paramedic relationship. It identifies that the paramedic functions as the agent of medical command, only provides care as authorized by a physician, and is accountable to that physician.

5. Describe the purpose and limitations of Good Samaritan Laws.

p. 41

The Good Samaritan Laws provide protection against negligence proceedings for those who render care at an emergency scene without compensation. The individual must act in good faith, within that person's scope of practice, and not be guilty of gross negligence. Some Good Samaritan Laws have been extended to municipal services. However, the constitutionality of all Good Samaritan Laws is being challenged.

6. Explain the need to know state motor vehicle laws that apply to emergency vehicles.

pp. 41 to 42

Special motor vehicle laws govern the operation of emergency vehicles. These laws grant special privileges and place certain responsibilities on the operator of an authorized emergency vehicle.

7. Define a "Living Will" and a "Durable power of attorney for Health Care."

p. 42

A **Living Will** is a legal document by which the patient requests that no heroic acts be provided if he or she succumbs to a terminal illness.

A **Durable Power of Attorney** is a legal document that designates another to make health care decisions for the patient.

8. Discuss the concept of "standard of care" as it applies to prehospital care.

p. 44

The standard of care is a standard against which a paramedic will be judged to determine negligence. It is the care a similarly trained and experienced paramedic would be expected to provide under similar circumstances.

9. List and define the four components required to prove negligence in a malpractice proceeding.

p. 44

Duty to act - the obligation to provide services by the nature of employment, other contract or, as with a volunteer service, by providing the service.

Breach of Duty - failure to meet the expected standard of care. The standard of care is the level of service expected by someone of equal preparation and experience, under similar circumstances.

Damages - actual injury or harm caused the plaintiff.

Proximate cause - the percentage harm experienced by the plaintiff which is attributed to the defendant.

10. Discuss the concept of *res ipsa loquitur*.

pp. 44 to 45

Res ipsa loquitur literally means it speaks for itself. Legally it means that damages would not have occurred had someone not been negligent. It places the burden on the paramedic to prove he acted properly rather than requiring the plaintiff to prove the paramedic acted inappropriately.

11. Discuss the following types of consent:

p. 45

Expressed consent occurs when a patient verbally, or in writing, gives permission to treat.

Implied consent is presumed from a patient who is unable to provide informed consent either due to inability to communicate or mental impairment.

Involuntary consent is consent for treatment issued by the court and against the patient's wishes.

12. Define the term "informed consent" and relate it to the practice of prehospital emergency care.

p. 45

Informed consent is given for treatment after the patient understands the nature, extent and risks of care to be offered.

In prehospital care, the patient must be informed of the need as well as the consequences and risks of care.

13. Define assault and battery, and give examples of each.

p. 46

Assault - any action that places a person in immediate fear of bodily harm. Approaching a patient with a catheter to start an IV without permission to treat might be grounds for assault charges.

Battery - the act of touching another without permission. The attempt to apply a traction splint without gaining the patient's permission might be grounds for battery.

14. Discuss the importance of the medical record.

p. 48

The ambulance run report is a permanent record of what happened during a call. Since legal action may occur years after an incident, the written report may be the only record of what happened. If it is incomplete or sloppy, it may be presumed that the care offered was incomplete or sloppy.

15. List several methods of protecting yourself from malpractice liability.

pp. 47 to 48

Practice good prehospital care.
Care for the patient as you would wish to be cared for if you were the patient.
Document all runs completely and appropriately.
Purchase and maintain malpractice insurance.

CASE STUDY REVIEW

Reread the case study in **PARAMEDIC EMERGENCY CARE** and then read the discussion below.

This call represents a realistic emergency medical response which has many elements of interest from a medical-legal point of view. It identifies a number of situations which put the paramedic legally at risk if proper consideration of the legal principles of emergency medical service are not observed.

Chapter 3 Case Study

The paramedics in this scenario respond to an "altered mental status" call and find a patient "staggering near the shoulder of the road." In this type of situation it is best to work in conjunction with the police rather than approach the patient without their help. It is very hard to anticipate the patient who may present with violent or assaultive behavior. The police have greater detainment power, equipment, and, in general, skill in handling violent individuals. They also may offer supporting testimony should the patient charge false imprisonment or assault.

Once at the patient's side the paramedics determine the patient is unconscious and presume implied consent. They assume he would consent to care had he been alert and understood the nature and severity of his problem. If the patient would have remained conscious, the paramedics would need to determine the patient's ability to understand and respond to his condition. The application of implied consent to a conscious but disoriented patient is a difficult judgment call.

The care they offer is prescribed by standing orders, part of the delegated practice of medicine which a paramedic is obligated to follow. The paramedic is acting as an agent of the physician and, as such, is responsible to the physician. Should the patient initiate legal proceedings against the paramedic for this action it is assured that the physician will also be named in the suit.

As the patient became conscious he then refused further care and transport to the hospital. While this is a patient's right, it is the obligation of the paramedic to inform the patient of the possible results of his refusal of continued care. This includes telling the patient that he has a serious medical problem, that the care they provided him is short term, and that he needs to be seen by a physician immediately. Should the paramedic fail to do this and the patient have a related problem shortly after the incident, the paramedic may be held negligent.

A patient's refusal to continue care must be documented. The paramedic must ask the patient to sign that he refused care against medical advice. If the patient is unwilling to sign, the paramedic should record the incident in written form and have someone at the scene witness the statement by signature.

One of the most important aspects of this call will be the documentation. The paramedic needs to record everything that happened during the response. This includes the actions of the patient before care was given, the events surrounding the detainment of the patient, the patient becoming unconscious, and the care rendered. The documentation must also include the patient's signed refusal and the refusal witnessed by one of the police officers. The documentation of the refusal should also contain a statement describing the information given the patient when he refused.

The report must be complete and thorough. It may be all that remains of this call five years later when the estate of the patient calls the paramedic into court to ask why he was released to drive his truck when he was acting irrational just minutes before.

The constitution of the United States guarantees all of us the right to sue when we feel we have been harmed. A suit may be filed for any reason whether just or not. It is in the best interest to treat the patient well, provide a good standard of emergency care, and to document each run neatly and completely.

READING COMPREHENSION SELF-EXAM

1. The principle which allows the paramedic to function in the field under the auspices and license of a physician is called ....

   A. *res ipsa loquitur.*
   B. medical command.
   C. the Good Samaritan principle.
   D. delegation of authority.
   E. none of the above.

   Answer D

2. As a paramedic, you may become involved in the legal system because of which of the following?
   1. as a witness in a criminal offense
   2. to testify in a civil matter
   3. you could be named in a malpractice suit
   4. to testify in a contract dispute

   Select the proper grouping.

   A. 1, 3
   B. 1, 4
   C. 2, 3, 4
   D. 1, 2, 3
   E. 1, 2, 3, 4

   Answer E

3. The Good Samaritan law was designed to protect EMS personnel against legal liability even if the care provider is grossly negligent.

A. True
B. False

Answer B

4. Generally, which circumstances require the paramedic to report an incident to law enforcement officials?
   1. child abuse
   2. abuse of the elderly
   3. rape or sexual abuse
   4. a shooting or stabbing
   5. physical assault

Select the proper grouping.

A. 1, 3, 5
B. 1, 2, 5
C. 1, 2, 4
D. 1, 2, 3, 4
E. 1, 2, 3, 4, 5

Answer E

5. If you respond to a home to find a patient who has a "do not resuscitate" order, you are obligated to provide Advanced Life Support to the limit of your training and ability.

A. True
B. False

Answer B

6. The principle of providing the same level of treatment as any other similarly trained individual would provide in a similar situation is called ....

A. negligence.
B. standard of care.
C. duty to act.
D. the prudent person principle.
E. proximate cause.

Answer B

7. In a malpractice suit the complaining party must prove ....
   1. the paramedic had a duty to act.
   2. the party was damaged or injured.
   3. failure to meet the standard of care (breach of duty).
   4. the paramedic's actions caused some of the damages.

Select the proper grouping.

A. 1, 3, 4
B. 1, 2, 4
C. 2, 3, 4
D. 1, 2, 3
E. 1, 2, 3, 4

Answer E

8. Caring for a patient without obtaining the proper consent is grounds for charges of ....

A. assault and battery.
B. malpractice.
C. negligence.
D. *res ipsa loquitur*.
E. B and C.

Answer A

9. Once a patient has given consent for care, he cannot refuse further care until he is attended by the physician. Allowing this to happen would subject the paramedic to abandonment.

A. True
B. False

Answer B

10. The permission to provide care obtained from the patient after the benefits and the risks of care are explained is called ....

A. the patient's right to know.
B. informed consent.
C. the duty to act.
D. implied consent.
E. none of the above.

Answer B

11. Which of the following patients would receive care based upon implied consent?
    1. the severe asthmatic who refuses transport
    2. the post-ictal epileptic who refuses care
    3. the unconscious drug overdose patient
    4. a seriously injured child with no parent present

Select the proper grouping.

A. 1, 2
B. 1, 3
C. 3, 4
D. 2, 3, 4
E. 1, 2, 3, 4

Answer C

12. The paramedic who releases a cardiac patient requiring a lidocaine drip to an EMT for transport is most likely guilty of ....

A. negligence.
B. failure to gain consent.
C. abandonment.
D. assault and battery.
E. malpractice.

Answer C

13. A patient's refusal to receive care and/or be transported should be ....

A. recorded in the run report.
B. signed by the patient.
C. witnessed by someone other than the EMS crew.
D. all of the above.
E. B and C only.

Answer D

14. Which type of patient presents the greatest threat for false imprisonment charges?

A. the overdosed adult who responds to Narcan
B. the psychiatric patient
C. the child patient, by the parents
D. the combative head injury patient
E. the mentally incompetent patient

Answer B

15. Recording false and malicious information on a patient's run report might subject the paramedic to legal action from a patient because of ....

A. libel.
B. medical control policy violation.
C. malpractice.
D. slander.
E. violation of the medical practices act.

Answer A

16. Compare and contrast the difference between negligence and *res ipsa loquitur* as they apply to the paramedic.

res ispa loquitar = is a form of negligence in which the nature of the events suggest that the paramedic caused harm to the patient. The burden to prove innocence becomes the responsible of the Paramedic

17. List the patient conditions in which care can be given even though patient consent cannot be obtained.

Optional:

The patient is unconcous
The patient is mentally impaired
The Patient unable to Comminicate
The Patent is a young Child

18. Reread the case study for this chapter and record the essential information which should be found in the narrative run report.

The Patient was observed Staggering near the Shoulder.
The Patient lunged at the Police
The Patient become unconcous
located a medic alert tag (diabetes)
assesmnt Identified a dextrose of 26mg by a dextrox stick.

SPECIAL PROJECTS

List your state's requirements for licensure of an advanced life support ambulance service.

Personnel requirements:

How many persons must respond with the ambulance?

What training must they have?

Vehicle requirements:

What type of vehicle is required?

Equipment requirements:

What emergency care equipment is required?

What radio equipment is required?

List the requirements and privileges of an authorized emergency vehicle in your state.

What is required in your state for authorization of a vehicle as an authorized emergency vehicle?

What conditions must exist before a vehicle can be operated as an authorized emergency vehicle?

What privileges are provided an authorized emergency vehicle and under what circumstances?

To park in the roadway

To operate regardless of traffic regulatory devices

To exceed the speed limit

What obligations are required of the operator of an authorized emergency vehicle?

This information should be confirmed with your instructor

4

EMS COMMUNICATIONS

Review of the Objectives for Chapter 4

After reading this chapter, you should be able to:

1. Describe the sequence of an EMS event.

pp. 52 to 53

Occurrence is the illness or injury which provides the need for the EMS response.
Detection is the recognition that there is a need for the EMS response.
Notification and response is when the emergency system is alerted and the dispatcher initiates the response. It may also occur as the police or other agency calls for medical assistance.
Treatment and preparation for transport is the phase of the emergency call in which the patient is assessed, managed and prepared for transport.
Transport and delivery is the loading, transport, and the delivery of the patient to the emergency department.
Preparation for the next event is the cleaning and restocking of the ambulance, and the completion of paperwork in preparation for the next EMS event.

2. Describe the five communications links in an EMS event.

pp. 53 to 54

Notification is the initial information which the dispatcher receives requesting a response.
Dispatch is the alerting and response of the EMS system to the scene.
Medical communications is the transmission of the results of patient assessment to the medical command physician, and a request for permission to employ care procedures.
Hospital arrival is the phase of communication in which the paramedic verbally informs the medical control physician of what was found in the field, what care was offered, what results came of the care, and gives a complete pertinent patient history.
In service is the notification to the dispatcher that the unit is again ready for an emergency response.

3. Define the following terms:

pp. 54 to 58

Base station is the principal transmitter and receiver of the system, located close to the antenna and usually operated by a remote unit found in the dispatch center.
Mobile two-way radio is a vehicle mounted radio unit with a lower transmit power than the base station.
Portable radio is a hand-held radio unit with less power and range than the mobile radio.
Repeater system is a series of radio base stations modified to re-transmit a radio broadcast so the area covered by the system can be increased. It is normally located strategically within the service area and tied to the dispatch center by either a telephone or radio link.

Voting is a process by which the repeater station receiving the strongest incoming signal is chosen to re-broadcast that signal.

Remote console is a unit designed to control the base station from a location some distance away from it.

Encoder is an electrical device which causes signals or tones to precede or to be superimposed on a radio transmission.

Decoder is an electrical device which listens to radio transmissions and recognizes only those which are encoded for it.

Trunking is a computer assisted radio system to maximize the use of available radio channels.

4. Describe the advantages of a repeater system over a non-repeater system.

pp. 55 to 56

The repeater system permits a communications network to be dependable over a large service area or through terrain which otherwise would limit communications. It assures better communications and will often allow communications even though one tower may be inoperative. It more dependably assures that weak transmissions from a mobile or portable unit will be heard.

5. List the two types of radio wave transmission.

p. 58

Amplitude modulation is the modification of a radio transmission by varying the amplitude of the signal. It is referred to as AM and has a relatively poor quality of transmission, though its range is good.

Frequency modulation is the modification of a radio transmission by varying the frequency of the signal. It is commonly known as FM and has very good quality of transmission, though its range is less than that of AM.

6. Define the following terms:

pp. 58 to 59

Hertz is the number of cycles of electrical activity per second in a radio signal.

Band is a group of radio frequencies close together in the electromagnetic spectrum.

Biotelemetry is the process of transmitting physiological data, such as an electrocardiograph, over distance, usually by radio.

Modulator is a device that electrically superimposes voice and telemetry on an electromagnetic transmission.

Demodulator is a device which recognizes a specific electromagnetic signal and withdraws from it previously modulated information.

7. Describe the 10 "Med Channels" and their usage.

p. 59

The ultra high frequency (UHF) channels designated as medical communications channels are duplex pairs designed for advanced life support service. Channels one through eight are paramedic - medical control physician communication only, while nine and ten are for dispatch.

8. Describe the most common causes of interference in biotelemetry communications.

p. 60

Muscle tremors, loose electrodes, 60 Hz interference
Fluctuation in transmitter power
Transmission of voice and EKG simultaneously

9. Describe briefly the functions and responsibilities of the Federal Communications Commission.

p. 61

The Federal Communications Commission is responsible for the overall operation and regulation of radio service. They approve equipment, allocate frequencies, license transmitters, license repair personnel, monitor the system, and spot-check station records.

10. Describe simplex, duplex, and multiplex transmissions and give examples of each.

pp. 60 to 61

Simplex is a one-frequency system which only allows the radio to transmit or receive at one time, not both, much like a push to talk intercom.

Duplex is a radio system design which uses two frequencies to permit two-way, simultaneous conversation. This allows the physician to interrupt the paramedic during a transmission or vice versa. It works like a telephone.

Multiplex is the simultaneous transmission of voice and telemetry over one frequency. It may be accomplished in either a duplex or simplex system. It is similar to a stereo radio.

11. Discuss the importance of communications equipment maintenance.

p. 61

Due to the expensive, fragile, and important nature of EMS communications equipment, proper care and maintenance are of high priority. The equipment should be regularly cleaned, and repaired if any malfunction is noted. Batteries need to be charged frequently, and spare ones readily available.

12. Define briefly the role of the EMS dispatcher.

pp. 61 to 62

The EMS dispatcher is responsible for gathering information from and calming the caller, instructing the caller in limited first aid procedures, directing the right resources (EMS, etc.) to the right location, monitoring the response to a call by the responding units, and monitoring the general radio communications.

13. Describe how the information necessary to initiate an EMS response is obtained.

pp. 62 to 63

The information needed for the emergency medical services response is gained from a person who has accessed the EMS system through the dispatcher. It may be the victim, a relative or friend of the victim, a bystander, or another member of the public safety service system, like a police officer. The caller is interrogated by the dispatcher to determine the nature of the call, the exact location, and any other pertinent information.

14. Describe the purpose of EMS radio codes, and give examples of local radio codes.

p. 63

Radio codes are designed to communicate a large amount of information quickly and accurately, or confidentially. The 10-codes are used frequently by police agencies. Some EMS systems use codes to describe circumstances which are better left confidential, as 10-99 designating intoxication or code blue to signify an incoming cardiac arrest.

15. List radio techniques that improve efficiency.

pp. 63 to 64

Listen before using a channel to ensure it is not in use
Key the microphone for one second before speaking
Speak close into the microphone or directly across it

Speak clearly and slowly
Do not convey emotion
Keep the message brief
Confirm reception of the message
Repeat important information back to sender
Do not use slang, salutations, or profanity

16. List the important components of the patient medical report.

pp. 64 to 66

Unit designation, personnel and level of certification
Scene description
Patient's name, age, sex, height, weight
The chief complaint/primary problem
Associated signs and symptoms
Results of secondary assessment
Brief history of current medical problem
Pertinent past medical history
Vital signs, level of consciousness
EKG, trauma score, Glasgow coma scale, etc.
Treatment rendered and results of care
Estimated time of arrival
Name of private physician

17. Discuss the importance of written medical protocols.

p. 66

Provide standard care process for various medical problems and situations
Reduce communication time
Backup for radio communications failure

18. Name five uses of the written EMS form.

p. 66

Record of the patient's initial condition
Legal record of prehospital care
Documentation of refusal of care
Information for billing, chart review, etc.
Defense against malpractice

CASE STUDY REVIEW

Reread the case study in **PARAMEDIC EMERGENCY CARE** and then read the discussion below.

This case review highlights some important aspects of radio communications during the emergency medical services response. The system is state of the art and the patient report to the medical command physician is an excellent example of how to organize the report and what it should contain.

Chapter 4 Case Study

Calling for an ambulance using computer aided dispatch (CAD) is becoming more and more prevalent in EMS. The information which the computer can provide is remarkable and efficient. Many CAD systems will print out the incident address, directions to the scene and any previously recorded information on the patient's medical status. The computer, coupled with a navigation system, can even locate ambulances during the dispatch and send the closest unit while tracking its response.

The assessment the paramedics provide in this case study is very thorough though it took only 60 to 90 seconds. The results reveal a patient who needs rapid transport and immediate care. The unconsciousness, inability on the part of the patient to protect his airway, and the evident head injury all call for intubation which the team performs by protocol even before anyone calls medical command. They load the patient and are en route before they contact medical command, thereby wasting little time in this rapid transport situation.

The paramedic making the radio report is concise and composes her message very well. She conveys a very complete and detailed picture of the patient's status, using a short amount of air time. She is no doubt reading her notes from the assessment, either made on a wide strip of adhesive tape on her thigh or recorded in a small note book. The information is factual and to the point. The description of the scene, the general description of the patient, the mechanism of injury, level of consciousness, vital signs, findings of the assessment, and care steps are presented in a well ordered fashion. This allows both the paramedic and physician to organize the information quickly and recognize the important points.

Place yourself in the position of the physician and read the report quickly. Do you get a sense of the severity of the injuries and the patient condition? Do you have faith in the paramedic because of the way the message is put together and because of its focus on the medically important information? It is essential that the paramedic presents the patient information in an accurate, understandable, and believable way. This will ensure that the receiving physician feels comfortable ordering patient care.

The result of this call is an important reality of emergency medical service. The patient died even though he was in the hands of good paramedics who did all they could to care for him. One of the hardest aspects of practicing prehospital emergency care is having a patient die. This death does not mean that the care givers did anything wrong or that more aggressive or different care procedures would have made a difference.

READING COMPREHENSION SELF-EXAM

1. Identify the appropriate sequence of communications and events in prehospital care.
   1. treatment and preparation for transport
   2. preparation for the next event
   3. occurrence and detection
   4. notification and response

   Select the proper grouping.

   A. 3, 4, 1, 2
   B. 2, 4, 1, 3
   C. 3, 4, 2, 1
   D. 1, 3, 4, 2
   E. 4, 3, 2, 1

   Answer A

2. The main transmitter of an EMS radio system is located close to the antenna, and is called the ....

   A. remote console.
   B. repeater.
   C. base station.
   D. satellite receiver.
   E. encoder module.

   Answer C

3. The normal range for the mobile transmitter, without a repeater, is about ....

A. 5 miles.
B. 10 to 15 miles.
C. 25 miles.
D. 50 to 100 miles.
E. about 125 miles.

Answer B

4. The device that receives a radio signal and re-transmits the message at a higher power level is the ....

A. portable radio.
B. mobile radio.
C. repeater.
D. remote console.
E. none of the above.

Answer C

5. The device that activates the radio to receive messages containing a certain signal or tone is called ....

A. a remote.
B. a satellite receiver.
C. an encoder.
D. a decoder.
E. none of the above.

Answer D

6. The type of radio transmission that is relatively line of sight, and less subject to interference is called amplitude modulation (AM).

A. True
B. False

Answer B

7. Which radio transmission design will allow the receiver to interrupt the caller while he or she is talking?

A. simplex
B. duplex
C. amplitude modulation
D. multiplex
E. none of the above

Answer B

8. The responsibilities of the Federal Communications Commission include ....
   1. approve radio protocols for EMS systems.
   2. license and allocate radio frequencies.
   3. monitor radio frequencies.
   4. check station licenses and station records.

Select the proper grouping.

A. 1, 3
B. 2, 3
C. 1, 2, 4
D. 2, 3, 4
E. 1, 2, 3, 4

Answer D

9. Which of the following are among the responsibilities of the EMS dispatcher?
   1. direct the appropriate vehicle to the appropriate address
   2. monitor and coordinate system communications
   3. obtain information necessary for the EMS response
   4. instruct the caller in first aid measures
   5. maintain records of the complete response

   Select the proper grouping.

   A. 1, 3, 4
   B. 1, 2, 3
   C. 2, 4, 5
   D. 2, 3, 4, 5
   E. 1, 2, 3, 4, 5

   Answer E

10. One of the more important skills of the paramedic is to gather essential patient information, organize it, and relay it to the medical control physician.

    A. True
    B. False

    Answer A

11. Which of the following is not appropriate for good emergency medical services communications?

    A. speak close to the microphone
    B. speak directly into or across the microphone
    C. talk in a normal tone
    D. speak without emotion
    E. take time to explain everything in detail

    Answer E

12. If the portable radio you are using does not transmit from your location, attempt to ....
    1. move to higher ground.
    2. touch the antenna to something metal while transmitting.
    3. speak louder into the microphone.
    4. move toward a window or away from structural steel.

    Select the proper grouping.

    A. 1, 2
    B. 1, 4
    C. 1, 2, 3
    D. 2, 3, 4
    E. 1, 2, 3, 4

    Answer B

13. Which of the following should be addressed by protocol?

    A. care steps for all major medical emergencies
    B. patients who refuse care
    C. non-EMS physicians on the scene
    D. "Do Not Resuscitate" orders
    E. all of the above

    Answer E

14. The time needed to send an adequate EKG strip via telemetry is about ....

A. 15 to 20 seconds.
B. 20 to 30 seconds.
C. 30 to 45 seconds.
D. about one minute.
E. none of the above.

Answer A

15. The written run report may become ....

A. a record of the patient's initial condition.
B. a legal record of prehospital care.
C. the source of essential information for billing, etc.
D. documentation of a patient's refusal of care.
E. all of the above.

Answer E

SPECIAL PROJECTS

The authoring of both the radio message to the receiving hospital and the written run report are two of the most important tasks you will perform as a paramedic. Read the following few paragraphs, compose a radio message, and complete the run report for this call.

The Call:

At 3:15 in the afternoon, your ambulance, unit 89, is paged out to an unconscious person at the local baseball field on a very hot (97°) Saturday. You are accompanied by Steve Phillips, an EMT, your partner for the day.

You arrive on scene at 3:22 to find a young male collapsed at third base. He is un-arousable, perspiring heavily, and his skin is cool to the touch. The pillow under the boy's head (placed by bystanders) is removed, the airway is clear, breathing is adequate, and the pulse is rapid and bounding. One of the bystanders said he was playing ball and just collapsed. Another young bystander identifies himself as the victim's brother, and states that "nothing like this has happened before." He says "his brother is 13 and is called John (Thompson), and lives about a mile away."

The rest of the assessment reveals no signs of trauma. The vitals are: blood pressure 136/98, pulse 92 and strong, the EKG traces normal sinus rhythm, and respirations are 24 and normal in depth and pattern (at 3:27). The young boy responds to painful stimuli but not to verbal command or his name. Pupils are noted to be equal and slow to react. Oxygen is applied at 4 liters by nasal cannula, and the patient is moved to the shade.

Receiving Hospital is contacted, and you call in the following report:

Unit 89 to Recieving Hospital - We are at the ballfield treating a 13 y/o M who collapsed while playing baseball. He is currently unresponsive to all but painful stimuli, cool to the touch & sweating profusely. Vitals are BP 136/98 pulse 92 and strong. Respirations 24 & regular and pupils equal & slow to react. ECG is showing NSR - No physical signs of trauma noted and past medical history is unknown. O'2 is applied 4l via nasal cannula. Expected ETA - 20 min.

Finish on last Page

Expected ETA is 20 minutes

Medical command at Receiving Hospital, the closest facility, orders you to start an IV line with normal saline run just to keep open. You repeat the orders to medical control and then begin your care. Your first IV attempt is unsuccessful on the right forearm; the second attempt (on the left forearm) gets a flashback and infuses well. You retake vitals. The patient is now responding to verbal stimuli, the BP is 134/96, pulse 90, EKG reads NSR, respirations 24. The patient is loaded on the stretcher at 3:37 and moved to the ambulance.

You contact medical command and provide the following update:

One IV in left forearm running TKO w N.S. Patient is now Responding to Verbal Stimuli. Vitals BP 134/96, pulse is 90 and strong. Respirations 24, ECG-NSR ETA 10 minutes

ETA 10 minutes

Enroute vitals (3:45) are BP 132/90, EKG reads NSR, pulse 88, respirations at 24. The patient is now conscious and alert though he cannot remember the incident. The trip is uneventful, and you arrive at the hospital at 3:57. You transfer the responsibility for the patient to the emergency physician, and restock and wipe out the ambulance. You report back in service at 4:15, grab a cup of coffee and sit down at the hospital to write the run report.

Complete the run report on the following page from the information contained in the narrative of this call.

Compare the radio communication and run report form which you prepare against the example in the answer key section of this workbook. As you make this comparison, realize that there are "many correct" ways to communicate this body of information. Ensure that you have recorded the major points of your assessment and care, and enough other material to describe the patient and his condition.

Sharon 468-6818

Date 5 / 3 / 94	Emergency Medical Service Run Report	Run # 911

Patient Information	Service Information	Times
Name: Thompson John	Agency: Unit 89	Rcvd 15 :15
Address: unknown	Location: Ball field	Enrt 15 :15
City: St: Zip:	Call Origin: Dispatch	Scne 15 :22
Age: 13 Birth: / / Sex: [X M][F]	Type: Emrg[X] Non[ ] Trnsfr[ ]	LvSn 15 :40
Nature of Call: Person collapsed.		ArHsp 15 :57
Chief Complaint: Unconcous possible Heat exhaustion		InSv 16 :15

Description of Current Problem:

The Patient collapsed while playing Baseball on a very Hot Sunny day. Pt. was found to be cool diaphoretic unresponsive to Verbal Stimuli and Responsive to painful Stimuli. Pupils were normal in size but slow to React. Physical assesment reveals no apparent signs of trauma or other medical Problem.

Medical Problems

Past		Present
[ ]	Cardiac	[ ]
[ ]	Stroke	[ ]
[ ]	Acute Abdomen	[ ]
[ ]	Diabetes	[ ]
[ ]	Psychiatric	[ ]
[ ]	Epilepsy	[ ]
[ ]	Drug/Alcohol	[ ]
[ ]	Poisoning	[ ]
[ ]	Allergy/Asthma	[ ]
[ ]	Syncope	[ ]
[ ]	Obstetrical	[ ]
[ ]	GYN	[ ]

Other:

Trauma Scr: n/A Glascow: 6

On Scene Care: provided O'2, Removed patient from Sun & heat—Attempted IV in left forearm (unsuccessful) Started IV in Ⓡ Forearm w/16ga NS. TKO

First Aid: pillow was placed under head

By Whom? bystanders

O2 @ 4 L 15:25 Via NC	C-Collar n/A :	S-Immob. n/:A	Stretcher 15 :37

Allergies/Meds: Unknown	Past Med Hx: Unknown

Time	Pulse	Resp.	BP S/D	LOC	EKG
15:27	R: 92 [X r][i]	R: 24 [s][l]	136/98	[a][v][X p][u]	NSR
Care/Comments: Pt unresponsive to All but painful Stimuli					
15:37	R: 90 [X r][i]	R: 24 [s][l]	134/96	[a][X v][p][u]	NSR
Care/Comments: Pt. became Responsive to Verbal Stimuli					
15:45	R: 88 [X r][i]	R: 22 [s][l]	132 / 90	[X a][v][p][u]	NSR
Care/Comments: Patient became full conscious alert + oriented.					
:	R: [r][i]	R: [s][l]	/	[a][v][p][u]	
Care/Comments:					

Destination: Recieving Hospital	Personnel: Certification
Reason:[ ]pt [X] Closest [ ] M.D[ ] Other	1. Cindy Robertson [X P][E][O]
Contacted: [X] Radio [ ] Tele[ ] Direct	2. Steve Phillips [P][X E][O]
Ar Status: [X] Better [ ] UnC[ ] Worse	3. n/A [P][E][O]

5

RESCUE OPERATIONS

Review of the Objectives for Chapter 5

After reading this chapter, you should be able to:

1. List the items required for personal and patient safety during a rescue.

pp. 70 to 73

Personal Safety

Helmet with a four-point suspension system and either a removable duck bill or none at all
Eye protection - vented goggles or industrial safety glasses
Hearing protection - multi-baffled or sponge-like ear plugs or the high-quality ear muff style
Respiratory protection - surgical or commercial dust masks
Gloves - leather work gloves
Boots - high-topped, steel-toed with coarse lug sole
Coveralls - brightly colored or with reflective bands, insulated for cold weather
Turnout - coat/pants, fire department issue, available to all paramedics
Specialty equipment - self contained breathing apparatus, hazardous material gear.

Patient Safety

Helmet - light duty
Eye protection - vented goggles
Protective blankets - vinyl tarps for water, aluminized for heat/fire, wool for cold
Hearing and respiratory protection - same as for rescuers
Protective shielding - back boards, special litters, etc.

2. Discuss the purpose of written safety procedures.

p. 73

Safety procedures identify the safety needs for each member of the rescue team in each particular circumstance. They are created to assure that each team member considers personal protection as an integral part of the rescue effort.

3. Describe the role of the safety officer.

p. 73

The safety officer is responsible for overviewing the scene and ensuring that all activities are conducted with safety in mind. The officer is responsible for approving all actions before they are begun.

4. Describe how pre-planning contributes to the safety and efficiency of a rescue operation.

pp. 73 to 74

Pre-planning identifies locations where rescue is likely to take place, and the types of rescue that may become necessary. It also identifies the particular equipment, manpower, and techniques that may be required, and allows the service to plan the skills before an emergency arises.

5. Describe the six phases of a rescue operation, and discuss the key elements of each rescue phase.

pp. 74 to 82

Assessment is the overall evaluation of the scene and circumstance to determine if and what type of rescue is needed. It rules out all hazards, or for those that exist, secures the scene. Assessment also determines the nature of the incident (mechanism of injury), and the number of patients and their location.

Gaining access is obtaining a direct access to the patient for the purpose of immediate assessment and, if necessary, life-saving care. It is the beginning of the technical rescue, and needs to be carried out with good coordination and planning.

Emergency care is the actual assessment, immediate care, management, and patient packaging. The assessment and patient management should provide emergency medical care within the confines of the rescue scene and physical constraints of the entrapment.

Disentanglement is the process which removes the vehicle, structure or debris from around the patient. It is the technical aspect of the operation, and employs the paramedic stabilizing and reassuring the patient as well as acting as the patient advocate to the rescue team leaders.

Removal is the technical removal of the injured patient. It involves concerns for the patient's injuries against the confines and constraints of the rescue scene. It is a time when the rescue crew and the paramedic need to coordinate and compromise.

Transport is transporting the patient to the appropriate medical facility. It is the final stage of the rescue operation, and may be as routine as just transporting the patient to the hospital via ambulance or traveling miles over rough terrain by foot.

6. List the types of hazards that might be encountered at a rescue scene.

pp. 75 to 76

Chemical spills, radiation, gas leaks.
Fire or explosion.
Electrical current.
Poisonous or caustic substances.
Biological agents or germ-infested materials.
Water hazards such as swift moving currents, floating debris, or poisonous contamination.
Confined spaces such as vessels, trenches, mines or caves.
Extreme heights, particularly in mountainous situations.

7. List the types of information, in addition to hazards, that a paramedic should get during scene assessment.

pp. 75 to 76

Nature of the situation - exactly what mechanism caused the patient injuries and the need for rescue
Number of victims - account for all the patients
Specific patient location - identify their exact locations

8. Describe the reasons a paramedic's technical capability must be guaranteed before he or she attempts to reach an entrapped patient.

p. 73

It is necessary that the paramedic have technical knowledge of the rescue process so he may remain the patient's advocate. This will allow recommendations and cautions to be offered to rescuers before the patient's condition is endangered by a procedure or approach. Technical knowledge of the rescue process will also ensure that the paramedic's and patient's safety are considered during the entire rescue.

9. List three special rescue operations that require special skills or equipment.

pp. 77 to 78

Vertical Rescue
Swift Water Rescue
Confined-Space Rescue

10. Name the three major responsibilities of a paramedic in providing on-scene medical care during a rescue.

p. 78

Initiate patient assessment and care as soon as possible
Maintain patient care during disentanglement
Accompany patient during removal and transport

11. List the two key goals of patient assessment in a rescue.

pp. 78 to 79

Identify and care for current patient medical problems
Anticipate future patient needs and changing condition

12. List five situations in which patients may have to be moved prior to complete stabilization.

pp. 79

Injured, stranded window cleaners, water/radio-TV tower workers, high-rise construction workers;
Victims of trench cave-ins;
Persons stranded in swift-running water;
Victims of vehicular entrapment with associated fire;
Persons overcome by life-threatening atmosphere.

13. Discuss how prolonged time in reaching - or in disentangling, removing, and transporting - a patient will necessitate modification of management protocols.

pp. 79 to 80

The paramedic must use the prolonged disentanglement time to provide care. That care should go beyond the rapid transport approach, and focus on attempting to stabilize and maintain the patient while at the scene.

14. List three responsibilities of the paramedic during patient disentanglement.

pp. 80 to 81

Knowledgeable about the technical aspects of rescue
Prepared and able to provide extended prehospital care
Knowledgeable about specialty-rescue resources

15. Identify elements of a thorough patient survey upon removal.

p. 81

Secure the airway
Check oxygen delivery
Control hemorrhage
Assure spine immobilization
Treat shock aggressively - IVs, PASG, etc.
Pharmacologic interventions as indicated
Monitor ECG
Dress wounds
Splint fractures

16. Explain how the method of patient transport is determined.

pp. 82

The patient transport mode must be well thought out in advance of the disentanglement to ensure that the patient travels rapidly to the proper facility. Consideration should be given to physical carry out, ground transport or air evacuation.

17. Identify some of the scenarios that an EMS unit should consider in compiling a rescue resource list.

pp. 77 to 78

Light and heavy vehicle extrication, hazmat, water rescue, high angle/vertical rescue, wilderness rescue, etc.

CASE STUDY REVIEW

Reread the case study in **PARAMEDIC EMERGENCY CARE** and then read the discussion below.

This case study identifies some of the logistical problems associated with the rescue. It also presents the different approach which must be taken when the nature of the rescue places the patient with the paramedic for a prolonged time.

Chapter 5 Case Study

This rescue demonstrates the lengthening of the normal emergency medical service response times often associated with entrapment or wilderness rescues. The travel time to the scene, the four-wheel-drive time to the cliff, and the time spent waiting for a vertical rescue team, leave the patient injured without care for more than one hour. The on-scene time of more than 25 minutes is prolonged compared to the rapid transport this patient would otherwise receive. The time to extricate and transport this patient will also increase the time the paramedic spends at the patient's side and the prehospital care which is required.

The need for teamwork is apparent. A specialized vehicle to get close to the scene and climbing equipment are just a few of the technical elements that must come together for this rescue to be successful. The rescue also requires various specialists, including the paramedics, the park ranger/guide, the vertical rescue team, and the air medical team. The two most important elements of any interdisciplinary rescue are cooperation and coordination.

Once at the patient's side, the paramedic must change from the framework of the rapid transport approach. The patient has been down for at least 40 to 60 minutes. The effects of the injuries are much more advanced than are normally seen in emergency medical service, and it will be a long time until the patient can be delivered to definitive care. In the face of these considerations, the paramedic must provide a complete assessment, stabilize the patient (including environmental protection), bandage and splint all apparent injuries, and package the patient for a vertical lift and transport by foot to the air medical landing zone.

Environmental concerns also enter the picture. Dehydration and moderate blood loss may leave the patient hypovolemic. Exposure on a cold cliff, with movement restricted, may leave the patient hypothermic. The body's compensatory mechanisms for shock may begin to fail. The paramedic needs to be conscientious in assessment and aggressive in care for the patient in these circumstances.

The paramedic must also consider the effects of long-term care on the patient. Normally, the aggressive administration of fluid therapy does not carry the dangers of fluid overload in the prehospital setting. The time from the initiation of an IV to arrival at the Emergency Department is short, too short, for massive fluid overload to occur. However, in this scenario there does exist a chance for this problem to arise. The attending paramedic must be very careful to monitor blood pressure, pulse, and other signs of circulatory adequacy as well as breath sounds to ensure that fluid administration compensates for losses, yet does not overload the patient.

Finally the paramedic and rescue team leader must plan the extrication. This involves the coordination of resources to ensure that the patient is safely but practically removed from the cliff ledge. The ideals of patient care, and the practicality of vertical lift must be weighed, and a compromise agreed upon.

If all elements of the rescue come together, it can be an effective process. It is essential that the paramedic and rescue team work together to pre-plan for the expected and unexpected rescue operations. Roles may be defined, a chain of command determined, and a catalog of resources may be created. This will ensure that the emergency medical services team and the rescue team work together at the rescue scene.

READING COMPREHENSION SELF-EXAM

1. Which of the following statements are true?
   1. rescue is the freeing of a subject from entrapment
   2. a paramedic can be trained in all types of rescue
   3. proficiency in all but a few rescue specialties is rare
   4. the paramedic and rescue team should plan before the rescue

   Select the proper grouping.

   A. 1, 4
   B. 2, 4
   C. 1, 2, 4
   D. 1, 3, 4
   E. 2, 3, 4

   Answer D

2. Protection for the patient should involve the use of which of the following safety equipment?
   1. helmet
   2. safety goggles with elastic band
   3. coveralls
   4. protective blankets (wool or aluminized)

   Select the proper grouping.

   A. 1, 2
   B. 1, 2, 3
   C. 1, 2, 4
   D. 2, 3, 4
   E. 1, 2, 3, 4

   Answer C

3. Elements of the rescue pre-plan include ....
   1. identification of likely locations for rescue.
   2. specific procedures for likely rescue scenarios.
   3. evaluation of hazards of likely rescue operations.
   4. specific expertise and resource needs.
   5. plans for efficient use of personnel.

   Select the proper grouping.

   A. 1, 3, 4
   B. 2, 3, 4
   C. 1, 3, 4, 5
   D. 2, 3, 4, 5
   E. 1, 2, 3, 4, 5

   Answer E

4. The best type of helmet is that of construction quality with two-point suspension and elastic supports.

A. True
B. False

Answer B

5. Every rescue operation must have a Safety Officer who has the authority to interrupt the rescue operation should something appear unsafe.

A. True
B. False

Answer A

6. Place the following phases of a rescue in order as they would occur.
   1. disentanglement
   2. gaining access
   3. emergency care
   4. removal and transport
   5. scene assessment

   Select the proper grouping.

A. 5, 2, 1, 3, 4
B. 5, 2, 3, 1, 4
C. 2, 5, 1, 3, 4
D. 2, 5, 3, 1, 4
E. 2, 3, 5, 1, 4

Answer B

7. In the rescue, scene assessment should provide you with which of the following items of information?

A. nature of the situation
B. specific patient locations
C. number of victims
D. scene hazards
E. all of the above

Answer E

8. The initial responding units to a rescue often overestimate their capability to handle a rescue situation. They are sometimes hesitant to request reserves or specialty teams.

A. True
B. False

Answer A

9. Which of the following conditions require the patient be extricated before care is offered?
   1. trapped radio tower worker
   2. vehicular entrapment with active fire
   3. patient entrapped in an industrial machine
   4. patient overcome by life-threatening atmosphere
   5. person stranded in swift-running, rising water

   Select the proper grouping.

A. 1, 3, 5
B. 1, 2, 4
C. 2, 3, 4, 5
D. 1, 2, 4, 5
E. 1, 2, 3, 4, 5

Answer D

10. The paramedic should approach the care of the entrapped patient identically to the normal trauma patient. If the patient presents with injuries requiring rapid transport, extrication must occur immediately regardless of the circumstances.

A. True
B. False

Answer B

11. How does care for the entrapped patient with an anticipated long rescue differ from normal patient care?

A. it does not differ
B. it involves greater patient stabilization skills
C. it involves protection from the environment
D. B and C
E. none of the above

Answer D

12. The prolonged rescue may call upon the paramedic to manage patient hydration, reposition dislocations, cleanse wounds, and manage hypothermia and pain.

A. True
B. False

Answer A

13. Generally, the responsibilities of the paramedic during the rescue include ....
   1. advising the team of the impact of procedures on the patient.
   2. providing primary and secondary assessment.
   3. ensuring patient safety.
   4. calming and reassuring the patient.
   5. providing environmental protection for the patient.

   Select the proper grouping.

A. 1, 2, 4
B. 1, 3, 5
C. 2, 4, 5
D. 1, 2, 4, 5
E. 1, 2, 3, 4, 5

Answer E

14. Which of the following are considered a special rescue operation?
   1. vertical rescue
   2. prolonged patient care
   3. confined space rescue
   4. swift water rescue

   Select the proper grouping.

A. 2, 4
B. 1, 4
C. 2, 3, 4
D. 1, 3, 4
E. 1, 2, 3, 4

Answer E

15. The role and responsibility of the paramedic in the rescue includes ....
   1. being properly outfitted with protective gear.
   2. training specific to their assigned rescue responsibilities.
   3. accessing the scene quickly.
   4. rapid patient removal under situational threats.
   5. continual reassessment and patient care during rescue.

   Select the proper grouping.

   A. 1, 3, 4
   B. 2, 3, 5
   C. 1, 2, 4, 5
   D. 1, 2, 3, 5
   E. 1, 2, 3, 4, 5

   Answer E

SPECIAL PROJECTS

SCENE ASSESSMENT EXERCISE

In the next two problems you are asked to look at the chapter openers in your textbook. Assess the scene and identify the hazards you would suspect at the scene and the special rescue equipment you may need.

Evaluate the photographs located on the pages listed and identify:

16. Page 792 (Chapter 25 Opener)

Hazards expected at the scene:	Special rescue needed:
Structural Collapse	Heavy equipment
Debris	Search Dogs
Confined Spaces	Confined-Space Rescue
Electrical Hazards.	
Explosion Hazards.	

17. Page 862 (Chapter 28 Opener)

Hazards expected at the scene:	Special rescue needed:
Fast water Rescue	water rescue
Potiential hypothermia	Dive Rescue
Potiential drowning	Rescue Boats
	multi-causualty Response.

6

MAJOR INCIDENT RESPONSE

Review of the Objective for Chapter 6

After reading this chapter, you should be able to:

1. Name the three categories of EMS response to a mass-casualty incident.

pp. 88 to 89

Level I Response is a multiple-casualty incident that can be handled locally.

Level II Response is a multiple-casualty incident that severely taxes or overwhelms local resources. It usually merits mutual aid from several outside agencies.

Level III Response is a multiple-casualty incident that severely taxes or overwhelms regional resources. It will often require the establishment of an EOC and significant interagency coordination.

2. Describe the need for controlling and organizing responding rescuers at a mass-casualty incident.

p. 90

The mass-casualty incident is an overwhelming incident in which the resources are outstripped by the number of injured. Only with organization, a chain of command, and an overall picture of what needs to happen can the incident be efficiently managed. The current approach to the mass-casualty incident is called incident command.

3. Identify the incident commander and explain how to contact him or her.

p. 90

The incident commander is the individual who has overall responsibility for managing the mass casualty incident. The incident commander is generally the highest ranking public safety service officer on-scene, identified as command via radio, and may be uniquely identified by hat, vest or other method. Command is transferred from the first arriving unit to the highest ranking officer, as they arrive.

4. Explain the responsibilities of an incident commander.

p. 90

Is briefed, assumes command, and sizes up the incident
Alerts dispatch to the nature and severity of the incident
Develops a plan to manage the scene, extricate, treat, and transport the patients
Establishes the needed sectors and coordinates their activity
Assigns arriving resources to sectors
Obtains updated reports on the rescue and care activities
Reassesses needs and reassigns available units and personnel
Coordinates the release of units as the incident concludes

5. Describe the transfer of command process for the incident commander and sector officers.

pp. 94 to 95

As a higher ranking officer arrives on the scene, the officer is briefed on the nature and current status of the incident. Once the briefing is concluded, the transfer of command occurs. It is announced via radio to the sector officers.

6. Describe the "sectors" that are used at mass-casualty incidents and explain the responsibilities of each sector.

pp. 95 to 102

Sectors are subdivisions of incident management identified by the particular responsibilities which occur there.

Extrication is responsible for the management of patients where they are found, until they can be extricated and moved to the treatment sector.

Triage is a sector which may be created between the extrication and treatment sectors to assess patients and determine what level of care they will receive.

Treatment is a sector designated for the treatment of the casualties, usually divided into critical and noncritical areas.

Transportation sector is the area where patients are treated and packaged for transport. From this location, the hospitals are alerted as to incoming patients.

Staging is an area designated for the arrival of resources. It is remote from the scene, keeping it uncongested. Resources are directed to their assignments from this sector by the incident commander.

Supply is established to receive and distribute medical and rescue supplies to the incident. It is located near the treatment sector.

7. Explain the need for triage and tagging at mass-casualty incidents.

pp. 102 to 103

Triage and tagging are essential at the mass-casualty incident because one patient will be cared for by many individuals. If a system is not employed, the patient will have to be assessed by each attending EMT or paramedic. Triaging will also ensure that the most appropriate patients receive the needed care first.

8. Explain the START method of triaging patients.

pp. 103 to 103

"Simple Triage And Rapid Treatment" is a system designed to address the problems of triaging the mass-casualty incident. The walking wounded are cleared from the scene, and then each remaining patient is given a quick assessment (under 60 seconds). The assessment focuses upon ventilation, perfusion/pulses, and level of responsiveness/consciousness.

9. Explain the communication system requirements at a mass-casualty incident, and describe how to use the system to direct rescuers and process information for decision making.

p. 104

Communications at the mass-casualty incident are essential. The incident commander receives reports and communications from the sector officers only. The rescuers within a sector must limit their radio communication and only communicate with the sector officer. When responders are communicating with other service members they should use "plain English."

10. Explain the importance of plans and procedures for response to mass-casualty incidents.
pp. 104 to 105

The development of compatible mass-casualty plans among agencies ensures that turf battles will not arise, and will bring the incident to a swift and effective conclusion. The plans should identify the chain of command and responsibilities for each anticipated responding service.

11. Cite some of the major duties of paramedics involved in a mass-casualty incident.
pp. 105 to 106

Provide patient care - at the direction of the extrication, triage, or treatment sector officer, provide assessment and care of the injured at the mass-casualty incident.

Act as a sector officer - at the direction of the incident commander, provide overall supervision of the designated sector (most likely the extrication, triage, or treatment sector), and keep incident command informed of resources needed and progress made during the incident.

Act as incident command - on rare occasions, a paramedic may assume and maintain the position of incident command. He or she must coordinate the overall incident activity and assure resources are directed appropriately to areas of need.

12. List essential items that help a commander and sector officers perform more effectively.
pp. 106 to 108

Clipboard with paper and pencils will allow incident command and sector officers to record and keep notes on the status of the various activities associated with the various sectors.

Sector vests and incident command vests will quickly identify those in charge to all members of the mass-casualty response.

CASE STUDY REVIEW

Reread the case study in **PARAMEDIC EMERGENCY CARE** and then read the discussion below.

This study presents a multi-casualty incident requiring interdisciplinary cooperation and coordination. It permits discussion of the size-up of the incident, the establishment and transfer of command, and the roles the paramedic may play at the incident. The responsibilities associated with the incident command are also viewed, including the logistics of multiple responding vehicles and personnel at the scene.

Chapter 6 Case Study

The charter bus accident presents the senior paramedic with a mass-casualty situation that could rapidly move to chaos. As the first-ranking public safety service official on the scene, he becomes command and informs the dispatch center. Instead of rushing to the first few patients, the incident commander determines the nature and severity of (sizes-up) the incident. The nature of the incident as well as its hazards are communicated to dispatch and, through dispatch, to the responding units. The number of injured and severity of injuries are reported as is the need for ten ambulances. The highway is ordered closed. All units are directed to a staging area rather than having them congest the scene.

If the paramedic had chosen to act as a paramedic and had begun caring for the injured, the system response and the overall coordination of response would have suffered. The patients would have had to wait longer for the arrival of enough EMS personnel to provide the needed care and even longer for enough vehicles to provide transport for the large number of seriously injured. While it is difficult to step back from the care of injured patients, in this incident the paramedic did what was best for all the patients.

The fire department and ambulances begin to arrive. The EMS supervisor arrives at the scene and begins to assume the responsibilities of incident commander. That transfer of responsibility is not completed until he is briefed on the overall circumstances of the incident including the number of injured, severity of the injuries, rescue attempts underway, resources on-scene and enroute, and personnel who are acting as sector officers. As the briefing concludes, the command change is communicated to all sector chiefs and dispatch.

It is unusual that a paramedic is the best choice for incident commander. The skills of the paramedic are best utilized at either the extrication or treatment sector. The incident commander is responsible for resource allocation and sector coordination, a role best filled by fire or rescue management personnel. Communications are kept to a minimum while the incident progresses. The incident commander is updated periodically by each sector chief. The updates include progress reports, any resource needs, and reports of the personnel and equipment which have been released to the staging area. Resources are reallocated as needed.

The paramedic moves to the treatment sector where care is offered to those patients who have just been extricated from the bus. Incident command directs ambulances from the staging sector to the treatment sector to load and transport patients to the hospital and return. Most bandaging, splinting, and other trauma equipment is quickly off-loaded for use at the treatment area. First Responders or police officers drive the ambulances, allowing the paramedics and EMTs to provide care at the scene or during transport.

As the incident comes to an end, command releases ambulances and fire trucks, and some of the extrication and EMS personnel. The fire department and the highway crews clean the scene and return the highway to a safe condition. Two weeks later the director of emergency operations calls an incident review. The evaluation of the incident finds that in general it was handled well. Dispatch procedures are updated to involve the new ambulance service to the north and the Fire Department has requested that all responding vehicles radio to the staging area on the mutual aid frequency three and five minutes before their arrival.

READING COMPREHENSION SELF-EXAM

1. The cornerstone of the incident command system is the requirement that the overall incident command responsibilities be fixed in one person.

   A. True
   B. False

   Answer A

2. The designation of an incident command officer should await the arrival of a ranking officer in the police, fire or emergency medical service. Premature designation of an incident commander may lead to confusion and chaos.

   A. True
   B. False

   Answer B

3. Once incident command is established it is essential to establish which of the following three sectors?

   A. triage, treatment, staging
   B. extrication, staging, transport
   C. rescue, resource, transport
   D. staging, triage, supply
   E. extrication, treatment, transport

   Answer E

4. The staging sector of a major incident is where ....

   A. resources are stored.
   B. incoming units await direction.
   C. patients await patient packaging.
   D. triage is performed.
   E. the incident command center is located.

   Answer B

5. It is the responsibility of the incident commander to develop a plan of action which ....
   1. stabilizes the scene.
   2. provides for extrication services and patient triage.
   3. provides for patient care.
   4. allows the commander to move about the scene.
   5. provides for patient transport.

   Select the proper grouping.

   A. 1, 3, 4
   B. 2, 3, 5
   C. 1, 2, 3, 5
   D. 1, 3, 4, 5
   E. 1, 2, 3, 4, 5

   Answer C

6. Which sector is normally the first established at the mass-casualty scene?

   A. triage
   B. treatment
   C. supply
   D. extrication
   E. transport

   Answer D

7. Triaging of patients at a mass-casualty incident may occur at which of the following locations?

   A. the extrication sector
   B. the treatment sector
   C. in a special triage sector
   D. all of the above
   E. A and B only

   Answer E

8. The treatment sector needs ....
   1. adequate space to provide care.
   2. fewer paramedics than the extrication sector.
   3. paramedics directed to critical, then delayed patients.
   4. one care provider per patient.

   Select the proper grouping.

   A. 1, 3
   B. 1, 3, 4
   C. 2, 3, 4
   D. 1, 2, 4
   E. 1, 2, 3, 4

   Answer B

9. The level of mass-casualty response that overwhelms local and regional resources and typically involves several sites is a ....

A. level I response.
B. level II response.
C. level III response.
D. command incident.
E. none of the above.

Answer A

10. The staging area should be located in close proximity to the extrication sector to enhance the response of needed units.

A. True
B. False

Answer B

11. The START system of triage examines which of the following?
1. potential for spine injury
2. ventilation
3. wounds and hemorrhage
4. perfusion
5. level of consciousness/responsiveness

Select the proper grouping.

A. 2, 5
B. 3, 5
C. 2, 4, 5
D. 1, 3, 4, 5
E. 1, 2, 3, 4, 5

Answer C

12. Categorize the patient below according to the START triage system. Severe head injuries with very rapid and deep gasping respirations, blood from ears and nose, present carotid pulse, and patient only responsive to painful stimuli.

A. critical/immediate
B. delayed
C. dead/non-salvageable
D. unable to determine priority
E. none of the above

Answer A

13. Categorize the patient below according to the START triage system. An entrapped patient is not breathing when rescuers arrive, the head is repositioned and spontaneous breathing begins at 22 breaths per minute. The patient has a pulse of 90 and awakens; appropriately responsive to questioning.

A. critical/immediate
B. delayed
C. dead/non-salvageable
D. unable to determine the priority
E. none of the above

Answer B

14. One rule which normally applies to the mass-casualty incident is that there are more patients than ambulances until well into the incident. Transportation therefore must remain a high priority.

A. True
B. False

Answer A

15. Categorize the patient below according to the START triage system.
A patient is found to be breathing at 24 times per minute. Neither a radial nor carotid pulse can be found.

A. critical/immediate
B. dead/non-salvageable
C. delayed
D. unable to determine the priority
E. none of the above

Answer A

List the personnel, equipment needs, and responsibilities for each of the following sectors of a mass-casualty incident.

16. Extrication:

fire Suppression
limited medical Personal Rescue
equipment.
light + heavy extrication Safety
limited medical equipment

Special Rescue
extrication equipment

Patients extricated to treatment
area + triaged there.

17. Treatment:

Paramedics
Emt's
most medical Personel
medical Supplies
Large Area for treatment
possible triaging

Protection from the enviorment
for Patients location of medical
treatment.

18. Staging:

Responding Units + Personel without
Assignment (Fire, police, Ems Rescue)
Units not yet needed Should be A

distance from the Scene So As not to
Congest or interfere with the incedent.
Location where they may Await Assignment.

19. Transport:

Located near treatment Sector.
Sufficient Space to Accept and load Ambu-
-lances + possible helecopters. Personel:
Sector officer and those help needed

to load Ambulances. Patient distributed
to hospitals: Hospitals told of #
And Nature of Patients enroute.

7

STRESS MANAGEMENT IN EMERGENCY SERVICES

Review of the Objectives for Chapter 7

After reading this chapter, you should be able to:

1. Define the term "stress."

p. 112

Stress is a nonspecific mental or physical strain. It induces a state of physical and psychological arousal. It is to some degree present in everyone.

2. Describe the stress reaction, including the various psychological and physiological components.

pp. 113 to 116

The body's response to stress is called the stress reaction. It is a series of physical and emotional responses which prepare the body to react to the stress. The emotional response affects the limbic system causing the strong feelings of fear, anger, rage, etc., and triggers the physical response caused by the hypothalamus. The physical response includes the release of epinephrine and norepinephrine, increasing the heart rate, blood pressure, blood glucose levels, muscle tension, etc. (the fight or flight response).

3. Describe the three stages of the body's response to stress.

p. 113

Alarm reaction is the initial response to stress. It includes increasing pulse and respiratory rate, blood pressure, pupillary dilatation, and catecholamine release.

Resistance is the stage at which the human system begins to adjust and adapt to stress. The pulse, blood pressure, etc., may return toward normal.

Exhaustion is a stage where the human system is no longer able to withstand the stressors and begins to return to the alarm reaction stage, though the response may now be irreversible.

4. Describe the term critical incident, and describe critical incident stress.

pp. 113 to 114

The **critical incident** is a particular event that impacts a rescuer. It may be a disaster, a particularly gruesome accident, or an incident involving a patient which reminds the care giver of someone who is personally close (father, daughter, etc.).

Critical incident stress is a reaction to a catastrophic event which has a powerful emotional impact on the rescuer. If unrecognized and left untreated, it may adversely affect the rescuer. The program designed to intervene is Critical Incident Stress Debriefing.

5. Describe the three types of stress reaction.

pp. 113 to 116

Acute Stress Reaction usually occurs immediately or shortly after a catastrophic event and has a powerful emotional impact. It will manifest with physical and psychological signs and symptoms shortly after the incident.

Delayed Stress Reaction (post-traumatic stress disorder) occurs days or as long as years after a catastrophic event. The individual may experience recurrent nightmares or recollections of the incident, be less responsive to the external world, as well as experience physical and cognitive symptoms.

Cumulative Stress Reaction (burnout) is due to recurring minor stressors and takes years to develop. The individual will experience boredom, apathy, fatigue, physical complaints, sleep disturbances, depression, irritability, paranoia, crying spells, poor job performance, problems with personal relationships, and sometimes, suicide.

6. Describe anxiety, and discuss its role in helping us to cope with various stressors.

pp. 116 to 117

Anxiety is an emotional state caused by stress that initiates defense mechanisms which, in turn, protect us from stress.

Anxiety alerts us to something stressful in our life. It heightens our awareness of the environment and prepares us to confront or withdraw (fight or flight response) from the stressor. Some stress, and consequently some anxiety, is normal. It helps us develop defense mechanisms to cope with everyday stress. If we are put in a new situation, such as starting work as a paramedic, we will experience stress as we assume the role. With time the anxiety will lessen, however we will always be under some anxiety due to the responsibility of the job. This on-alert stress level is a protective mechanism.

7. Name common causes of job stress for the paramedic.

pp. 117 to 118

multiple role responsibilities
unfinished tasks
angry and confused citizens
continuous time constraints
absence of challenge
excessive demand on time, energy, ability, or emotions
restrictions on practice
unpredictable changes in the work place
lack of recognition
limited career mobility
abusive patients and dangerous situations
critically ill or dying patients

8. List techniques the paramedic can use to deal with stress.

pp. 118 to 120

Identification of stressors

What is really happening?
Are you to blame?
Are expectations realistic?

Seek support

individual communication
group communication (CISD)

Life style

adequate rest and sleep
leave the job at work
balancing work and recreation
accept that certain things are beyond your control

9. Describe the purpose of Critical Incident Stress Debriefing.

p. 120

CISD is intended to defuse the stress associated with a major incident which has the ability to impact the rescuers. Examples are an infant or child severely injured or killed, a fellow paramedic dying in the line of duty, a severely gruesome accident or a multi- or mass-injury situation. The CISD is intended to allow the participants to vent their anger, frustration, disappointment, and other strong emotional responses to avert delayed stress syndrome.

10. Describe the stages of the grief process.

pp. 120 to 121

Denial and isolation - when the individual withdraws into himself and insulates himself from the stressor.

Anger - when the individual strikes out with anger and frustration because of the stressor. Other people are often targets, not the source of the stress.

Bargaining - when the individual attempts to bargain in attempts to hold off the inevitable.

Depression - when the individual reacts to the loss or impending loss by depression and solitude.

Acceptance - when the patient has accepted the inevitable. It may be a stage of relief or one absent of feelings.

11. Describe the needs of the dying patient, the family of the dying patient, and the EMT-P.

p. 121

Patient

The opportunity to bring up the subject of death
Honest and supportive care givers
A truthful description of the circumstances if asked

Family

Honest, supportive and reassuring care givers
If the patient has died, the family becomes the patient
The use of accurate terms, not euphemisms (passed away, expired, moved on, etc.)
A gentle voice, reassuring touch and non-verbal communication

Paramedic

Recognize that death is often an occurrence we can do little to stop
Be realistic about personal expectations
Recognize the need to talk about stressful situations

CASE STUDY REVIEW

Reread the case study in **PARAMEDIC EMERGENCY CARE** and then read the discussion below.

The case study described in this chapter addresses the severe impact that violence, which draws Emergency Medical Services into operation, can have upon care providers. It also identifies the importance of recognizing the need for seeking help.

Chapter 7 Case Study

Three care providers, Bill, Cathy, and the student, are presented with a hostage situation and some of the more dramatic stressors found in Emergency Medical Service. As health care providers, they are prepared to offer help, yet in this scenario they are unable to provide any care. They are exposed to a hostile and angry environment, to severe and brutal trauma inflicted by one individual on others, and are unable to contribute any real service other than identifying that nothing can be done.

This circumstance is one of the more devastating scenarios one could experience in EMS. The personal reactions which occur are intense. Bill is obviously affected by the incident, especially since the murdered child is about the same age as one of his own. He is reacting to the stress by repressing his feelings of anger and frustration. If these feelings are not eventually identified and released, chances are good they will have a negative effect on Bill's career, leading either to his leaving EMS or to experiencing burnout.

The Critical Incident Stress Debriefing is a good mechanism for venting stress and the pent-up feelings one may hold after a devastating incident. Bill finally opens up and allows the impact of the incident to surface where he can recognize and deal with it. It is evident that this and the follow-up debriefings were effective enough to keep Bill, Cathy, and the student from delayed stress syndrome and burnout.

It is also important to develop situational support from EMS partners and peers. While this incident was dramatic, many of the minor or common frustrations of prehospital care are not appropriate for the CISD session. The support of other crew members who understand the stressors and can empathize with your feelings can make an EMS career worthwhile and psychologically healthy.

READING COMPREHENSION SELF-EXAM

1. Stress is an inherent aspect of emergency medical services. Prehospital personnel must learn to manage stress, as well as the particular stressors that cause it.

   A. True
   B. False

   Answer A

2. The body, in response to stress, generally goes through which of the following stages?

   A. alarm
   B. resistance
   C. exhaustion
   D. all of the above
   E. A and C above

   Answer D

3. Which of the following signs and symptoms indicate acute stress reaction requiring corrective action?

A. decreased alertness to surroundings
B. seriously slowed thinking
C. elevated blood pressure
D. crying spells
E. all of the above

Answer E

4. Post traumatic stress syndrome is an immediate result of a terrible incident that impacts the care provider and renders him or her unable to function at the emergency scene.

A. True
B. False

Answer B

5. Which of the following is true of cumulative stress reaction (burnout)?
1. it is best treated by prevention
2. it is the end result of failure of coping mechanisms
3. it is manifest by overreaction to patient needs
4. the paramedic no longer cares about the job
5. appears only while at work
Select the proper grouping.

A. 1, 2, 5
B. 1, 2, 4
C. 2, 3, 4, 5
D. 1, 2, 3, 4
E. 1, 2, 3, 4, 5

Answer B

6. Anxiety is a sympathetic nervous system response to danger. It maintains all potential resources, emotional and physical, in readiness for emergencies. Anxiety is based upon the individual's perception of the environment around him or her.

A. True
B. False

Answer A

7. Which of the following are effective elements of stress control?
1. leaving the job at work
2. physical activity
3. trying to reduce coping mechanisms
4. balancing work and recreation
Select the proper grouping.

A. 1, 4
B. 2, 3
C. 1, 3, 4
D. 1, 2, 4
E. 1, 2, 3, 4

Answer D

8. Critical Incident Stress Debriefing is or does all **except** which of the following?

A. psychotherapy and psychological treatment
B. designed to reduce the impact of the critical incident
C. structured group meetings
D. accelerates normal recovery
E. allows rescue personnel to openly discuss their feelings

Answer A

9. The step in the grieving process in which the patient formulates an agreement which, the patient thinks, will postpone the inevitable.

A. isolation
B. acceptance
C. denial
D. bargaining
E. depression

Answer D

10. In caring for the family of a patient who has just died, phrases like expired, passed away, or moved on, are preferred to words like dead or died.

A. True
B. False

Answer B

11. Which of the following are signs or symptoms that might normally be caused by anxiety?
   1. chest tightness or pain
   2. abdominal cramps and nausea
   3. increased blood pressure
   4. life threatening dysrhythmias
   5. frequent urination

Select the proper grouping.

A. 1, 3, 5
B. 2, 3, 4
C. 1, 4, 5
D. 1, 2, 3, 4
E. 1, 2, 3, 5

Answer E

12. Cumulative stress reaction or burnout is often associated with a single event which strongly affects an individual, persistently nags at the individual, and results in a disinterest in life.

A. True
B. False

Answer B

13. The acute stress reaction is the impact that follows a catastrophic event. The process designed to deal with this stress and prevent post-traumatic stress disorders is called ....

A. alarm defusing.
B. critical incident stress debriefing.
C. peer support counseling.
D. constructive stress management.
E. Kubler-Ross sessions.

Answer B

SPECIAL PROJECTS

Prehospital Environment Crossword Puzzle

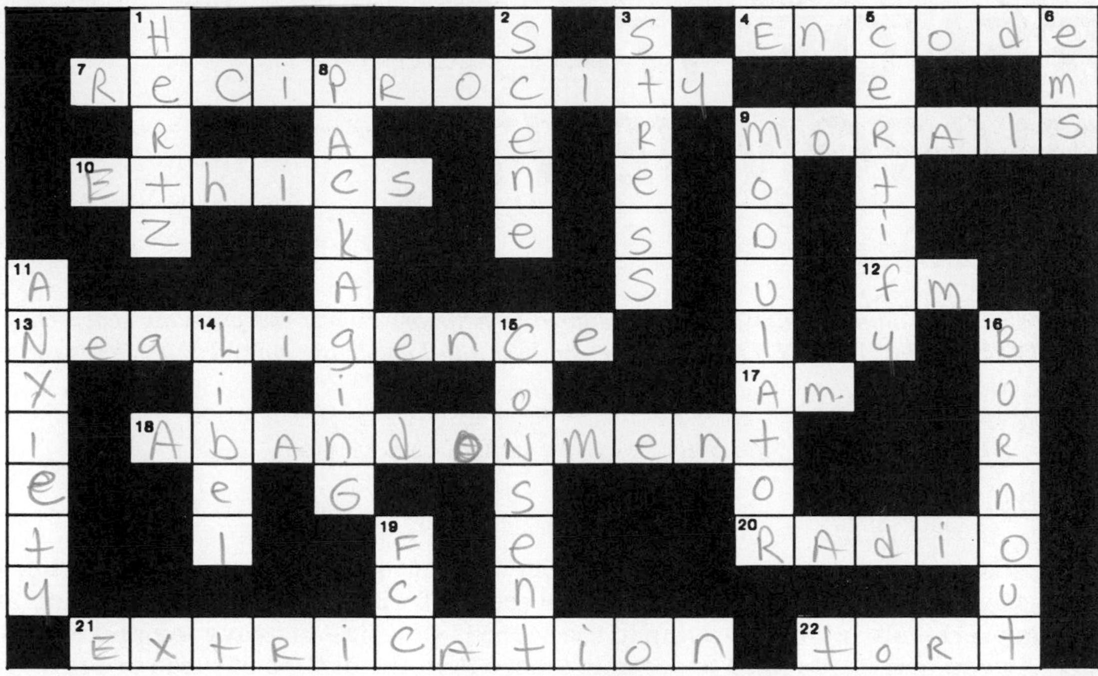

The crossword puzzle above addresses the vocabulary of chapters 1 through 7.

ACROSS

4. The process of superimposing a signal on another radio signal.
7. The granting of licensure or certification based upon meeting someone else's standards.
9. The principles of right and wrong governed by an individual's conscience.
10. The rules or standards of conduct for a profession or group.
12. The radio design which modulates the signal frequency to transmit voice.
13. A deviation from the accepted standard of care which cases harm to a patient.
17. The radio design which modulates the signal amplitude to transmit voice.
18. The termination of health care without assurance that an equal or greater level will continue.
20. The device which receives and transmits signals in the electromagnetic spectrum to allow voice communication.
21. The use of force to disentangle an entrapped patient.
22. A branch of civil law concerning civil wrongs between two parties.

DOWN

1. One cycle of electrical activity per second.
2. The location of a medical or traumatic emergency.
3. A nonspecific mental or physical strain.
5. The recognition process which identifies that an individual has met an agency's standards.
6. The initials commonly associated with the prehospital emergency care system.
8. The preparation of a patient for removal from a rescue scene.
9. A device which converts sound waves into radio waves.
11. An emotional state caused by stress.
14. The act of injuring a person's name or character by false or malicious writings.
15. The granting of permission to treat, by a patient to a health care provider.
16. The failure of normal coping mechanisms to buffer job-related stress.
19. The initials of the federal agency responsible for licensing and monitoring the EMS radio system.

DIVISION REVIEW

PREHOSPITAL ENVIRONMENT

Chapters 1 through 7

The following scenario-based questions are designed to help you review the previous seven chapters of **PARAMEDIC EMERGENCY CARE**. *They combine the knowledge gained thus far through your reading and course work.*

Scenario I

Dispatch calls your paramedic ambulance to an accident at the interstate exit ramp. Police are on the scene and have reported a three car accident with numerous patients and at least four persons seriously injured. Driving to the scene is slow due to heavy fog and very limited visibility. As you arrive, it's hard to see much more than the outline of three or four wrecked cars and the lights of several police cars.

1. As a result of your survey of the scene you should do which of the following?
   1. call for additional EMS units
   2. establish your unit as incident command
   3. assure the highway and ramp are closed to traffic
   4. request fire service for possible fire suppression
   5. request rescue and extrication services

   Select the proper grouping.

   A. 1, 3, 4
   B. 2, 4
   C. 1, 2, 3
   D. 1, 3, 4, 5
   E. 1, 2, 3, 4, 5 — Answer E

2. When you leave the ambulance, you will do which of the following?
   1. look for hazards
   2. begin to provide patient care
   3. identify the number of patients
   4. identify the location of patients
   5. determine the need for additional resources

   Select the proper grouping.

   A. 1, 3, 4, 5
   B. 2
   C. 1, 4, 5
   D. 3, 5
   E. 1, 2, 3, 4, 5 — Answer A

You quickly walk through the scene and find twelve seriously injured patients in the three cars. Four or five patients may be trapped and at least one appears dead. The police have the scene well secured and have cleared the ramp for emergency vehicle entry. The local fire department arrives as does the EMS supervisor from your service.

3. While both the fire chief and your supervisor wish to be incident command, the best choice is the local fire chief.

   A. True
   B. False

   Answer A

4. During your walk through the scene you have assessed some of the patients. Since you have now left those patients, are you liable for abandonment?
   1. you have not established a patient-care provider relationship
   2. the multiple-casualty incident requires a different approach to assessment and care
   3. while performing triage you will assure all patients are cared for in order of priority
   4. you are abandoning the patients and may be held liable

   Select the proper grouping.

   A. 1, 3
   B. 1, 2, 3
   C. 2, 3
   D. 1
   E. 4

   Answer B

5. Which of the following should be communicated to the hospitals in the area?
   1. The existence of a multi-casualty incident.
   2. The number of expected patients.
   3. A listing of each patient and their injuries.
   4. The nature of injuries.
   5. The seriousness of injuries.

   Select the proper grouping.

   A. 3
   B. 1, 4
   C. 2
   D. 1, 2, 5
   E. 1, 2, 4, 5

   Answer D

6. As you surrender incident command you should do all **except** which of the following?

   A. Relinquish your authority and leave to begin patient care immediately.
   B. Relate the number of injured patients to the new incident commander.
   C. Identify the resources requested and en route to the new incident commander.
   D. Identify the sectors which are established to the new incident commander.
   E. Provide the new commander with a list of units in the staging sector.

   Answer A

You surrender incident command and report to the extrication sector where you are asked to assume the role of safety officer.

7. You immediately notice that two of the crew members are without gloves while working around broken window glass. You should halt the operation immediately and assure they don gloves.

A. True
B. False

Answer A

You notice that one of your paramedics is just standing and trembling with a horrified look on his face. He has just found a very young child who is lifeless under the dash of a wrecked car.

8. The paramedic is most likely experiencing ....

A. anxiety.
B. delayed stress syndrome.
C. paranoia.
D. acute stress reaction.
E. denial and isolation.

Answer D

9. The death of a child, and the response of the paramedic to it, suggest that this incident should be followed by a Critical Incident Stress Debriefing.

A. True
B. False

Answer A

10. This paramedic and the rest of the crew are candidates for delayed stress reaction.

A. True
B. False

Answer A

Scenario II

A known heart patient has called 911 for assistance due to severe chest pain. The police arrive and find the patient unconscious, apneic, and pulseless. They begin mouth to mask ventilation, cardiac compression, and attach their automatic defibrillator. The machine charges and shocks twice. The patient gasps for a breath and begins to move about as you arrive with advanced life support.

11. The type of response described here is ....

A. multiphasic.
B. dual.
C. tiered.
D. duplex.
E. none of the above.

Answer C

12. The patient in this emergency was treated in accordance with ....

A. expressed consent.
B. implied consent.
C. informed consent.
D. involuntary consent.
E. none of the above.

Answer B

13. The training for a dispatcher which would prepare him or her to instruct the caller in care procedures is called an integrated care/dispatching system.

A. True
B. False

Answer B

You attach electrodes and find the patient to have a normal sinus rhythm with frequent premature ventricular contractions. Following protocol you provide the patient with oxygen, establish an IV of D_5W, and administer a bolus of lidocaine. Shortly thereafter you call medical control to update them on the patient's condition and send the current ECG. The doctor interrupts you during your report and orders a second bolus of lidocaine.

14. Protocol which allows you to begin advanced life support care before contacting a physician is called ....

A. direct medical control.
B. indirect medical control.
C. delegated practice.
D. licensure.
E. none of the above.

Answer B

15. The radio you used to contact medical control is which of the following?
1. simplex
2. duplex
3. multiplex
4. FM
5. AM

Select the proper grouping.

A. 1, 5
B. 2, 5
C. 2, 4
D. 3, 4
E. 3, 5

Answer D

16. The principle which permits you to initiate advanced and invasive procedures under the license of the medical control physician is called ....

A. implied consent.
B. indirect medical control.
C. delegation of authority.
D. extended practice.
E. *res ipsa loquitur.*

Answer C

8

MEDICAL TERMINOLOGY

Review of the Objectives for Chapter 8

After reading this chapter, you should be able to:

1. Locate at least 10 medical terms in a medical dictionary.

p. 125

The medical dictionary is an essential tool of the practicing paramedic. It provides an opportunity to investigate the meanings of new terms and to confirm spellings for documentation.

2. Identify common root words and define their meaning.

pp. 125 to 129

Root words are the essence of medical terminology. They identify the object of the term and are modified by the attachment of prefixes or suffixes.

3. Identify and define common suffixes and prefixes.

pp. 130 to 133

Prefixes and suffixes modify root words and provide the flexibility of medical terminology. To a degree, they are used interchangeably, allowing a person to dissect an unknown term and decipher its meaning.

4. Identify and determine the meaning of common medical terms.

pp. 125 to 133

Medical terminology represents the language of medicine and is a hallmark of the health care professional. Terminology allows the paramedic to communicate very specific information very quickly with the accuracy essential to emergency care.

5. Identify common medical abbreviations.

pp. 134 to 139

Medical abbreviations enhance efficiency in the recording of common signs, symptoms, medical information, and care procedures. They greatly reduce the time and space needed to record patient and care information on the run report.

CASE STUDY REVIEW

Reread the case study in **PARAMEDIC EMERGENCY CARE** and then read the discussion below.

This case study highlights the language of medicine and its importance to you as you care for a patient and interact with the medical community.

Chapter 8 Case Study

The crew of Air 1 responds to a pre-arranged transport of a cardiac patient from a rural community hospital to a large urban hospital for definitive care. The circumstances of an interfacility transfer commonly bring the paramedic to communicate both with the transferring and receiving hospital staff.

If you are placed in this role, you will be expected to take (and understand) the report from the sending physician. This will certainly be communicated in the terms associated with medicine.

Some of the terminology used in this case study can be examined to reveal the root words, suffixes, and prefixes commonly used in emergency medicine. The patient is on a *thrombolytic* which is a word combining thrombo, meaning clot, and lytic, meaning destruction or loosening (a clot buster). The nurse uses the word *retrosternal* to describe the patient's pain. The word is made up of the prefix retro, meaning backward or behind, and the root, sterno, which describes the sternum. Hence the pain is behind the sternum. She also uses the words *dyspnea* (dys - difficult, pnea - breathing), *hypertension* (hyper - over or excessive, tension - pressure), *angioplasty* (angio - blood vessel, plasty - molding or surgical forming), *cholecystectomy* (chole - bile or gall bladder, cyst - stone or cyst, ectomy - a cutting out), and *endoscopic* (endo - within, scopic - examination with an instrument), *polypectomy* (polyp - pedicle or foot, ectomy - a cutting out).

The nurse also uses some terminology in her report. *EKG* stands for electrocardiogram (the K is from the original German spelling) and *CABG* refers to a coronary artery bypass graph performed during open heart surgery. Medical abbreviations will also be extensively used when the paramedics go to document the call. Abbreviations save space and yet quickly and accurately convey medical information. Knowledge of common terminology and proper medical abbreviations will help you throughout your career as a paramedic.

MEDICAL TERM DISSECTION

Identify the meaning of the root word, prefix, and suffix (as appropriate) for each of the medical terms listed below.

Please note that often root words, prefixes, and suffixes are used interchangeably.

	Prefix	Root	Suffix
1. myasthenia	—	muscle	weakness.
2. cephalgia	—	Head	Pain
3. percuss	through	Shake Violently	—
4. cyanosis	—	Blue	Condition
5. hyperflexion	over	bending	—
6. pathology	—	disease	Study.
7. tachypnea	Rapid	breathing	—
8. rhinorrhea	—	nose	flow.
9. dysuria	difficult	Urination	—
10. hypertrophy	over	nourishment	—
11. osteocyte	—	bone	Cell
12. hypoxemia	low	oxygen	—

13. adrenal	toward	Kidney	—
14. hepatomegaly		liver	enlarged
15. abduct	AWAY	guide	—
16. otoscope	—	EAR	examine
17. perinatal	AROUND	Birth	—
18. antecubital	before	elbow	—
19. dissect	twice	cutt	—
20. epicardium	Above	heart	—
21. postpartum	After	Birth	—
22. intervertebral	between	Spinal Bones.	—
23. neuroplasty	—	nerve	Repair
24. hemothorax	blood	thorax	—
25. polyphagia	frequent	eating	—

Identify the meaning of these common medical abbreviations.

26. abd. Abdomen

27. ARDS Adult Respiratory distress Syndrome.

28. ASCVD Atherosclerotic Cardiovascular Disease

29. AMA Against medical Advice

30. BBB Bundle branch Block.

31. b.i.d. twice per day

32. C/C Chief Complaint

33. CHF Congestive heart failure

34. COPD Chronic obstructive Pulmonary disease

35. CSF Cerebral Spinal Fluid

36. Dx diagnosis

37. DPT Diphtheria Pertussis Tetnas Vaccine.

38. ETOH ethanol alcohol

39. fx fracture

40. GSW gunshot wound

41. GU Genito – Urinary

42. Hct. hematocrit

43. Hx history

44. IPPB Intermittent Positive Pressure Breathing

45. JVD Jugular Vein distension

46. MVA motor vehical Accident

47. NPO nothing by mouth

48. PRN as needed.

49. pt. patient

50. Rx Care or Remedy.

51. S/S Signs or Symptons

52. S.O.B. Shortness of breath.

53. T.K.O. to Keep open.

54. y.o. years old.

55. wt. Weight

Locate the following words in a medical dictionary.

autoantigen

kyogenic

contralateral

eudiaphoresis

canthorrhaphy

divulsion

retroperitoneal

prodromal

vulnerate

thrombasthenia

mesosystolic

vesicostomy

9

ANATOMY AND PHYSIOLOGY

Review of the Objectives for Chapter 9

After reading this chapter, you should be able to:

1. Define the following terms:

p. 142

Anatomy is the study of the structure of the human body.
Physiology is the study of the function of the human body.
Biochemistry is the study of chemical events occurring within a living organism.
Biophysics is the application of the principles of physics to body mechanics.

2. Describe the hierarchy of the human body.

p. 143

The human body consists of billions of cells which are organized into tissues, organs, organ systems, and finally, the entire organism.

3. Define the following:

pp. 143 to 146

The **cell** is the basic unit of life and the most elemental component of the human body.
A **tissue** is a group of cells which perform a similar function.
An **organ** is a group of tissues which function together.
An **organ system** consists of organs which work together to perform essential and coordinated functions.
An **organism** is the collection of cells, tissues, organs, and organ systems which work together to maintain life.

4. List the four types of tissue.

p. 144

Epithelial tissue lines the surfaces of the body and provides protection and specialized functions such as secretion, absorption, diffusion, and filtration.
Muscle tissue has the ability to contract with force. There are three types: cardiac, smooth, and skeletal.
Connective tissue provides support, connection, and insulation. It is the most abundant tissue in the body.
Nerve tissue is a very specialized tissue designed to conduct electrical impulses throughout the body.

5. List the major body organ systems and describe their functions.

pp. 145 to 446

The **cardiovascular system** transports oxygen, carbon dioxide, nutrients, and waste products within the human body.

The **respiratory system** draws in oxygen and expels carbon dioxide and other waste products.
The **gastrointestinal system** takes in, digests and absorbs nutrients, and eliminates unneeded materials and waste products.
The **genito-urinary system** plays an important role in fluid regulation and electrolyte balance.
The **reproductive system** is responsible for reproduction of the organism and production of hormones which make the sexes distinct.
The **nervous system** controls virtually all bodily functions, and is the intellect and the essence of being.
The **lymphatic system** plays an important role in disease fighting, filtration of blood, and removal of waste.
The **endocrine system** is a system of controls which effect the body's function by the release of chemical messengers into the bloodstream.
The **muscular system** is responsible for movement, posture, and heat production.
The **skeletal system** provides support, shape, protection, and movement for the body.

6. Define homeostasis, and give an example of a homeostatic response.

p. 146

Homeostasis is the tendency of the body to keep the physiologic environment fairly constant. Examples include sweating to lose excess heat when the body temperature rises, or breathing faster and deeper after exercise to eliminate CO_2 and metabolic acids.

7. List the topographical anatomy terms frequently used in Emergency Medical Services and give an example of each.

p. 159

(see the matching questions in this chapter of the workbook)

8. Describe in topographical terms the locations of various lines on the chest.

p. 160

Mid-axillary line is a line separating the anterior and posterior chest drawn from the middle of the axilla downward.
Mid-clavicular line is an imaginary line drawn downward from the mid-point of each clavicle.
Mid-sternal line is a vertical line drawn downward from the middle of the manubrium.
Mid-spinal line is a vertical line drawn down the center of the spine.
Mid-scapular line is a vertical line drawn through the middle of the scapula on each side of the posterior chest.

9. Describe, in anatomical terms, a wound on the chest and abdomen which tells the medical control physician the precise location of the lesion.

p. 160

Any location on the chest can be described in terms of the intersection of the mid-sternal, mid-clavicular, mid-axillary, mid-scapular or mid-spinal lines and the corresponding rib or intercostal space.

10. Describe the four anatomical divisions of the abdomen and list the organs within each.

pp. 161 to 162

The abdomen is divided by a vertical and horizontal line intersecting at the umbilicus and forming four quadrants: the right upper, the left upper, the right lower, and the left lower.

Right upper quadrant - liver, gall bladder, pancreas, duodenum, right kidney, and colon

Left upper quadrant - spleen, pancreas, stomach, left kidney, and colon
Right lower quadrant - appendix, ascending colon, small intestine, right ovary, and right fallopian tube
Left lower quadrant - small intestine, descending colon, left ovary, and left fallopian tube

11. List the major body cavities and the important organs in each.

pp. 160 to 163

The **cranium** contains the brain (cerebrum, cerebellum, and brainstem).
The **thoracic cavity** contains the lungs, heart, and structures of the mediastinum.
The **abdominal cavity** contains the liver, gall bladder, stomach, pancreas, spleen, intestines, kidneys, and adrenal glands.
The **pelvic cavity** contains the bladder, ovaries, rectum, fallopian tubes, and uterus.
The **spinal cavity** contains the spinal cord.

CASE STUDY REVIEW

Reread the case study in **PARAMEDIC EMERGENCY CARE** and then read the discussion below.

This case study identifies the need for a method of describing precise anatomical locations to the medical command physician. It also identifies the significance that an accurate description has to the awaiting medical team.

Chapter 9 Case Study

The injuries presented in this case study penetrate the chest and certainly damage the structures within. The wounds are obvious to the attending paramedics though they must be described to the medical control physician, who cannot view them. The use of anatomical landmarks, body planes, and descriptive terminology can present a picture over the radio which is concise and specific.

The information conveyed by Steve identifies the specific locations of the three entrance wounds by the use of the anatomical lines of the chest. Steve could be even more effective if he also identified the locations of the exit wounds. That information would give a better picture to the emergency physician of the path of travel of the projectiles and suggest which internal organs have been affected. Steve should also relate the type of weapon used and the range from which it was fired. Nonetheless, Dr. Johnson is able to identify potential surgical procedures needed to determine the exact organ injuries the gunshot wounds have likely caused, and repair the damage.

This case study demonstrates the immediacy of penetrating injuries to the chest, and abdomen. In these types of injuries the paramedic is unable to effectively stabilize the patient in the field and best serves the patient by expediting transport and initiating what care can be offered in the moving ambulance. The initiation of an IV is accomplished quickly without any time lost in delivering the patient to the emergency department. Note that the use of the PASG is contraindicated in the patient with penetrating trauma to the chest.

The patient is quickly moved from the ambulance to the emergency department and then to surgery. While the outcome of this patient scenario is unknown, the delivery of care was expeditious and appropriate based upon the information communicated by the paramedics to the medical control physician.

Once the transport has been completed, Steve will be responsible to record the elements of this call on the run report form. He will use medical terminology and abbreviations to document patient injuries, condition and pertinent history. The terminology and abbreviations he uses are commonly used by the hospitals in his area, and serve to help record all the information in the limited space of the report form.

Steve also uses anatomical terms to describe the precise locations of the entrance and exit gunshot wounds. He knows full well that there is a good chance he will be called to testify in the criminal charges against the gunman. If his documentation is complete and professional, he will appear to have done his job well when in front of the jury or judge.

READING COMPREHENSION SELF-EXAM

1. The basic unit of life is the ....

   A. cell.
   B. organ.
   C. tissue.
   D. organism.
   E. mitochondria.

   Answer A

2. A group of cells which perform a similar function are called ....

   A. an organ.
   B. a tissue.
   C. an organ system.
   D. organelles.
   E. muscles.

   Answer B

3. The natural tendency of the body to maintain a physiologically constant environment is termed ....

   A. biochemistry.
   B. biophysics.
   C. homeostasis.
   D. physiologic stability.
   E. none of the above.

   Answer C

4. The vertical anatomic line located anteriorly on the thorax between the sternum and the mid-axillary line is the ....

   A. mid-scapular line.
   B. anterior axillary line.
   C. mid-mamillary line.
   D. posterior axillary line.
   E. none of the above.

   Answer E

5. Which of the following organs can be found in the right upper quadrant of the abdomen?
   1. right kidney
   2. spleen
   3. appendix
   4. descending colon
   5. gall bladder

   Select the proper grouping.

   A. 1, 5
   B. 1, 2, 4
   C. 2, 3, 5
   D. 2, 3, 4, 5
   E. 1, 2, 3, 4, 5

   Answer A

SPECIAL PROJECTS

Matching: **Anatomical terms relating to direction** *(some answers may be used more than once)*

A. toward the front
B. toward the back
C. toward the mid-line
D. on or near the surface
E. well below the surface
F. inside the body
G. outside the body
H. nearer the trunk
I. further from the trunk
J. away from the mid-line
K. toward the tail or bottom
L. toward the top or head

---

distal	6. I	ventral	12. A	superficial	18. D
craniad	7. L	superior	13. L	posterior	19. B
deep	8. E	caudal	14. K	external	20. G
internal	9. F	medial	15. C	inferior	21. K
anterior	10. A	dorsal	16. B	cephalad	22. L
lateral	11.____	proximal	17. H		

Matching: **Anatomical terms relating to body position**

A. lying on the side
B. head of bed elevated greater than 45 degrees
C. lying horizontal with face upward
D. lying horizontal with feet higher than head
E. lying horizontal with face downward
F. lying face up, legs flexed, thighs abducted
G. head of bed elevated less than 45 degrees

Trendelenburg position 23. D
semi-Fowler's position 24. G
lateral recumbent position 25. A
Fowler's position 26. B
prone position 27. E
lithotomy position 28. F
supine position 29. C

Short Answer: **Anatomical terms relating to body movement**

a movement away from the body 30. Abduction
rotating the arm, bringing the palm facing down 31. PRONAtion
the act of bending 32. flexION
a movement toward the body 33. Adduction
the act of straightening 34. extension
rotating the arm, bringing the palm facing up 35. SupinAtion

10

PATIENT ASSESSMENT

Part I - (pages 166 to 176)

Objective Review for Chapter 10

After reading this chapter, you should be able to:

1. Identify information gathered in each of the six phases of patient assessment.

pp. 167 to 200

Dispatch Information Review
location of the call
nature of the call
what equipment may be needed
what skills may be needed
what other units are responding

Survey of the Scene
hazards to personal and patient safety
mechanism of injury
number of patients
additional resources needed

Primary Assessment
identify life threatening injuries/problems
correct life threatening injuries/problems
determine transport status

Secondary Assessment
head to toe evaluation for the signs of injury
verbal questioning for symptoms
gathered by inspection, palpation, auscultation, and percussion

Determination of Vital Signs
pulse rate and quality
respiratory rate, depth, and effort
blood pressure
temperature - core and peripheral

Patient History
history of chief complaint
previous medical history
medications
allergies
personal physician

2. List some of the potential scene hazards that need to be ruled out before patient care can occur.

p. 169

traffic hazards
electrical hazards
fire hazards

explosion hazards
toxic chemicals (inhalation, contamination or burns)
adverse surface conditions (debris, oil, etc.)
adverse weather conditions
structural collapse

3. Explain the A, B, C, D, and E of the primary assessment.

pp. 171 to 174

A - **Airway and cervical spine control** - is the spine stabilized and is the airway clear of obstruction?
B - **Breathing** - are respirations adequate in volume and rate?
C - **Cardiovascular function** - is capillary refill more than 3 seconds, is the skin cool and clammy, are pulses rapid and weak or are distal pulses absent?
D - **Disability (neurologic)** - is the patient conscious, alert, and oriented (AVPU); is there any sign of neurologic deficit?
E - **Expose and Examine** - for any signs of potentially life threatening injury, including hemorrhage or head, neck, chest or abdominal injury.

4. Compare and contrast the results of the primary assessment for the medical and trauma patients.

pp. 174 to 176

Trauma Patient
The trauma patient is assessed through the primary survey to determine whether he or she would be best served by rapid transport or on-scene care. The survey examines the mechanism of injury and the status of airway, breathing, circulation, and the signs or symptoms of serious internal or external injury.

Medical Patient
The medical patient is assessed to determine any immediate life threat. Many circumstances like cardiac arrest require on-scene care while there are some which demand immediate transport, like ectopic pregnancy. In the medical emergency you must determine the problem affecting the patient through signs, symptoms, and patient history, since the mechanism of injury may not be apparent.

CASE STUDY REVIEW

Reread the case study in **PARAMEDIC EMERGENCY CARE** and then read the discussion below.

This case study examines an auto accident and applies the elements of response which have been addressed within this chapter. Included in the first part of this case study are the dispatch information, scene survey, primary assessment, and the determination of the need for rapid transport or on-scene care.

Chapter I0 Case Study

This study demonstrates the importance of a complete patient assessment, even though an apparent cause for the problem might be suspected. A complete and orderly approach is the only way to assure that all elements of a complete patient physical evaluation and history are addressed and that no important items are overlooked.

The dispatch information should allow the responding paramedics to prepare their trauma equipment for arrival at the scene. They might wish to ready a 1000 ml bag of lactated Ringer's solution and ready an IV start kit with large-bore catheters. The splinting and bandaging equipment may be located and loaded on the stretcher as may the trauma bag, PASG, and long spineboard.

Once within view of the scene, the paramedic must evaluate for hazards. Electrical sources, fire, and debris are all concerns. The unit is parked well away from the scene and the crew does not approach the auto until the scene is safe. They are concerned for the safety of others and cordon off the area. They locate what appears to be the only patient and instruct him not to move. As the fire department arrives, the scene is secured, the power is shut off and safety measures (the charged line and blocked vehicle) are taken. The mechanism of injury is assessed, as is the history of the event and the evidence describing it. Before they approach the patient, the paramedics know something is wrong. The absence of skid marks and the description of a swerving vehicle reflect problems before the impact. The primary assessment is completed as the spine is immobilized and the airway, breathing, and circulatory status are secured. The patient has a decreased level of consciousness, and based upon that alone, he is considered for rapid transport.

READING COMPREHENSION SELF-EXAM

1. Place the elements of patient assessment in proper order.
   1. secondary assessment
   2. vital signs
   3. survey of the scene
   4. primary assessment
   5. dispatch information review

   Select the proper grouping.

   A. 4, 1, 3, 2, 5
   B. 2, 4, 1, 3, 5
   C. 5, 3, 4, 1, 2
   D. 3, 5, 4, 1, 2
   E. 3, 4, 1, 5, 2

   Answer C

2. The patient assessment is completed in the first few minutes while at the patient's side. If done correctly, it never needs to be repeated nor updated.

   A. True
   B. False

   Answer B

3. A relatively complete patient assessment needs to be employed with both medical and trauma patients for many reasons, including ....
   1. trauma may be caused by a medical problem.
   2. an apparent medical problem may have a traumatic origin.
   3. medical problems may have significant physical signs.
   4. pre-existing medical problems increase the impact of trauma.

   Select the proper grouping.

   A. 1, 4
   B. 1, 2, 4
   C. 2, 3
   D. 2, 3, 4
   E. 1, 2, 3, 4

   Answer E

4. All elements of the scene survey should be evaluated before the paramedic arrives at the patient's side.

   A. True
   B. False

   Answer A

5. The survey of the scene should include all except which of the following ....

A. identification of mechanism of injury.
B. identification of hazards.
C. assessment of the patient for life-threatening problems.
D. locating all potential patients.
E. determination of any additional assistance needed.

Answer C

6. What percentage of trauma patients are in need of rapid transport to the hospital?

A. less than 5%
B. less than 10%
C. less than 20%
D. less than 25%
E. less than 50%

Answer B

7. The first step of the primary assessment is ....

A. airway assessment.
B. breathing assessment.
C. circulatory function assessment.
D. airway assessment with cervical spine control.
E. cervical spine stabilization.

Answer D

8. Which of the following are characteristics of normal respiration?
1. volume of 500 ml
2. rate of 12 to 20 / min
3. irregular pattern
4. quiet and unobtrusive
Select the proper grouping.

A. 1, 2
B. 2, 3
C. 1, 2, 4
D. 1, 3, 4
E. 1, 2, 3, 4

Answer E

9. Airway and breathing are not always as easy to evaluate in the initial assessment as one would first believe. Only with careful and conscious effort can the paramedic determine if the airway is indeed clear and breathing adequate.

A. True
B. False

Answer A

10. Which of the following pulses would be the last to be lost as a patient moves into shock?

A. brachial
B. radial
C. carotid
D. temporal
E. tibial

Answer C

11. Place the following in order from completely conscious to deeply unconscious.
    1. unresponsive
    2. responds to verbal stimuli
    3. responds to painful stimuli
    4. alert

Select the proper grouping.

A. 1, 3, 2, 4
B. 2, 3, 4, 1
C. 3, 2, 1, 4
D. 4, 2, 3, 1
E. 4, 3, 2, 1

Answer D

12. The "Expose" of the primary assessment examines the patient to determine ....

A. if significant external hemorrhage is occurring.
B. if there is potential respiratory compromise.
C. if there are any other life-threatening injuries.
D. all of the above.
E. none of the above.

Answer D

13. Under what conditions is the trauma patient considered for rapid transport?
    1. threat to respiratory function
    2. signs or symptoms of shock
    3. neurologic deficit

Select the proper grouping.

A. 1
B. 2
C. 3
D. 1, 3
E. 1, 2, 3

Answer E

14. A soft tissue injury will quickly (in a few seconds) develop the "black and blue" discoloration of ecchymosis, making it easy for the paramedic to identify during the primary and secondary assessment.

A. True
B. False

Answer B

15. During the auscultation process you should ....

A. warm the disc or bell before application.
B. explain the procedure to the patient.
C. apply the bell or disc gently.
D. all of the above.
E. none of the above.

Answer E

SPECIAL PROJECTS

The authoring of both the radio message to medical command and the written run report are two of the most important tasks you will perform as a paramedic. Read the following information, reread the case study in your textbook, compose your initial and updated radio messages, and then complete the run report for this call.

The Call:

At 6:32 p.m. unit 21 is paged through dispatch and enroute to a one-car accident at the corner of Elm and Wildwood Lane. One patient is reported unconscious and the fire department is also en route. You and your partner, Mike Grailing (a paramedic), arrive with the ambulance at 6:45 and stand-by awaiting arrival of the fire department and the securing of the scene.

Once the scene is safe, your partner applies cervical immobilization while you apply the cervical collar (6:50) and begin the assessment. Oxygen is administered at 12 L per minute, the patient awakens and initial vitals (including a respiratory rate of 30 with audible wheezes) are taken at 6:52. The EKG displays normal sinus rhythm. Based upon protocol, you initiate the IV run T.K.O. in the right forearm while the patient is being immobilized and moved to a long spineboard. The patient is found to be 28 years old.

Medical command is contacted and you call in the following:

Unit 21 to medical Controll, we Are Attending A male victim of A one-car Accident. He was initially unconcous, but is now conscous, alert and oriented. He has A small Contusion on his forehead And A small welt on his neck. He was stung by A bee And has had A previous Allergic Reaction. Vitals are BP 120/76 pulse 90 And Strong respirations 30 And O'2 saturation of 98%. There Are wheezes Audible And he is Complaining of A lump in the throat He is on 12L of O'2 via NBreather mask And has one IV of LR Running TKO. A Cervical collar has been applied and Spinal Imobilization is underway.

Orders for Epinephrine (1:1,000) and Benadryl are received and they are administered at 6:55. Just prior to movement (6:59) to the ambulance, the patient is monitored and found to have the following vitals: B.P. 118/88, pulse 78 strong and regular, respirations 20 and regular with clear breath sounds, an EKG showing a normal sinus rhythm, and a pulse oximetry reading of 99%.

The patient history, which is taken at the scene and during transport, reveals that he is William Sobeski, 28 years old, and lives at 2145 East Brookline Drive, in Rochester City. The patient denies any allergy except to bee stings. He was stung by a bee two years ago and was rushed to the emergency department because he "couldn't catch his breath." He denies any headache, visual disturbances, and any numbness and tingling. He requests Community Hospital because his sister works there. En route vitals are B.P. 122/78, pulse of 68 strong and regular, respirations 22 and regular, and a pulse oximetry reading of 98%, all taken at 7:02.

Contact medical command and provide the following update:

0.3mg of Epi SQ & 50mg Benedryl IM Have Been Administered
Current vitals are BP 122/78 pulse 68 and Strong, Respirations
22 and Regular O_2 Saturation 98% patient states that lump
in throat is gone, wheezes have disappeared, ETA 10 minutes

ETA 10 minutes.

The final vitals, taken just before arrival, are blood pressure 122/80, pulse 86, saturation of 98%, and respirations at 24 and regular. The EKG still displays normal sinus rhythm, and the patient is conscious and oriented.

The trip is uneventful and the patient is delivered to the emergency department at 7:25. The patient responsibilities are transferred to the staff, and the attending physician is given the final patient update. The vehicle is re-stocked, cleaned, and you are ready for service at 7:55 p.m.

Using the information contained in the Case Study and this additional narrative, complete the run report on the following page.

Compare the radio communication and run report form which you prepared against the example in the answer key section of this workbook. As you make this comparison, realize that there are "many correct" ways to communicate this body of information. Ensure that the information you have recorded contains the major points of your assessment and care, and enough other material to describe the patient and his condition to the receiving physician and anyone else who might review the form. Remember that this document may be the only record of your assessment and care for this patient. When you are done, it should be a complete account of your actions.

Date 5/10/94 | Emergency Medical Service Run Report | Run # 912

Patient Information		Service Information	Times
Name: William Sobeski		Agency: Unit 21	Rcvd 18:32
Address: 2145 E. Brokline Dr.		Location: wildwood + Elm	Enrt 18:32
City: Rochester	St: NY Zip: 70645	Call Origin: Dispatch	Scne 18:45
Age: 28 Birth: 11/29/63	Sex: [M][F] (M circled)	Type: Emrg[X] Non[ ] Trnsfr[ ]	LvSn 19:02
Nature of Call: One CAR Accident			ArHsp 19:25
Chief Complaint: Head injury – Allergic Reaction, Bee Sting			InSv 19:55

Description of Current Problem:
Pt was Apparently Stung by a bee, Then Struck a tree In his Auto, Found Unconscious, then Awoke. Contusion on his forehead where it hit the windshield & a small welt on his neck. Patient complains of a lump In his throat + mild dyspnea – mild Wheezes on Auscultation. Pt Reports previous life threatening Allergic Reaction, has prescribed Kit Assesment otherwise Remarkable.

Trauma Scr: 16 Glascow: 15

Medical Problems	Past	Present
Cardiac	[ ]	[ ]
Stroke	[ ]	[ ]
Acute Abdomen	[ ]	[ ]
Diabetes	[ ]	[ ]
Psychiatric	[ ]	[ ]
Epilepsy	[ ]	[ ]
Drug/Alcohol	[ ]	[ ]
Poisoning	[ ]	[ ]
Allergy/Asthma	[X]	[X]
Syncope	[ ]	[ ]
Obstetrical	[ ]	[ ]
GYN	[ ]	[ ]

Other:

On Scene Care: O2 – C-collar, Spinal Imm IV-TKO D5W w/16ga R Forearm 0.3mg Epi SQ, 50mg Benedryl IM.

First Aid: None

By Whom?

O2 @ 12 L 18:52 Via non R | C-Collar 18:50 | S-Immob. 18:58 | Stretcher 18:59

Allergies/Meds: Be Sting/no other Allergies Known

Past Med Hx: Bee Sting And Reaction 2 yrs Ago no other history noted.

Time	Pulse	Resp.	BP S/D	LOC	EKG
18:52	R: 90 [r][i]	R: 30 [s][l]	110/76	[a][v][p][u]	NSR
Care/Comments: IV Initiated by Protocall – 16ga R Forearm.					
18:59	R: 78 [r][i]	R: 20 [s][l]	118/88	[a][v][p][u]	NSR
Care/Comments: Epi + Benedryl Administered, SaO2 99%, wheezes gone					
19:02	R: 68 [r][i]	R: 22 [s][l]	122/78	[a][v][p][u]	NSR
Care/Comments: SaO2 98%					
19:20	R: 86 [r][i]	R: 24 [s][l]	122/80	[a][v][p][u]	NSR
Care/Comments: Wheezes Reduced, SaO2 98%					

Destination: Comunity Hospital

Reason: [X]pt [ ] Closest [ ] M.D [ ] Other

Contacted: [X] Radio [ ] Tele [ ] Direct

Ar Status: [X] Better [ ] UnC [ ] Worse

Personnel:	Certification
1. Cindy Robertson	[P][E][O]
2. Dave Impson	[P][E][O]
3. Joe Carren	[P][E][O]

10

PATIENT ASSESSMENT

Part II - (pages 176 to 205)

Objective Review for Chapter 10

After reading this chapter, you should be able to:

5. List, by anatomical area, the each of the signs examined during the secondary assessment. **pp. 178 to 190**

Head
- Battle's sign
- bilateral periorbital ecchymosis (raccoon eyes)
- Cerebrospinal Fluid (CSF) drainage
- pupillary response and tracking
- instability, crepitation
- swelling, discoloration, hemorrhage, wounds

Neck
- jugular vein destination
- tracheal deviation
- crepitation
- swelling, discoloration, hemorrhage, wounds

Chest
- symmetry, bilateral excursion
- retraction, paradoxical movement, sucking chest wounds
- auscultate for rales, rhonchi, wheezes, stridor or unequal breath sounds
- respiratory rate, depth, and pattern
- instability, crepitation
- swelling, discoloration, hemorrhage, wounds

Abdomen
- symmetry, pulsation
- diaphragmatic breathing
- palpated for tenderness, rebound tenderness, guarding or distention
- swelling, discoloration, hemorrhage, wounds
- evisceration

Pelvis
- crepitation, instability
- swelling, discoloration, hemorrhage, wounds

Genitalia
- swelling, discoloration, hemorrhage, wounds, discharge

Lower Extremities
- distal pulse, capillary refill or neurologic deficit
- instability, crepitation
- swelling, discoloration, hemorrhage, wounds

Upper Extremities
- distal pulse, capillary refill or neurologic deficit
- instability, crepitation
- swelling, discoloration, hemorrhage, wounds

6. List the four vital signs and explain their significance to patient evaluation.

pp. 191 to 194

Pulse

Rate and strength may suggest stress, shock, head injury or other problem.

Respirations

Rate, volume, and pattern will determine the effectiveness and efficiency of respiratory effort.

Blood Pressure

Systolic and diastolic pressure will suggest the effectiveness of the circulatory system.

Temperature

Reflects the body's ability to generate and dissipate heat to maintain a standard internal environment at 37° C.

7. Cite some of the important information that can be obtained by a thorough evaluation of the chief complaint.

pp. 197 to 199

Location - What is the exact location of the pain or discomfort? Is it moving or radiating?
Quality - How is the pain described by the patient? Is it gnawing, cramping, dull, sharp, etc.?
Intensity - How severe is the pain, assessed by the patient's description and their reaction to it?
Duration - How long has the discomfort or pain affected the patient? Is it an acute problem or one which developed over time?
Onset - What events, actions or circumstances might be related to the onset of pain or discomfort?
Alleviating/aggravating factors - What circumstances either increase or decrease the pain or discomfort of the chief complaint?

8. Identify the important details gained by questioning the patient about medications, medical history, allergies, and personal physician.

pp. 199 to 200

Medications - What medications does the patient have prescribed, what are they for, and could they be contributing to the current problem?

Medical History - What pre-existing medical problems does the patient have and which are pertinent to the current problem?

Allergies - What substances, or medications, is the patient allergic to and could they be a contributing factor?

Personal Physician - Who is the patient's physician and what is the physician's specialty?

9. Demonstrate a complete patient assessment - from evaluation of dispatch information, to documentation of the call.

pp. 166 to 204

The complete assessment of an ill or injured patient includes the skills of dispatch information review, survey of the scene, the primary assessment, the secondary assessment, vital sign determination, and the gathering of a complete and pertinent patient history. The paramedic must observe, listen, and feel carefully to determine everything wrong with the patient and support that suspicion with signs, symptoms, and observation.

(Attempt patient assessment under the supervision of your instructor.)

CASE STUDY REVIEW (cont.)

Reread the case study in **PARAMEDIC EMERGENCY CARE** and then read the discussion below.

This case study examines an auto accident and applies the elements of response which have been addressed within this chapter. Included in the second part of this case study review are the secondary assessment, vital signs, and important elements of the medical history.

Chapter 10 Case Study (cont.)

The secondary assessment should be applied quickly in this case, if at all. However, the information provided as the patient awakens identifies an explanation for the incident. The vital signs support patient stability though blood pressure is a late sign in shock's development and may be misleading with head injury. The allergic reaction becomes a primary concern as does the possibility of head injury. The paramedic will continue to question and examine for other causes and injuries.

The patient is provided with oxygen, which could have been given earlier, and a prophylactic IV is started with a large bore catheter. This is done just in case rapid fluid infusion is required. Epinephrine and Benadryl are ordered and administered while the patient is prepared for transport. The on-scene time is kept to a minimum, though most care is provided at the scene.

During transport the paramedics continue their evaluation and care of the patient. The allergic reaction may compromise the airway very quickly. Intubation equipment must be ready for use. The history of unconsciousness might suggest a possible head injury. This could also compromise the patient's airway and breathing.

The attending paramedics must be very careful in communicating the events of this call to the emergency department personnel and in documenting the call on the run sheet. The circumstances at the scene: the lack of skid marks, the bystanders - description of the events prior to impact, and the paramedic's description of the scene - all will help to justify the initial care rendered. The information given by the patient, the description of the lump on the neck, and the wheezes will help establish the credibility of an allergic reaction as the cause of the incident. If this information is described carefully it will support the care steps taken. If it is not documented, or documented poorly, it may leave the medical control physician wondering what was done at the scene and why.

READING COMPREHENSION SELF-EXAM

16. The order of the steps of the secondary assessment is not important, though the paramedic must be sure to provide a complete survey.

    A. True
    B. False

    Answer A

17. Battle's sign is reflective of what medical problem?

    A. periorbital ecchymosis
    B. basilar skull fracture
    C. cerebrospinal fluid leak
    D. cerebral concussion or contusion
    E. none of the above

    Answer B

18. Pin-point pupils suggest which of the following medical problems?

    A. opiate overdose
    B. hypertension
    C. heat stroke
    D. all of the above
    E. A and C

    Answer A

19. Distended jugular veins are suggestive of which of the following conditions?

A. congestive heart failure
B. cor pulmonale
C. tension pneumothorax
D. cardiac tamponade
E. all of the above

Answer E

20. In caring for a patient with a traumatic chest injury, the trachea is found to deviate away from the injured side. What problem would you suspect?

A. flail chest
B. tension pneumothorax
C. airway obstruction
D. cardiac tamponade
E. all of the above

Answer B

21. As you palpate the chest you perceive a crackling sensation much like crushing "Rice Krispies" beneath the skin. This finding would lead you to suspect ....

A. tension pneumothorax.
B. pericardial tamponade.
C. flail chest.
D. tracheal deviation.
E. none of the above.

Answer A

22. Which of the following sounds heard during auscultation of the airway is generally the quietest?

A. stridor
B. rhonchi
C. wheezes
D. rales
E. none of the above

Answer D

23. The pain experienced during palpation of the abdomen which occurs as you release gentle pressure is called ....

A. Cullen's sign.
B. Grey Turner's sign.
C. rebound tenderness.
D. guarding.
E. none of the above.

Answer C

24. Your assessment may reveal a pelvic fracture exists when pressure is applied to the iliac crests. This fracture may present with ....

A. pain.
B. crepitation.
C. instability.
D. any of the above.
E. A and B only.

Answer D

25. If no distal pulse can be located, which of the following should be used to evaluate distal perfusion?

A. skin temperature
B. skin color
C. capillary refill
D. all of the above
E. A and C

Answer D

26. The Glasgow Coma Scale will give the conscious and alert patient a maximum score of ....

A. 12.
B. 10.
C. 15.
D. 25.
E. 100%.

Answer C

27. Hypotension is a very helpful sign in predicting shock. Blood pressure falls as the body begins to compensate for blood loss; hence it is a reliable and early predictor of impending shock.

A. True
B. False

Answer B

28. A systolic blood pressure of 120 mm. Hg. ....

A. is considered normal in a healthy adult.
B. may indicate hypertension in a patient.
C. may indicate hypotension in a patient.
D. all of the above.
E. none of the above.

Answer D

29. Blood pressure taken by palpation is expected to be lower than a normal reading by about ....

A. 10 mm Hg.
B. 20 mm Hg.
C. 30 mm Hg.
D. 50 mm Hg.
E. 75 mm Hg.

Answer A

30. If a patient's pulse rate rises by more than 15 beats per minute when moved from a supine to a seated position, it generally indicates a blood loss of more than ....

A. 100 ml.
B. 250 ml.
C. 500 ml.
D. 1000 ml.
E. 1250 ml.

Answer C

31. Normal body temperature, or core temperature, is about ....

A. 37 ° C.
B. 35 ° C.
C. 25 ° C.
D. 76 ° F.
E. none of the above.

Answer A

32. At which temperature does the body's normal warming mechanisms cease to function?

A. 98 ° F
B. 93 ° F
C. 89 ° F
D. 70 ° F
E. 35 ° F

Answer B

33. A well oxgenated patient will normally generate a pulse oximetry reading of ....

A. 75%.
B. 85%.
C. 90%.
D. 94%.
E. 98%.

Answer E

34. Conditions where the pulse oximeter may give false or inconsistent readings include ....
   1. low red blood cell count (anemias).
   2. hyperventilation.
   3. high concentrations of oxygen.
   4. carbon monoxide inhalation.

Select the proper grouping.

A. 1, 4
B. 2, 3
C. 2, 4
D. 1, 3
E. 1, 2, 3

Answer A

35. In some cases of prolonged extrication, blood may be drawn from the patient and rushed to the hospital to be typed and cross-matched. This may permit whole blood to be available for the patient immediately upon arrival at the emergency department.

A. True
B. False

Answer A

36. That which causes the patient (or someone else) to call for assistance is the chief complaint and is defined as the ....

A. discomfort.
B. pain.
C. dysfunction.
D. all of the above.
E. none of the above.

Answer D

37. During the patient assessment, the paramedic must carefully listen to what the patient says. Too often we anticipate the patient's problem and then suffer tunnel vision. We fail to look for other signs, symptoms, or conditions which could account for the patient's presentation.

A. True
B. False

Answer A

38. The words crushing, oppressive, gnawing are best categorized under ....

A. intensity of the pain.
B. quality of the pain.
C. duration of the pain.
D. location of the pain.
E. quantity of the pain.

Answer B

39. A sleep disturbing dyspnea which is associated with congestive heart failure is called ....

A. paroxysmal nocturnal dyspnea.
B. the blue bloater syndrome.
C. Biot's respirations.
D. pulmonary edema.
E. ascites.

Answer A

40. The objective of radio communication between the paramedic and medical control is the conveyance of just enough information to support the request for care and to allow the emergency department to prepare for the patient's arrival.

A. True
B. False

Answer A

41. Identify information that can be gained from the dispatcher.

Type of medical Emergency — Best Scene Approach
Vehical Placement
Seriousness
Skills + equipment needed

42. Identify information that the survey of the scene may provide.

mechanism of Injury — Haz mat Problems.
Scene hazards — Police needed.
number of Patients
location of Patients
Additional resources needed

SPECIAL PROJECTS

Patient Assessment Crossword Puzzle

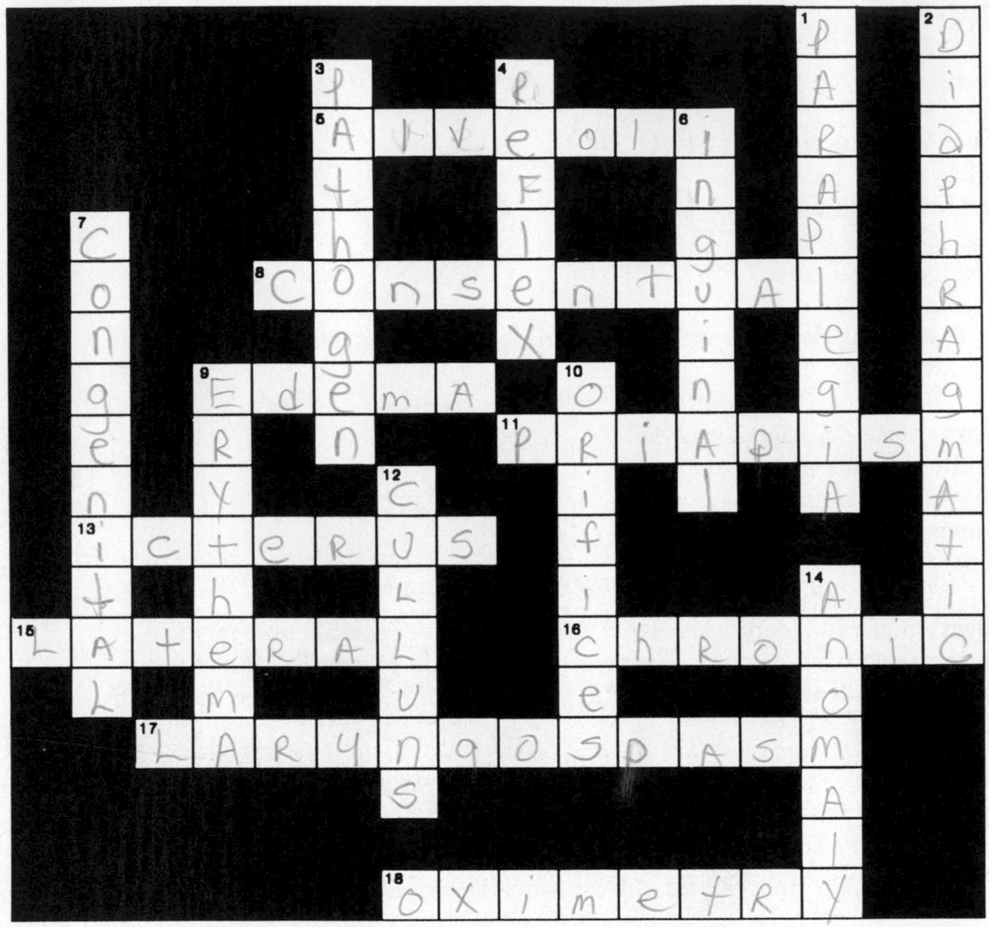

The crossword puzzle above addresses the vocabulary in chapter 10.

ACROSS

5. A microscopic chamber of the lung.
8. Moving together. Frequently used to describe eye movement.
9. An accumulation of fluid in the tissue.
11. A painful and prolonged erection of the penis.
13. A yellow discoloration of the mucus membranes, due to failure of the body to rid itself of bile.
15. To the side.
16. A condition which begins or progresses slowly.
17. A spasm of the vocal folds which may occlude the airway.
18. An assessment modality which evaluates the oxygen saturation of arterial blood.

DOWN

1. Paralysis of the lower extremities.
2. Pertaining to the diaphragm.
3. A disease-producing micro-organism.
4. A neurological response to stimuli, occurring without conscious thought.
6. Pertaining to the groin region.
7. Occurring at or about birth.
9. A red discoloration of the skin due to inflammation or irritation.
10. Openings found within the human body.
12. A bluish discoloration around the umbilicus.
14. A deviation from the norm or average.

II

ADVANCED AIRWAY MANAGMENT AND VENTILATION

Part I - (pages 208 to 228)

Review of the objectives for Chapter II

After reading this chapter, you should be able to:

1. Describe the anatomy of the upper airway, including:

pp. 209 to 212

The **mouth** or oral cavity is a single cavity which serves as an auxiliary air passage. The posterior upper surface is the soft palate which moves upward and closes off the passages from the nose to the pharynx during swallowing.

The **nose** is a hollow two-sided chamber, lined with mucous membranes which warm, filter, and humidify air as it enters the respiratory system. Its openings are the nares; or nostrils.

The **pharynx** plays the role of both food and air passage. It is the throat and functions as the transitional area for food and air between the nose and mouth and between the esophagus and larynx.

The **epiglottis** is a flap-like structure covering the opening of the trachea, the glottis. It closes during swallowing to prevent food or fluids from entering the trachea and respiratory system.

The **larynx** is the tubular structure which begins the lower airway. It consists of the thyroid and cricoid cartilages, the vocal cords, the arytenoid folds, and the upper portion of the trachea. It is the "Adam's apple," located in the anterior neck.

2. Name the three regions of the pharynx.

p. 210

The pharynx can be subdivided into the naso-, oro-, and laryngo-pharynx. Each is the portion of the throat which is most closely associated with the nasal cavity, oral cavity or larynx, respectively.

nasopharynx **oropharynx** **laryngopharynx (or hypopharynx)**

3. Identify the relationship between the larynx and the tongue, pharynx, esophagus, and vocal cords.

pp. 210 to 211

The **tongue** is found well above the larynx.
The **pharynx** is the airway chamber found directly above the larynx.

The **epiglottis** is the flap of tissue which covers the glottic opening of the larynx.
The **esophagus** is found directly posterior to the larynx.
The **vocal cords** are found within the larynx and form the glottic opening.

4. Discuss the following functions of the respiratory system.

pp. 214 to 216

Mechanics of Ventilation

Respiration is the exchange of gases between a living organism and its environment. The lungs are stretched as the thoracic cage expands due to the muscular activity of the diaphragm, intercostal muscles, and other accessory muscles. Gravity and the elasticity of the lungs causes the air drawn in to be expired.

Pulmonary Circulation

The right ventricle pumps blood depleted of its oxygen to the pulmonary artery. The blood is directed to the respective lungs through the right and left pulmonary arteries which then divide, ultimately to the pulmonary capillaries. The blood returns through the pulmonary veins to the left atrium.

Gas Exchange in the Lungs

The air brought into the lungs contains 21% oxygen and very little carbon dioxide. It mixes with the gases leaving the bloodstream and is then exhaled, containing about 14% oxygen and 5% carbon dioxide.

Diffusion of Respiratory Gases

The oxygen of the inspired air diffuses into the alveolar space and then through the alveolar wall and the pulmonary capillary membrane where the oxygen attaches to the hemoglobin. Carbon dioxide diffuses from the blood plasma in the reverse direction.

5. Describe oxygen transport in the blood, and cite factors that affect it.

pp. 216 to 217

Oxygen is transported by the hemoglobin found in the red blood cell. As it passes a well oxygenated alveolus, 97% of the red blood cells are saturated. Very little oxygen is carried in the plasma of the blood. As the oxygenated blood passes the body's cells, the hemoglobin releases the oxygen. The following factors affect oxygen transport.

Inadequate alveolar ventilation

If the available oxygen at the alveolar level is reduced it will affect the oxygen saturation. This may be caused by low oxygen levels in the air, respiratory muscle paralysis, chronic obstructive pulmonary disease, asthma or pneumothorax.

Decrease alveolar diffusion

Pulmonary edema is a condition where fluid enters the space between the interior of the alveoli and the capillary. This increases the distance the oxygen must diffuse and hampers effective exchange.

Ventilation/perfusion mismatch

If some of the alveoli are without air exchange (as in atelectasis) some of the blood will pass alveoli which are not oxygenated and then mix with the oxygenated blood from other areas of the lung. If the circulation is obstructed to some of the alveoli (as in pulmonary embolism) a significant amount of blood is prevented from reaching the alveolar/capillary membrane.

6. Discuss carbon dioxide transport in the blood and list factors that affect it.

pp. 217 to 218

Approximately 66% of the carbon dioxide is transported in the blood as bicarbonate, 33% is transported attached to the hemoglobin and about 1% is dissolved in the plasma. Factors which affect carbon dioxide transport include the following.

Increased CO_2 production

The production of CO_2 is increased by the following actions; fever, muscle exertion, shivering, and metabolic acidosis.

Decreased CO_2 elimination

Decreased alveolar ventilation will result in decreased CO_2 elimination and may be caused by drug induced respiratory depression, airway obstruction, COPD, and impairment of respiratory muscles.

7. Describe the neurological control of respiration.

pp. 218 to 219

Respiration is controlled by the involuntary nervous system through the use of stretch receptors in the tissue of the lungs and through chemoreceptors which monitor the oxygen and carbon dioxide levels in the blood and the pH of the cerebrospinal fluid. An increase in carbon dioxide, a decrease in oxygen or a decrease in pH will increase the stimulus to breath. Stretching the lung tissue, as with a deep breath, will decrease the stimulus to breath.

8. Describe the various measures of respiratory function, and give the average normal values for each.

pp. 219 to 220

Tidal volume (V_T) is the average volume of air inspired (or expired) with each breath, about 500 ml.

Dead air space (V_D) is the portion of the tidal volume which does not reach the alveoli and is unavailable for gas exchange, about 150 ml.

Alveolar volume (V_A) is the amount of air that reaches the alveoli which each breath, about 350 ml.

Minute volume (V_{min}) is the amount of air moved by the respiratory system with each breath (tidal volume x respiratory rate).

Functional reserve capacity (FRC) is the maximum amount of air a person can move between a maximum inhalation and a maximum exhalation, about 4.5 liters.

9. Describe assessment of the airway and the respiratory system.

pp. 221 to 226

Assessment of the airway is an integral part of both the primary and secondary assessment. During the primary assessment, the focus is directed at detecting any potentially life threatening airway problems. If the patient is not conscious, alert, and speaking, the airway and respiration are closely evaluated. The rate, depth, and symmetry of respiration are noted as is the presence of any unusual respiratory sounds. During the secondary assessment the focus is on the finer details of respiratory evaluation including skin color, auscultation of breath sounds, abnormal breathing sounds, palpation of the thorax, and the use of pulse oximetry and/or capnography.

10. Discuss pulse oximetry and end-tidal carbon dioxide detection, and describe the prehospital use of both.

pp. 224 to 226

Pulse oximetry is a non-invasive monitoring of the arterial oxygenation of the skin. It accurately reflects the oxygen delivery to the end organs, giving an ongoing evaluation of circulation and respiration. In prehospital care, the oximeter is quick and easy to use and provides an accurate and constant evaluation of the cardio-respiratory system.

End tidal CO_2 detection (capnography) is accomplished either by a disposable device or an electronic sensor which affixes to an endotracheal tube. The units measure the amount of CO_2 in the exhaled gas. The disposable unit will change color while the electronic detector will register a reading. In prehospital care, the presence of CO_2 reflects proper endotracheal tube placement. However, in patients without effective circulation the CO_2 levels may be very low.

11. Describe the common causes of airway obstruction, and detail the special considerations of each.

pp. 226 to 228

Tongue - the most common cause of airway obstruction is the tongue. In the unconscious person the lack of muscle tone allows the tongue to rest against the posterior pharynx, and thereby obstruct the airway.

Foreign body - large, poorly chewed food and aspirated objects in children commonly account for airway obstruction. The victim will often grasp his or her throat which has become a universal distress signal.

Trauma - physical injury to the structures of the upper airway may result in loose objects such as the teeth or tissue and blood obstructing the airway. Further, blunt or penetrating trauma may result in collapse of the airway due to fracture or displacement of the larynx or trachea.

Laryngeal spasm or edema - the glottis is the smallest part of the airway and may be responsible for obstruction secondary to spasm or swelling. Spasm may be caused by anaphylaxis, epiglottitis, and inhalation of toxic substances, superheated steam, or smoke. Edema may be caused by trauma.

Aspiration - vomitus, blood, teeth, etc. may be aspirated by the adult and result in obstruction. Fluids may also accumulate in the lung tissue (pulmonary edema) and reduce the ability of oxygen to travel from the alveoli to the blood.

CASE STUDY REVIEW

Reread the case study in **PARAMEDIC EMERGENCY CARE** and then read the discussion below.

The paramedics in this case study are presented with a patient who requires airway maintenance and ventilation, as part of the advanced level care for cardiac arrest. While many aspects of emergency care are involved, the focus of this study is airway care and ventilation.

Chapter II Case Study

This particular presentation is common in prehospital emergency care. The patient is unresponsive and not breathing. The advanced procedures which PARAMEDIC EMERGENCY CARE teaches must be preceded by the basic emergency skills. In this case, the patient is not breathing and is initially cared for with head positioning. If trauma is not suggested by the scene survey, the head may be positioned some by the head tilt/chin lift. If spine injury is possible, the modified jaw thrust maneuver may be used. It may have been more appropriate for the paramedic to use the head tilt/chin lift, as it is better able to move the tongue out of the airway. The procedure does not restore spontaneous breathing. The oral airway is inserted to maintain the airway while the bag valve mask is employed. The BVM is used with the reservoir to ensure close to 100% oxygen at a flow of 12 to 15 liters per minute.

Pulselessness is treated with CPR as well as cardiac monitoring and the placement of an IV access route (the endotracheal tube may be used for some drugs). Advanced life support benefits from the advantage of the endotracheal tube to secure the airway. Otherwise, regurgitation provides the chance of pushing the gastric contents down the trachea, making ventilation and patient recovery more difficult. The endotracheal tube provides a direct and secure passageway for air to the lungs and prevents aspiration. It does carry some dangers. The placement of the tube too deep, as with this patient, will pass the tube beyond the left mainstem bronchus and allow inflation only of the right lung. The paramedics check for and identify the problem. Simply easing the tube back a few centimeters corrects the problem and provides good ventilation of both lung fields. The tube is secured well with tape and the depth of the tube is noted by the position of its markings (in centimeters) as they meet the upper teeth. Chest excursion and breath sounds are monitored frequently to verify tube placement throughout the resuscitation effort.

While the energy expended in this resuscitation attempt was not effective, the paramedics performed well and practiced their advanced life support skills. The prognosis for a patient found in cardiac arrest is not good. Many attempts will be unsuccessful, yet the careful application of these skills will provide the best chance for success. The paramedics of Medic 1 review their call, find just a few items they might improve next time, and prepare for their next call.

READING COMPREHENSION SELF-EXAM

1. The nasal cavity is responsible for ....
   1. warming the air.
   2. deoxygenating the air.
   3. humidifying the air.
   4. cleansing the air.

   Select the proper grouping.

   A. 1, 2
   B. 3, 4
   C. 1, 2, 4
   D. 1, 3, 4
   E. 1, 2, 3, 4

   Answer D

2. The space located between the tongue and the epiglottis is called the ....

   A. vallecula.
   B. cricoid.
   C. arytenoid fold.
   D. epiglottic fossa.
   E. none of the above.

   Answer A

3. Place the following in order as air would pass during **inspiration**.
   1. larynx
   2. nares
   3. nasopharynx
   4. laryngopharynx
   5. trachea

   Select the proper grouping.

   A. 2, 4, 3, 5, 1
   B. 2, 3, 4, 1, 5
   C. 5, 1, 4, 3, 2
   D. 4, 3, 1, 2, 5
   E. 3, 5, 2, 4, 1

   Answer B

4. The amount of air moved with one normal breath is called ....

   A. minute volume
   B. alveolar air
   C. tidal volume
   D. dead air space
   E. vital capacity

   Answer C

5. The oxygenated circulation that provides perfusion for the actual lung tissue flows through the ....

A. pulmonary arteries.
B. pulmonary veins.
C. bronchial arteries.
D. bronchial veins.
E. none of the above.

Answer ______

6. The percentage of carbon dioxide in air is approximately ....

A. 10%.
B. 4%.
C. 0.4%.
D. 0.04%.
E. none of the above.

Answer ______

7. Most of the carbon dioxide carried by the blood is ....

A. carried by the hemoglobin.
B. dissolved in the plasma.
C. transported as bicarbonate.
D. found as free gas in the blood.
E. bicarbonate, carried in the blood.

Answer ______

8. Which of the following conditions can cause reduced inspiratory volumes?
1. pneumothorax
2. asthma
3. respiratory muscle paralysis
4. emphysema

Select the proper grouping.

A. 1, 3
B. 2, 4
C. 2, 3, 4
D. 1, 3, 4
E. 1, 2, 3, 4

Answer ______

9. The normal oxygen saturation of hemoglobin in blood as it leaves the lungs is about ....

A. 75%.
B. 85%.
C. 90%.
D. 95%.
E. 97%.

Answer ______

10. The primary center controlling respiration is located in the ....

A. medulla.
B. pons.
C. spinal cord.
D. cerebrum.
E. cerebellum.

Answer ______

11. Which of the following would increase the production of carbon dioxide?
    1. fever
    2. airway obstruction
    3. shivering
    4. obstructive lung disease

    Select the proper grouping.

    A. 1, 2
    B. 1, 3
    C. 2, 3
    D. 2, 4
    E. 1, 3, 4

    Answer B

12. The reflex which responds to the stretch of the lungs by inhibiting respiration is the ....

    A. apneustic reflex.
    B. pneumotaxic reflex.
    C. Frank-Starling reflex.
    D. Hering-Breuer reflex.
    E. baroreceptor response.

    Answer D

13. Which of the following is the primary stimulus that causes respiration to occur?

    A. increase in pH of the blood
    B. decrease in pH of the blood
    C. increase in pH of the cerebrospinal fluid
    D. decrease in pH of the cerebrospinal fluid
    E. reduced oxygen in the blood

    Answer D

14. Which of the modified forms of respiration listed below is designed to expand the alveoli, which may have collapsed during periods of inactivity or rest?

    A. cough
    B. sneeze
    C. hiccup
    D. grunting
    E. none of the above

    Answer E Sigh

15. Hypoxia may be caused by which of the following?
    1. smoke or toxic gases
    2. high altitude
    3. airway obstruction
    4. asthma, pneumonia or emphysema
    5. shock or blood loss

    Select the proper grouping.

    A. 2, 4, 5
    B. 1, 3, 4
    C. 1, 3, 4, 5
    D. 2, 3, 4, 5
    E. 1, 2, 3, 4, 5

    Answer E

SPECIAL PROJECTS

Airway Obstruction

List the five causes of airway obstruction and identify the mechanism that causes each problem.

Tongue

The Absence of sufficient muscle Tone.

Foreign Body

Swallowing a Toy or marble.

Trauma

Large Poorly Chewed pieces of food: Alcohol or dentures have alot to do with this.

Laryngeal Spasm or Edema

anaphylaxis, Epiglottis, Inhalation of Super heated air, Smoke or Toxic Substances.

Aspiration

Dentures, teeth, vomitus

Normal Respiratory Values

Identify the normal values for each of the items listed below

	Inspired Air	Expired Air
% Oxygen	21%	14%
% Carbon dioxide	0.04	5%

PaO_2 80-100 $PaCO_2$ 35-45

Normal Respiratory Rates Volume:

Infant 40 to 60 Child 18 to 24 Adult 12 to 20

Tidal Volume 500ml Dead Space Volume 150ml

Alveolar Volume 350ml Minute Volume 4,500ml

II

ADVANCED AIRWAY MANAGEMENT AND VENTILATION

Part II - *(pages 228 to 287)*

Review of the objectives for Chapter II

After reading this chapter, you should be able to:

12. Describe the procedures used to open the airway manually.

pp. 228 to 230

Head-tilt/chin-lift places one hand on the forehead gently tilting the head back, while the other is on the mandible, displacing it anteriorly.

Jaw-thrust (or the triple airway maneuver) places both hands on the lateral mandible, displacing it inferiorly and anteriorly. If spinal injury is suspected, the head should not be tilted backwards (the modified jaw-thrust).

Jaw-lift places the rescuer's thumb into the mouth where the jaw and tongue are grasped between the thumb and fingers and are displaced anteriorly. Care must be exercised to ensure that the patient does not clench his teeth against the rescuer's thumb. Do not tilt the head with this maneuver if spinal injury is suspected.

Head-tilt/neck-lift maneuver places the rescuer's hand on the patient's forehead and under the neck. The head is tilted back while the neck is displaced anteriorly. (This technique is no longer recommended.)

13. Discuss indications, contraindications, and methods for insertion and use of the following mechanical airways.

pp. 231 to 233

The **Oropharyngeal Airway** is designed to maintain an airway by displacing the tongue anteriorly. It should not be used for patients who are conscious or have an intact gag reflex. It is inserted by displacing the tongue forward and inserting it with a tongue blade along the base of the tongue. It may also be inserted by placing it backwards into the oral cavity to the base of the tongue and then rotating it 180 degrees and continuing the insertion. The oral airway should be used when the patient is ventilated by any mechanical device.

The **Nasopharyngeal Airway** is designed to be inserted into the nasopharynx in the unconscious or semiconscious patient. It is a soft rubber tube which is lubricated and inserted posteriorly in the largest nostril. It is indicated in the semiconscious patient or as the oral airway would be used. It should be used with care in the patient with possible skull fracture.

The **Esophageal Obturator Airway** (EOA) is a blunt tube which is inserted into the esophagus. Its large, soft, low pressure cuff is inflated to occlude the esophagus and prevent both air from entering the stomach and materials from entering the airway. It is inserted blindly in a patient with the head and neck in the neutral or slightly flexed position. It should only be used in persons between five to six and one half feet tall and who do not have a history of esophageal disease, alcoholism or caustic ingestion.

The **Esophageal Gastric Tube Airway** (ETGA) is a modified EOA which has an opening for the passage of a gastric tube. It will allow for gastric suctioning or relief of gastric distention secondary to positive pressure ventilation. Its indications and contraindications are the same as for the EOA.

The **Pharyngeo-Tracheal Lumen Airway** (PTL) is a multi-tube device which isolates the oro- and nasopharynx and a second tube and cuff which will seal off either the trachea or esophagus. If the trachea is intubated, the lumen of the tube is used for ventilation. While the PTL airway has many applications, it may be difficult to determine whether the distal tube is located in the esophagus or trachea.

The **Esophageal Tracheal Combitube Airway** (ETC) is similar to the PTL airway except that it is designed to be inserted into either the trachea or esophagus. It will then occlude the passageway and the oral pharynx. The result is that the trachea is isolated from the esophagus. As with the PTL, EOA, and EGTA, the biggest drawback to this device is that the user must determine which tube the airway is in to assure the patient will be adequately ventilated.

14. List the equipment used to perform endotracheal intubation.

pp. 239 to 243

Laryngoscope handle and pre-selected blade
Magill forceps
endotracheal tube - selected size (and one larger and one smaller)
10 ml syringe
stylet (if desired)
bite block
suction
tape or commercial tie down
bag valve mask

15. Recall the indications, contraindications, and alternatives of endotracheal intubation.

pp. 243 to 245

Indications - Endotracheal intubation is the method of choice for the patient who is unable to protect his or her airway. It may also be considered for the patient who is expected to lose the airway due to swelling such as occurs with the inhalation injury, trauma patient, or one who is in need of assisted ventilation.

Contraindications - Endotracheal intubation is an advanced skill and should only be attempted by someone with extensive training in the technique. The skill is also contraindicated in the pediatric patient with possible epiglottitis unless respirations are worsening.

Alternatives - Alternatives to endotracheal intubation include EOA, EGTA, naso- or oropharyngeal airway or the PTL airway.

16. Explain the need for rapid placement of the endotracheal tube.

pp. 261 to 262

The indications for endotracheal intubation are a very high priority in emergency medical care. The process of its placement denies the patient oxygen via ventilation. Hence it is essential that the tube be placed correctly and rapidly.

17. Describe the methods used to assure correct placement of the endotracheal tube.

pp. 247 to 248

The most definitive confirmation of tube placement is seeing the tube pass through the vocal cords. However, it is essential to auscultate both lung fields to assure bilateral breath sounds and the epigastric area to ensure there are no gastric sounds immediately after tube placement and frequently during patient care.

18. List and demonstrate the steps in performing endotracheal intubation.

pp. 245 to 248

Assure the patient is being well ventilated by other means.
Assemble equipment including laryngoscope and blade, endotracheal tubes, tape, stylet, suction, BVM, 10 ml syringe, and Magill forceps.
Test equipment, including laryngoscope light and tube cuff.
Hyperventilate the patient.
Insert the laryngoscope and visualize the vocal cords.
Pass the endotracheal tube between the cords and advance it one-half to one inch beyond the cuff. Ventilate through the tube and auscultate both lung fields and epigastrium.
Inflate cuff with 5 ml to 10 ml of air.
Tape the tube securely in place and note the depth in centimeters.
Re-auscultate the lung fields and epigastric area.

19. State the precautions that should be used when intubating a trauma patient.

pp. 256 to 258

The trauma patient may have sustained spinal injury: all airway care must be provided with limited (if any) movement of the head and neck. In addition to the cervical collar, the head should be held in a neutral position manually by an EMT while intubation is attempted. Oro- or nasotracheal intubation may be tried or lighted stylet or digital techniques.

20. Identify the indications, contraindications, and methods of performing cricothyrotomy and percutaneous transtracheal ventilation.

pp. 272 to 276

Cricothyrotomy is an incision through the cricothyroid membrane to allow the passage of air. It is employed only when no other means of ventilating the patient is possible. A 6 mm tracheostomy tube may be used to maintain the opening.

Percutaneous transtracheal catheter ventilation (or needle cricothyrotomy) is used only for severe, partial, or complete, airway obstruction above the vocal cords which is not correctable by other methods. A needle is inserted through the cricothyroid membrane and attached to a high-pressure, high-volume oxygen line. Oxygen is passed through the large (14 ga or larger) catheter and then is allowed to escape. Expiration should take twice as long as inflation. If the chest does not deflate, a second needle or cricothyrotomy may be needed.

21. Discuss the indications, contraindications and methods of performing suctioning.

pp. 277 to 278

Suctioning is the use of pressures less than atmospheric to draw fluids and semifluids out of the airway. It should be used any time it can effectively remove material from the airway. Continuous suctioning should be avoided because it draws against the patient's ventilation attempts and generally interrupts ventilation in the apneic patient. It can be provided by electric or mechanical device.

22. Discuss indications, contraindications, and methods for using the pocket mask, bag-valve devices, demand valve resuscitator, and automatic ventilator.

pp. 282 to 286

The **pocket mask** is an adjunct to mouth-to-mouth ventilation which provides some protection against direct contact with the patient and the patient's exhaled air. It is a mask which is simply sealed to the patient's face with the rescuer's hands and held in place during ventilation. It is recommended anytime mouth-to-mouth ventilation is needed.

Bag-valve devices are mechanical devices which provide positive pressure ventilation. Its mask is sealed to the patient's face by one hand while the other hand squeezes the bag. It is best used for the intubated patient because the volume of air and the pressure delivered to the patient is low. If the patient is not intubated, the air exchanged may not be enough to sustain life. Any time the BVM is used it should have the oxygen reservoir attached and oxygen flowing at 12 to 15 liters per minute.

Demand valve resuscitators are oxygen-powered ventilation devices which will ventilate the patient with a flow of oxygen when a button or bar is pushed. It can be used with face mask, EOA, EGTA, PTL airway or endotracheal tube. It provides the patient with 100% oxygen. However, the pressures it uses may cause gastric insuflation or lung tissue damage. It is not recommended for patients who are intubated or the pediatric patient.

Automatic ventilators provide a patient with ventilation with 100% oxygen at a rate and volume determined by the user. Recent advances in technology make automatic ventilators compact and dependable for field use. They are not recommended for children under the age of 5 years and are dependent upon a good airway.

READING COMPREHENSION SELF-EXAM

16. In the head tilt/chin lift, the fingers under the chin should apply a firm pressure to ensure the jaw is displaced forward effectively.

A. True
B. False

Answer B

17. Which of the airway adjuncts act primarily by displacing the tongue anteriorly?
    1. oropharyngeal airway
    2. PTL airway
    3. endotracheal tube
    4. nasopharyngeal airway
    5. esophageal gastric tube airway

    Select the proper grouping.

A. 3
B. 1, 4
C. 2, 5
D. 1, 2, 4
E. 2, 3, 5

Answer B

18. The EOA and EGTA have which of the following advantages?
 1. They are inserted blindly.
 2. They may be inserted without spinal extension.
 3. They are dependably inserted into the esophagus.
 4. They are inserted without other equipment.
 5. They will not cause harm if inserted in the trachea.
 Select the proper grouping.

 A. 1, 3
 B. 2, 4, 5
 C. 3, 4, 5
 D. 1, 2, 4
 E. 1, 2, 4, 5

Answer D

19. The cuff of the esophageal obturator or gastric tube airway is designed to occlude the esophagus and should be filled with a maximum of ....

 A. 5 mm of air.
 B. 10 mm of air.
 C. 15 mm of air.
 D. 35 mm of air.
 E. 50 mm of air.

Answer D

20. During the insertion of the EOA or EGTA, the patient's head and neck should be in the ....

 A. hyperflexed position.
 B. flexed position.
 C. neutral position.
 D. extended position.
 E. B or C.

Answer E

21. The intent behind employing "Sellick's Maneuver" is to ....

 A. displace the diaphragm.
 B. increase venous return.
 C. prevent regurgitation.
 D. clear an airway obstruction.
 E. none of the above.

Answer C

22. In which of the respiratory arrest patients listed below should the EOA or EGTA be used with caution?
 1. cardiac arrest
 2. drug overdose
 3. electrocution
 4. hypoglycemia
 Select the proper grouping.

 A. 1
 B. 3
 C. 2, 4
 D. 1, 3
 E. 1, 2, 3

Answer C

23. Which of the following are features of the PTL airway?
   1. It can be inserted blindly.
   2. It can seal off the nasal and oral cavities.
   3. Whether the tube is in the trachea or esophagus, the patient can be ventilated.
   4. It can be inserted without displacing the spine.

   Select the proper grouping.

   A. 1, 4
   B. 2, 3
   C. 1, 3, 4
   D. 2, 3, 4
   E. 1, 2, 3, 4

   Answer E

24. Which of the following are benefits of the use of endotracheal intubation to secure the airway?
   1. gastric distention is prevented
   2. complete airway control is achieved
   3. the trachea can be easily suctioned
   4. medications can be introduced

   Select the proper grouping.

   A. 2, 3
   B. 1, 4
   C. 1, 2, 4
   D. 2, 3, 4
   E. 1, 2, 3, 4

   Answer E

25. The light of the laryngoscope should be a bright yellow and flicker slightly when pressure is placed on the blade.

   A. True
   B. False

   Answer B

26. The tip of the curve of the MacIntosh laryngoscope blade is designed to fit into which anatomic structure?

   A. the nasopharynx
   B. the glottic opening
   C. the vallecula
   D. the arytenoid fossa
   E. none of the above

   Answer C

27. The major purpose for using a malleable stylet during endotracheal intubation is to ....

   A. maintain a pre-set curve in the tube.
   B. keep the tube's lumen open.
   C. stiffen the tube so it can be pushed through the glottis.
   D. prevent foreign matter from entering the tube.
   E. none of the above.

   Answer A

28. When using the stylet for intubation, the tip of the device ....

A. should extend 3 mm beyond the end of the endotracheal tube.
B. should be even with the end of the endotracheal tube.
C. should be recessed one-half inch from the tube end.
D. is moved in or out during the intubation attempt as needed.
E. none of the above.

Answer C

29. To confirm the proper placement of the endotracheal tube, the paramedic should ....

A. watch the tube pass through the glottic opening.
B. auscultate the epigastric area during ventilation.
C. auscultate the left lung field.
D. auscultate the right lung field.
E. all of the above.

Answer E

30. Which of the following are true regarding endotracheal intubation?
1. the laryngoscope is held in the right hand
2. the laryngoscope is inserted in the right side of the mouth
3. the straight blade lifts the epiglottis
4. the curved blade lifts the epiglottis
5. advance the tube into the glottis, one half to one inch beyond the tube cuff

Select the proper grouping.

A. 1, 4
B. 2, 4
C. 1, 4, 5
D. 2, 3, 5
E. 1, 2, 3, 5

Answer D

31. Dangers to the patient inherent in endotracheal intubation include ....
1. damage to teeth.
2. soft tissue damage to the oropharynx.
3. patient hypoxia during intubation attempts.
4. bronchial intubation.
5. esophageal trauma.

Select the proper grouping.

A. 2, 3, 5
B. 1, 2, 4
C. 2, 3, 4, 5
D. 1, 2, 3, 4
E. 1, 2, 3, 5

Answer E

32. Upon placing the endotracheal tube, the paramedic can only auscultate breath sounds on the right side. He or she should ....

A. withdraw the tube a few centimeters.
B. withdraw the tube completely.
C. pass the tube a few centimeters further.
D. secure the tube and ventilate more aggressively.
E. none of the above.

Answer A

33. Upon the placement of an endotracheal tube you hear very faint breath sounds and some gurgling over the epigastric region. You should do which of the following?

A. advance the tube slightly.
B. withdraw the tube slightly.
C. inflate the cuff and auscultate again.
D. ventilate more forcibly.
E. place a second endotracheal tube.

Answer E

34. Rapid sequence intubation is indicated in a patient who has a gag reflex, clenched teeth, and may be combative, yet who has trouble maintaining his or her airway.

A. True
B. False

Answer A

35. The duration of action of Succinylcholine (Anectine) is ....

A. 1 to 2 minutes.
B. 2 to 3 minutes.
C. 3 to 5 minutes.
D. 4 to 6 minutes.
E. 10 to 15 minutes.

Answer C

36. Which of the following is not an advantage of nasotracheal intubation?

A. it is well tolerated by a semiconscious patient
B. it is easier and quicker to perform than oral intubation
C. it can be placed without displacing the patient's head
D. the tube cannot be bitten
E. the tube can be easily anchored

Answer B

37. Indications for nasotracheal intubation include which of the following?

1. a patient with a potential spine injury
2. a patient with a basilar skull fracture
3. a patient with maxillofacial injuries
4. a severely obese patient
5. a patient with clenched teeth

Select the proper grouping.

A. 1, 2, 4
B. 2, 4, 5
C. 1, 3, 5
D. 1, 3, 4, 5
E. 1, 2, 3, 4, 5

Answer D

38. In attempting digital intubation, the fingers of the rescuer must reach to the ....

A. epiglottis.
B. posterior nares.
C. back of the tongue.
D. laryngeal opening.
E. none of the above.

Answer A

39. Blind nasotracheal intubation requires which of the following?
   1. slight extension of the patient's neck
   2. a generally quiet environment
   3. a strong malleable stylet
   4. a patient who is breathing

   Select the proper grouping.

   A. 1, 2
   B. 1, 3
   C. 2, 4
   D. 1, 2, 4
   E. 1, 2, 3, 4

   Answer C

40. A danger to the rescuer associated with digital intubation is that the patient may bite down or clench his teeth during the process and injure the care giver.

   A. True
   B. False

   Answer A

41. The use of a laryngoscope, and the passage of an endotracheal tube, may cause a child's heart rate to drop dramatically. This may reduce cardiac output and blood pressure.

   A. True
   B. False

   Answer A

42. In small children and infants, it is recommended that the paramedic use ....
   1. a cuffed endotracheal tube.
   2. an uncuffed endotracheal tube.
   3. a straight laryngoscope blade.
   4. a curved laryngoscope blade.

   Select the proper grouping.

   A. 1, 3
   B. 1, 4
   C. 2, 3
   D. 2, 4
   E. 1 only

   Answer C

43. The smallest catheter recommended for use when performing adult percutaneous transtracheal catheter ventilation is a ....

   A. 14 gauge.
   B. 16 gauge.
   C. 18 gauge.
   D. 20 gauge.
   E. 22 gauge.

   Answer A

44. The reason behind penetrating the cricothyroid membrane with a catheter attached to a syringe with 1 to 2 ml of saline is to infuse the solution to slow any residual bleeding.

   A. True
   B. False

   Answer B

45. Which of the devices listed below delivers the highest concentration of oxygen to the patient?

A. nasal cannula
B. simple face mask
C. non-rebreather mask
D. venturi mask
E. all deliver about the same concentration

Answer C

46. Which of the devices below delivers the most controlled concentration of oxygen to a patient?

A. nasal cannula
B. simple face mask
C. non-rebreathing mask
D. venturi mask
E. all deliver about the same concentration

Answer D

47. The percentage of oxygen delivered to the patient when using the demand valve resuscitator is about ....

A. 40 %.
B. 50 %.
C. 75 %.
D. 90 %.
E. 100 %.

Answer E

48. Bag-valve-devices should not feature a pop-off valve except when used in pediatric ventilation.

A. True
B. False

Answer A

49. Hazards of using the demand valve to ventilate a patient include all except which of those listed below?

A. oxygen toxicity
B. gastric distention
C. pulmonary barotrauma
D. pneumothorax
E. subcutaneous emphysema

Answer A

50. Advantages of automatic ventilators include ....
1. freeing a rescuer when patient is not breathing.
2. convenience and ease of use.
3. dependability.
4. use in children below age 5.
Select the proper grouping.

A. 2, 3
B. 1, 2, 3
C. 2, 3, 4
D. 1, 3, 4
E. 1, 2, 3, 4

Answer B

SPECIAL PROJECTS

Problem Solving - Airway Maintenance

You have been called to a report of a man down and arrive with one EMT and another paramedic. You find bystanders doing CPR on a male in his mid-fifties in a parking lot. You take the patient's head and determine the bystanders are doing a fine job of ventilating the patient. You get out your airway bag and prepare to place an endotracheal tube.

What equipment would you prepare?

Suction | Stethoscope
Laryngoscope 10ml syringe | et tube
Stylette | water soluble gel
Tape | magill forceps.

How would you check your equipment?

Laryngoscope - check blade - light bright white and non-flickering
Tube cuff - inflate with 10ml - will it hold air
one larger and one smaller tube available

What would you ask the ventilator to do prior to your attempt?

Hyperventilate the patient

Identify the steps of the procedure you're about to attempt.

1. Fill syringe w/10-15ml air
2. Position the patient's head.
3. Grasp the handle in L hand.
4. Insert blade R side mouth.
5. Displace tongue to (L)
6. Insert blade to epiglottis
7. Lift laryngoscope along axis of handle.
8. Visualize the vocal folds of glottis.
9. Grasp tube + pass it between the cords.
10. Inflate the cuff. + auscultate.

You place the endotracheal tube. What actions would you take to ensure it is properly placed?

1. Visualize, with the laryngoscope, the tube passing through the vocal folds.

2. Check the depth of the tube against the mouth.

3. Auscultate all lung fields for bilaterally equal breath sounds

4. Auscultate epigastrium for gurgling sounds.

You place the endotracheal tube and notice no chest rise with the first breath. Auscultation reveals diminished breath sounds and gurgling over the epigastric area. What actions would you take?

If the tube is placed in the esophagus, leave it in place, hyperventilate the patient and attempt to place another tube in the trachea, Reauscultate and assure the tube is poorley placed.

12

PATHOPHYSIOLOGY OF SHOCK

Part I - (pages 291 to 310)

Review of the Objectives for Chapter 12

After reading this chapter, you should be able to:

1. Identify the body's major fluid compartments and the proportion of total body water they contain.

p. 291

Total body water (TBW) accounts for 60% of the body weight, or about 42 liters in the 70 Kg person. It is divided between two compartments.

Intracellular fluid (ICF) accounts for 75% of body fluid.

Extracellular fluid (ECF) accounts for 25% of body fluid and is subdivided into two compartments: the interstitial and the intravascular.

Interstitial fluid remains outside the cells, yet not within the vascular space. It accounts for about 17.5% of body fluid.

Intravascular fluid is the fluid contained within the circulatory system. It accounts for 7.5% of body fluid.

2. Describe the states of hydration, their common causes, and effects on the human system.

pp. 292 to 293

Homeostasis is the balancing of all the activities of the human body to maintain a constant environment within. In body fluid dynamics, it means that the intake and output are maintained by a system of checks and balances.

Dehydration is the net loss of body fluid caused by vomiting, diarrhea, disorders of absorption, fever states, diaphoresis, seeping wounds or third space losses. Dehydration can leave the cardiovascular system without the medium (plasma) to transport essential body materials effectively.

Overhydration is the net accumulation of fluid caused by the inability of the person to eliminate fluid (as in kidney failure) or an excessive intake (as in aggressive intravenous fluid administration). The excess fluid flows out of the vascular space into the interstitial spaces and lungs.

3. List the major electrolytes and the role they play in maintaining a fluid balance within the human body.

pp. 293 to 294

Sodium is the chief extracellular cation (positively charged particle) and plays a role in regulating the distribution of water.

Potassium is the chief intracellular cation and plays a major role in the transmission of electrical impulses.

Chloride is the body's chief anion (negatively charged particle) and plays an important role in kidney function and fluid balance.

4. Define diffusion, osmosis, active transport, and facilitated diffusion and explain the roles they play in human fluid dynamics.

pp. 294 to 296

Diffusion is the tendency of molecules within a solution to move toward an equilibrium. This process keeps the fluids within the various body compartments consistent in mixture within that compartment.

Osmosis is the movement of solvent (body water) from an area of lesser particle concentration to one of greater concentration. This process causes body water to follow the various electrolytes into the intracellular, intravascular, and interstitial spaces.

Active transport is the biochemically powered movement of a substance across a cell's membrane, often against an osmotic gradient. It is much faster than osmosis or diffusion, though it requires cell energy. It is an essential activity of the cell membrane, which allows the body to control movement of electrolytes and essential molecules.

Facilitated diffusion is an assisted transport across the cell membrane. It is the mechanism by which glucose is brought into the body's cells.

5. Identify the major elements of the blood and describe their purpose.

pp. 296 to 297

Plasma is the fluid portion of the blood which is predominantly made up of water (92%). It also contains proteins, clotting factors, electrolytes, etc. It is the medium of transport for the blood cells.

Erythrocytes are the red blood cells, and make up 99% of the remaining portion of the blood (the formed cells). They contain hemoglobin and are responsible for the transport of oxygen to the body cells. The ratio of red blood cells by volume to plasma is the hematocrit.

Leukocytes are the white blood cells which identify and consume pathogens in the human body.

Thrombocytes, known also as platelets, are the bodies which play an essential role in the clotting process.

6. Explain the ABO blood typing system and its significance to emergency medical care.

pp. 297 to 298

The ABO blood typing system identifies two antigens which commonly occur on red blood cells. A person either has one, both, or neither, and hence is classified as A, B, AB or O (which is without). Since a person without an antigen will have an antibody of that type and will react to blood with the antigen, typing is essential to ensure compatibility. The AB patient has both antigens and can accept any AB classification (the universal recipient) while the O patients have neither antigen and their blood can be given to any ABO classification recipient (the universal donor). Because of the potential incompatibility of blood types, it is impractical to administer whole blood in the field.

7. List the various fluid replacement products and relate the advantages and disadvantages of field use.

pp. 298 to 302

Whole blood is the most ideal fluid replacement when blood is being lost. However, it is a very precious commodity and carries with its administration the risk of reaction or disease transmission.

Blood products are very valuable in resuscitation of the patient who has lost fluid. However, as with whole blood, they too carry the risk of reaction or transmission of disease.

Colloids are solutions containing proteins or other large molecules which tend to remain in the vascular space for extended periods of time. They draw water from the interstitial space and expand the vascular volume. They tend to be expensive and have a relatively short shelf life.

Crystalloids are solutions of electrolytes which have greater (hypertonic), the same (isotonic), or lesser (hypotonic) osmotic concentration than plasma. They remain in the vascular space for a relatively short time but are inexpensive, are practical to store, and have limited side effects. Isotonic fluids are used most commonly in the field. These include lactated Ringers solution, normal saline, and 5% dextrose in water.

8. Describe the acid-base balance system and its impact on the human body as it applies to shock and fluid use.

pp. 302 to 306

Three systems help mediate the pH of the human system. They are the buffer system, the respiratory system, and the urinary system. The buffer system chemically reduces the effect of adding or removing hydrogen ions. The respiratory system removes or retains CO_2, which forms a weak acid when dissolved in water. Lastly, the kidneys will either retain or excrete bicarbonate, an alkali, to raise or lower the pH. Failure of these systems can lead to acid-base disorders. Hypoventilation may lead to respiratory acidosis while hyperventilation may produce respiratory alkalosis. Metabolic problems (such as failure of the circulatory system to deliver oxygen to the cells) or diarrhea, vomiting or medications may cause a metabolic acidosis. Alkalosis may be caused by medications or prolonged vomiting. A variation in pH of just 0.4 from the normal range of 7.35 to 7.45 may result in death.

9. Illustrate the structure and function of the cardiovascular system.

pp. 306 to 310

The cardiovascular system is a system of interconnected tubes which direct blood to the essential organs and tissues of the body. The system is powered by the central pump, the heart, and contains the fluid, blood. If any part of the system fails, the body is at risk. Failure can occur when the tubes relax and can no longer direct the flow; when the fluid is lost to hemorrhage or plasma loss; when the fluid is no longer effective in its delivery of vital material, such as oxygen; and when the pump fails to provide the power to move blood to essential tissues. Fluid therapy is designed to supplement the volume of the vascular system and thereby assist the vessels and heart in delivering the needed resources to the body cells.

CASE STUDY REVIEW

Reread the case study in **PARAMEDIC EMERGENCY CARE** and then read the discussion below.

This case study presents an example of aggressive and appropriate care for a patient who, by mechanism of injury alone, is suspected for the development of shock. It highlights both the elements of shock assessment and care.

Chapter 12 Case Study

Arriving on the scene, Bob is presented with a situation which contains no noticeable hazards, one patient and a mechanism of injury which indicates the potential for serious internal bleeding. The bulldozer turning over and trapping the patient's legs and pelvis may have fractured the pelvis and femurs. These injuries are frequently associated with severe internal blood loss and shock.

Bob is suspicious that as the vehicle is lifted off the patient internal bleeding will occur rapidly. In preparation he ensures good oxygenation and assesses the portion of the patient which is visible. He gathers a baseline set of vital signs (all of which indicate that the patient is not yet in shock) including a pulse oximeter reading. He starts two IV lines using 1000 ml bags of lactated Ringer's solution and trauma tubing. He places pressure infusers over the bags, just in case they are needed. The PASG is set out on the long spineboard so the patient can be moved in one step to the board and immediately have the PASG applied. Bob and his fellow rescuers converse with the patient not only to calm and reassure but also to maintain a continuous assessment of the patient's level of consciousness and determine a patient history.

As the bulldozer is removed, the patient is quickly assessed and then moved to the awaiting backboard. The pelvic, femur, and tibial fractures suggest shock will develop so the PASG is inflated immediately, not only to stabilize the fractured pelvis and femurs but to tamponade the internal hemorrhage expected with these injuries. The IVs are run wide open and the patient is prepared for rapid transport.

Normally, fellow care providers would slow the IVs en route, however, the patient is becoming restless, the pulse rate is increasing and the oximetry reading is dropping. These herald the progression of shock and require continued aggressive care. The hospital is updated on the patient's condition so they can prepare O negative blood. Whole blood or packed red cells are required because the replacement of blood lost through hemorrhage with crystalloid dilutes the number of red blood cells available.

The hospital personnel are ready and waiting for the patient as the ambulance backs into the emergency department bay. The blood is already hung and connected, and infusion is begun. The trauma surgeon makes his quick assessment and the patient is en route to surgery in minutes.

If any one of a number of critical steps in the care of this patient had not been completed, this patient probably would not have survived the trip to the hospital. Bob moved quickly and decisively, performing those skills which maintained his patient yet not focusing on all care which would be provided, had he not been critical. The paramedic must, through experience, be able to quickly distinguish the patient who needs rapid transport and aggressive care from the patient who is best benefited by meticulous care at the scene and during transport.

READING COMPREHENSION SELF-EXAM

1. The intravascular fluid accounts for what percentage of the total body water?

A. 7.5%
B. 15%
C. 35.6%
D. 45%
E. 75%

Answer 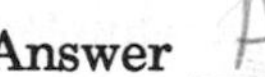

2. Dehydration classically presents with which of the following signs?
   1. rapid pulse rate
   2. decreased blood pressure
   3. excessive thirst
   4. poor skin turgor
   5. sunken anterior fontanelle (infants)

Select the proper grouping.

A. 1, 2, 3
B. 2, 4, 5
C. 1, 3, 5
D. 2, 3, 4, 5
E. 1, 2, 3, 4, 5

Answer E

3. The most prevalent extracellular cation is which of the following?

A. potassium
B. sodium
C. calcium
D. chloride
E. bicarbonate

Answer B

4. The process by which a solvent travels through a semi-permeable membrane from a lesser concentration of solute particles to a greater concentration is called ....

A. diffusion.
B. active transport.
C. osmosis.
D. facilitated transport.
E. facilitated diffusion.

Answer C

5. A solution which has a similar electrolyte concentration as plasma is called ....

A. hypertonic.
B. homeostatic.
C. hypotonic.
D. isotonic.
E. none of the above.

Answer D

6. The process which causes a solute to distribute itself equally throughout a solvent is called ....

A. osmosis.
B. diffusion.
C. active transport.
D. facilitated diffusion.
E. none of the above.

Answer B

7. The percentage of the blood which consists of red blood cells is referred to as ....

A. its type.
B. viscosity.
C. erythrocytic count.
D. hematocrit.
E. none of the above.

Answer D

8. The red blood cells account for what percentage of the formed cells of the blood?

A. 65%
B. 75%
C. 85%
D. 99%
E. none of the above

Answer D

9. If a patient has type A antigen and antibody B, he can generally be expected to safely receive which blood types?

A. A and O
B. B and O
C. A and AB
D. B and AB
E. A only

Answer A

10. If a patient has type O blood, she can safely receive which blood types?

A. A and O
B. B and O
C. AB and O
D. A, B, AB, and O
E. O only

Answer E

11. Which of the fluid replacement choices would be most desirable for the patient who is losing blood through internal bleeding?

A. packed red blood cells
B. fresh frozen plasma
C. whole blood
D. colloids
E. crystalloids

Answer C

12. If a patient is in need of blood and there is not time to type and cross-match, he should be given ....

A. O negative blood.
B. O positive blood.
C. AB negative blood.
D. AB positive blood.
E. fresh frozen plasma.

Answer A

13. You are transporting a patient who is receiving typed and cross-matched blood. She begins to display fever, tachycardia, and hypotension. You should ....

A. warm the blood.
B. administer epinephrine.
C. slow the administration rate.
D. mix the blood before continuing.
E. none of the above.

Answer E

14. A solution for intravenous administration which contains proteins or other large molecules is referred to as a(n) ....

A. crystalloid.
B. colloid.
C. isotonic solution.
D. hypotonic solution.
E. hypertonic solution.

Answer B

15. Most of the solutions used in prehospital care for infusion are ....

A. hypotonic colloids.
B. isotonic colloids.
C. hypertonic colloids.
D. hypotonic crystalloids.
E. isotonic crystalloids.

Answer E

16. Which of the fluids listed below is commonly used in prehospital care?
1. Dextran
2. normal saline
3. Plasmanate
4. lactated Ringer's solution
5. 5% dextrose in water
Select the proper grouping.

A. 1, 3, 5
B. 2, 3, 5
C. 2, 4, 5
D. 1, 3, 4, 5
E. 1, 2, 3, 4

Answer C

17. Increasing the pH value from 7.4 to 7.6 represents an increase in the strength of the acidity of a solution.

A. True
B. False

Answer B

18. The normal pH range for the human system is from ____ to ____ .

A. 7.00 to 7.50
B. 7.35 to 7.45
C. 6.90 to 7.65
D. 6.95 to 7.05
E. none of the above

Answer B

19. Which of the following systems is the first to respond to an increase in acidity and moderates the trend?

A. the respiratory system
B. the urinary system
C. the buffer system
D. the hepatic mediator system
E. none of the above

Answer C

20. A patient who was hypoventilating for quite some time would be expected to have which of the following?

A. metabolic acidosis
B. metabolic alkalosis
C. respiratory alkalosis
D. respiratory acidosis
E. none of the above

Answer D

12

PATHOPHYSIOLOGY OF SHOCK

Part II - (pages 311 to 336)

Review of the Objectives for Chapter 12

After reading this chapter, you should be able to:

10. Define shock, explain the shock process and describe some of the body's compensatory mechanisms.

pp. 311 to 313

Shock is inadequate tissue perfusion. It is the inability of the human system, through the cardiovascular system, to supply the body's cellular needs. The shock process has three distinct stages. They are:

Compensated shock is the initial response of the body to fluid loss. The blood vessels constrict, the heart rate and strength of contraction increase, and blood is directed from less critical structures such as the skin to the internal and vital organs. If the loss is not controlled, compensated shock will progress into uncompensated shock.

Uncompensated shock is a state where the cardiovascular system is not receiving enough oxygenated circulation to maintain a compensatory state. The blood vessels relax, the heart can no longer forcibly contract and the blood pressure and circulatory flow drop precipitously. If immediate aggressive intervention does not occur, the patient will move into irreversible shock.

Irreversible shock is a state where cell death has begun and the cardiovascular system is no longer capable of sustaining life. Even if the lost fluid is replaced in its entirety (or the primary problem is corrected), the damage is irreversible.

The human body compensates for lost cardiovascular volume by increasing cardiac output, increasing heart rate, increasing peripheral vascular resistance, and reducing the vascular space (progressive vasoconstriction). The body further shunts blood to the vital organs and away from the skin.

11. Describe pathophysiology of hypovolemic, cardiogenic, and neurogenic shock.

pp. 313 to 314

Hypovolemic shock is shock secondary to the loss of intravascular fluid, either blood or plasma. This type of shock can be caused by internal or external hemorrhage or fluid loss due to burns, vomiting, diarrhea, diabetic ketoacidosis, excessive sweating, poor fluid intake, pancreatitis, liver failure, peritonitis or bowel obstruction.

Cardiogenic shock is shock due to the inability of the heart to pump effectively. It may be due to heart muscle or electrical system damage secondary to the myocardial infarction. It may be secondary to valvular damage or disorder, or to an excessively high workload such as in congestive heart failure. It may also occur due to physical restraint of the heart such as in pericardial tamponade.

Neurogenic shock is a reduction in the ability of the blood vessels to direct the flow of blood and control blood pressure. It is most commonly associated with injury to the spinal cord and results in the body's inability to control blood vessel function. Neurogenic shock may also result from septicemia, from a bacterial infection, an anaphylactic reaction, insulin overdose, and adrenal gland disorders (Addison's disease).

12. Describe the assessment of the shock patient.

pp. 315 to 317

The assessment of the shock patient should progress as it would for any patient. During the assessment the paramedic should look for the indications of shock. Respirations should be observed for rate and depth with rapid, shallow breathing suggestive of shock. The pulse should be carefully and deliberately assessed. If it is rapid and weak, and especially if distal pulses are absent, shock should be suspected. The skin color, temperature, and capillary refill times may reveal the reduced peripheral perfusion, an early sign of shock. Assessment of the level of consciousness may reveal either reduced faculties, confusion, disorientation or agitation. Any of these should raise the index of suspicion for shock, especially if they are not accounted for by the mechanism of injury. During the rest of the primary survey, the body cavity, pelvis, and extremities are quickly scanned for signs of injury which might contribute to shock. If shock is suspected as the primary survey ends, the patient is prepared for rapid transport. If shock is not suspected, the secondary assessment may continue at the scene. However, a constant and continuous vigil must be maintained to recognize the early signs of shock.

13. Describe the management of the shock patient.

pp. 318 to 322

The care of the potential shock patient revolves around the ABC's. The Airway must be secured and the patient provided with high flow oxygen. Breathing must be adequate or be assisted. Any significant identifiable blood loss must be quickly controlled. Circulation must be maintained by replacement of the volume lost (fluid infusion) and by directing the circulation to the critical organs (the application of the PASG). The patient should be placed in the shock position. Continue to identify and treat the causes of the developing shock throughout prehospital emergency care.

14. Identify the indications, contraindications, and application process for the PASG.

pp. 322 to 324

Indications - the PASG is indicated for any patient who displays internal or external hemorrhage in the lower abdomen, pelvis or lower extremities. It is recommended for the stabilization of any pelvic and/or femur fractures or for the signs and symptoms of shock.

Contraindications - PASG should not be used in the patient who is experiencing pulmonary edema or has a head or penetrating chest injury. It should be used with caution on any patient who is experiencing dyspnea due to the pressure it may place against the diaphragm. The abdominal section should not be employed if the patient is in the third trimester of pregnancy, has an abdominal evisceration or an impaled object in the abdomen.

Application - Prior to application of the PASG the patient's blood pressure, pulse rate and strength, and level of consciousness should be assessed and recorded. The abdomen, lower back, and lower extremities should be visualized to ensure that no sharp debris is present which could harm either the patient or the garment. The garment may be applied in many ways. One should be chosen which considers the patient's injuries and position. The lower extremity chambers must be inflated prior to or simultaneously with the abdominal chamber. Inflation should follow local protocol and be guided by patient condition. Ideally, the device should be inflated until the patient improves slightly and then inflated in increments to maintain that patient level.

15. Explain the indications for, and the initiation of, intravenous therapy.

pp. 303 to 305

Indications - the indications for intravenous therapy include the need for administration of intravenous medications, replacement of fluid loss, and obtaining venous blood sampled for analysis.

Initiation - the initiation of an IV begins with identification of an appropriate site, followed by the application of a venous tourniquet and the cleansing of the site for cannulation. A catheter is selected, tape is torn to secure the catheter, and an IV solution and administration set are connected and prepared. The skin is pierced, the vein is entered (as denoted by flashback) and the catheter is advanced. The needle is withdrawn and the administration set is connected.

16. List the equipment commonly used for intravenous therapy and explain the purpose and use of various items.

pp. 305 to 307

A **venous tourniquet** is used to obstruct the venous return, thereby dilating the vein and making cannulation easier.

Cleansing agents, such as Alcohol or Betadine are used to cleanse the site to reduce the chance that infectious agents will enter the skin and blood vessel with cannulation.

Catheters are most commonly of the over-the-needle variety and range from 24- to 14-gauge (smallest to largest). They are used to enter the skin and vessel and then the catheter is threaded into the vein and the needle is withdrawn.

Tape is torn prior to cannulation and used to secure the catheter, the connection between the catheter and the administration set, and the first few inches of administration set tubing.

The **administration set** is the tubing which carries the solution from the solution bag to the catheter. It contains a drip chamber and control valve that allow for controlling the rate of fluid administration. Sets normally come in 60 (mini) and 10 (macro) drops per milliliter versions.

Intravenous fluid is used to replace fluid a patient has lost and/or provide a carrier for drug administration. The most common for field use are lactated Ringer's solution, normal saline, and dextrose 5% in water.

17. Identify the common complications of intravenous therapy and the process of preventing or correcting those complications.

pp. 329 to 330

Infiltration - some pain is associated with cannulation. It may also be due to extravasation of fluid. Ensure the catheter is within the vein.

Hematoma - needle movement damage or delicate veins can lead to internal hemorrhage. Withdraw the catheter and apply direct pressure.

Pyrogenic reaction occurs when agents within the solution react with the patient's blood, and results in fever, nausea, vomiting, chills, and backache. If it is suspected, the IV should be discontinued immediately and saved.

Catheter shear may occur when a catheter is drawn back over a needle which has been inserted into the vein. Never withdraw the catheter over the needle.

Air embolism occurs when air is allowed to enter the vein through the administration set and catheter. Completely clear the administration set of air and ensure that your IV solution does not run out.

READING COMPREHENSION SELF-EXAM

21. Which of the following can cause shock?
    1. heart attack
    2. infection
    3. spinal injury
    4. allergic reaction
    5. hemorrhage

    Select the proper grouping.

    A. 1, 3, 4
    B. 2, 4, 5
    C. 1, 3, 4, 5
    D. 1, 2, 3, 4
    E. 1, 2, 3, 4, 5

    Answer E

22. Adequate perfusion is dependent upon which of the following elements?

    A. the pump (heart)
    B. the volume (blood)
    C. the container (blood vessels)
    D. all of the above
    E. B and C

    Answer D

23. The mechanism which accounts for a greater force of cardiac contraction when the heart is forcefully filled with blood and the myocardium is stretched is called the ....

    A. cardiac contractile force.
    B. Frank-Starling mechanism.
    C. Hering-Breuer reflex.
    D. rubber band syndrome.
    E. none of the above.

    Answer B

24. Under normal conditions the blood passing the alveoli will be oxygenated to what percentage?

    A. 65 to 70
    B. 75 to 85
    C. 90 to 95
    D. 97 to 100
    E. less than 65

    Answer D

25. Place the following stages of shock in the order of their occurence.
    1. irreversible
    2. compensated
    3. uncompensated

    Select the proper grouping.

    A. 1, 2, 3
    B. 2, 3, 1
    C. 2, 1, 3
    D. 3, 2, 1
    E. 3, 1, 2

    Answer B

26. Tissue perfusion is dependent upon which of the following?
   1. cardiac output
   2. peripheral resistance
   3. respiratory adequacy
   4. adequate preload
   5. blood volume

   Select the proper grouping.

   A. 1, 2, 4
   B. 3, 4, 5
   C. 1, 3, 4, 5
   D. 2, 3, 4, 5
   E. 1, 2, 3, 4, 5

   Answer E

27. The intent behind the mechanisms which compensate for shock is to ....

   A. reduce blood loss.
   B. reduce the vascular space.
   C. conserve oxygen.
   D. perfuse vital organs.
   E. all of the above.

   Answer E

28. Which of the following can cause hypovolemic shock?
   1. bowel obstruction
   2. pancreatitis
   3. diabetic ketoacidosis
   4. ascites
   5. peritonitis

   Select the proper grouping.

   A. 2, 4, 5
   B. 1, 3, 5
   C. 1, 2, 4, 5
   D. 1, 2, 3, 4
   E. 1, 2, 3, 4, 5

   Answer E

29. The color, temperature and general appearance of the skin can indicate shock before there are changes in the blood pressure.

   A. True
   B. False

   Answer A

30. Normally the color of a blanched finger will return when the pressure has been released (capillary refill) in under ....

   A. one second.
   B. two seconds.
   C. three seconds.
   D. four seconds.
   E. thirty seconds.

   Answer B

31. The reduction in tissue perfusion which accompanies shock may cause hypoperfusion of the brain which in turn may cause which of the following?
    1. unequal pupils
    2. fever
    3. agitation
    4. disorientation

    Select the proper grouping.

    A. 1, 2
    B. 3, 4
    C. 1, 3, 4
    D. 1, 2, 3
    E. 1, 2, 3, 4

    Answer B

32. The preferred position for the shock patient would be ....

    A. supine with head elevated slightly.
    B. on the left side (left lateral recumbent).
    C. supine with legs elevated 10 to 12 inches.
    D. supine.
    E. on the right side.

    Answer C

33. The PASG is believed to benefit the shock patient by ....
    1. increasing blood pressure.
    2. reducing chest wound hemorrhage.
    3. stabilizing pelvic fractures.
    4. increasing blood flow to the heart, brain, and lungs.

    Select the proper grouping.

    A. 3, 4
    B. 1, 2
    C. 2, 3, 4
    D. 1, 3, 4
    E. 1, 2, 3, 4

    Answer D

34. Which of the following is(are) specific concern(s) when applying the PASG in a very cold outside environment?

    A. the inability to remove the clothing before application
    B. the danger of the PASG cracking due to cold temperature
    C. the danger of a pressure increase as the suit warms
    D. increased volume of air needed to inflate the device
    E. all of the above

    Answer C

35. Which of the following is a benefit of having an intravenous line in a patient?
    1. easy administration of medications
    2. ability to draw blood samples
    3. ability to directly monitor cardiac output
    4. route to replace fluids

    Select the proper grouping.

    A. 1, 2
    B. 1, 3
    C. 2, 4
    D. 1, 2, 4
    E. 1, 2, 3, 4

    Answer D

36. The volume of fluid infused using the macrodrip administration set is usually ....

A. 5 drops per milliliter.
B. 10 drops per milliliter.
C. 25 drops per milliliter.
D. 40 drops per milliliter.
E. 60 drops per milliliter.

Answer B

37. If you have inserted an intravenous catheter, achieved flashback and the IV does not flow, which of the following might be the cause?
1. the catheter opening is up against a valve.
2. the IV bag may not be high enough.
3. the venous tourniquet has not been removed.
4. there is an administration set valve closed.
Select the proper grouping.

A. 1, 3
B. 2, 4
C. 1, 3, 4
D. 2, 3, 4
E. 1, 2, 3, 4

Answer E

38. If the drip chamber is completely filled with fluid the paramedic should ....

A. invert the bag and chamber, and squeeze the chamber.
B. apply pressure to the bag and let the fluid flow.
C. run fluid through the chamber; the problem will self correct.
D. discontinue the IV and start again.
E. replace the administration set.

Answer A

39. A patient you are attending, who has an IV in place and running, experiences fever, chills, nausea, and backache. She is probably experiencing ....

A. catheter shear.
B. pulmonary emboli.
C. an overhydration reaction.
D. a pyrogenic reaction.
E. none of the above.

Answer D

40. Which of the following actions is likely to cause catheter shear?
1. excessive movement of the catheter once in place
2. withdrawing the catheter over the needle
3. using too large a catheter for the vein
4. running fluid too fast
Select the proper grouping.

A. 2
B. 1, 2
C. 2, 4
D. 1, 3, 4
E. 1, 2, 3, 4

Answer A

Short Answer Questions:

Explain why these classic signs of shock occur.

Cool & clammy skin Peripheral vasoconstriction reduces blood flow to the Skin.

Agitation Cerebral hypoxia due to reduced Circulation to the brain & reduced levels of oxygen because of reduced efficiency of respiration and oxygen Capability of the blood.

Rapid pulse A Cardiovascular Compensatory mechanism to maintain blood pressure and perfusion when Cardiac preload is reduced due to hypovolemia

Dropping blood pressure A late Sign of Shock occuring when Compensatory mechanism fail and the heart and arterial System Cannot maintain blood pressure & Circulation

Ashen or cyanotic skin As the Body Compensates for Volume loss, it Shunts blood from the Skin and results in deoxygenation of the blood Still within the Skin & the ashen & Cyanotic colors.

Explain why the blood pressure drops late during shock.

Blood pressure drops late in the Shock process because the Compensatory mechanisms Compensate for blood loss and maintains the blood pressure. This includes vasoconstriction, increased heart rate and Shunting of blood to the critical organs only.

SPECIAL PROJECTS

Problem Solving - Shock Care

You are at the emergency scene described in the case study for this chapter. Why did you anticipate shock in the patient trapped by the bulldozer when he displayed normal vital signs and none of the classic signs of shock?

mechanisms of injury – Pelvic fracture, bi lateral femur

Identify the equipment you would prepare for IV initiation.

alcohol Swabs – betadine

tape

Administration Set

venous tourniquet

IV Solution

CAtheter

List the steps you would take for IV initiation.

1. Apply the Venous Tourniquet
2. locate the vein for CAnnulation
3. Clense Site
4. Insert CAtheter & enter the vein
5. obtAin Flash back
6. AdvAnce CAtheter
7. withdrAwl needle
8. Attach Administration Set.
9. Begin fluid Resuscitation
10. Secure cAtheter + Set

13

EMERGENCY PHARMACOLOGY

Part I - (pages 336 to 352)

Review of the Objectives for Chapter 13

After reading this chapter, you should be able to:

1. Define the following terms.

pp. 336 to 341

Pharmacology - the study of drugs and their effects on the human body.
Drug - chemical agent used in the diagnosis, treatment, and prevention of disease.
Pharmacodynamics - the study of drug action on the body.
Pharmacokinetics - the study of how drugs enter the body, reach their site of action and how they are eventually eliminated.

2. List four drug sources, and give an example of a drug derived from each source.

p. 336

Plant - atropine, used in the treatment of heart blocks and bradycardia, is a plant derivative.
Animal - insulin is extracted from the pancreas of cattle and used to treat diabetes.
Mineral - sodium bicarbonate is a mineral used to combat metabolic acidosis in the cardiac arrest patient.
Synthetic - lidocaine is a synthetic drug used to treat cardiac dysrhythmia.

3. Name three federal legislative acts that regulate drugs.

p. 337

Federal Food, Drug, and Cosmetic Act of 1938 - requires packaging to list the ingredients.
Harrison Narcotic Act - regulates the sale and manufacture of the opium plant and its derivatives.
Controlled Substances Act - regulates addictive drugs and defines the five schedules of controlled substances.

4. List the five addictive drug schedules and give an example of a medication from each.

pp. 337 to 338

Schedule I - these drugs have a high potential for abuse and have no medical indications. Heroin is an example.
Schedule II - these drugs have a high potential for abuse yet also have accepted medical indications. Morphine and Demerol are examples of schedule II drugs.
Schedule III - drugs in this schedule have a reduced potential for abuse and accepted medical indications. An example is acetaminophen and codeine (Tylenol #4).

Schedule IV - these drugs have a low potential for abuse, but may cause a physical or psychological dependence. Such drugs include valium.

Schedule V - drugs in this schedule have a low potential for abuse, yet contain small quantities of narcotics. Several cough medications are included in this schedule.

5. List the four names that can be used to identify a drug.

p. 338

Chemical name　　Generic name　　Trade name　　Official name

6. Describe three common drug references, and know how to find a medication in one of these references.

p. 338

AMA Drug Evaluations provides drug information on groups of drug including their recommended dosage, side effects, indications, and contraindications.

Physicians' Desk Reference (PDR) is a compilation of manufacturer's drug information on the most current drugs on the market. It contains photographs showing the actual size, shape, and color of many of the drugs. It is published yearly.

Drug Inserts accompany most drugs and supply the manufacturer's recommendations for use and much other information.

7. List several examples of both liquid and solid drugs.

pp. 338 to 339

LIQUIDS

Solutions are preparations in which the drug is dissolved in a solvent, usually water. Normal saline is an example.

Tinctures are drug preparations in which the drug was extracted with the use of alcohol. An example is tincture of iodine.

Suspensions are drugs which do not dissolve in the solvent but are rather suspended in solution and will separate if not frequently shaken. An example is amoxicillin, an antibiotic.

Spirits are volatile drugs dissolved in alcohol. Spirits of ammonia is one example.

Emulsions are mixtures of an oily substance and a solvent. They do not dissolve and, as with suspensions, must be shaken before administration.

Elixirs are preparations of a drug in alcohol with a flavoring added. Tylenol elixir is an example.

Syrups are drugs mixed with sugar, water, and flavoring, such as cough syrup.

SOLIDS

Pills are drugs shaped for easy swallowing. A vitamin is a common example of a pill.

Powders are a drug in powder form, usually intended for mixing with another agent.

Capsules are gelatin containers which contain the drug. As the gelatin dissolves in the intestinal tract, the drug is released. Dalmane capsules are an example.

Tablets are composed of powder pressed into an easily swallowed form. Aspirin is an example of this.

Suppositories are drugs mixed with a base that dissolves at body temperature. They are placed rectally or vaginally and dissolve, allowing the surrounding tissue to absorb the drug.

8. Define "parenteral drugs."

p. 339

Parenteral medications are introduced through routes other than the digestive system, such as intravenous, intramuscular, and subcutaneous. Most drugs used in emergency medical service are of this type.

9. Define the following terms.

p. 339

Ampule is a glass or plastic single-dose containers which must be broken to obtain and use the drug.
Vial is single or multiple-dose containers which are sealed with a rubber cap. The drug is obtained by withdrawing it with a needle and syringe.
Prefilled syringe is a single-dose preloaded administration device. It is rapid to use and is common in emergency medical service.

10. Define important pharmacological terminology.

p. 340

Antagonism is an opposition between the actions of two drugs.
Bolus is a single, often large dose of medication.
Contraindications are medical or physiological reasons against the use of a drug.
Cumulative action is the result of administering several small doses and achieving an increasing effect, usually due to increasing blood levels of the drug.
Depressant is a medication which decreases a body function or activity.
Habituation is a psychological or physiological dependence on a drug.
Hypersensitivity is an exaggerated reactivity to a drug.
Idiosyncrasy is an individual reaction to a drug which is very different from what is expected.
Indication is a medical condition for which the drug has a proven therapeutic value.
Potentiation is the enhancement of one drug by the administration of another.
Refractory is a condition of failure of a drug to provide the therapeutic action desired for the patient.
Side effects are unavoidable and undesirable effects of a drug even in therapeutic doses.
Stimulant is a drug that increases a bodily function or activity.
Synergism is a combination of two drugs which together perform better than the sum of their isolated effects.
Therapeutic action is the intended action of a drug.
Tolerance is the reduction in the obtained effects of a dosage of a drug over time.
Untoward effect is a harmful side effect of a drug.

11. Define a drug's mechanism of action.

p. 341

The chain of biochemical events that eventually lead to the physiological changes desired.

12. List four factors that influence the concentration of a drug at its site of action.

pp. 341 to 344

Absorption is the entrance of the drug into the cardiovascular system.
Distribution is movement of the drug to the site where it is to be used.
Biotransformation is the conversion of the drug into its active form.
Elimination is the withdrawal of the drug from the cardiovascular system and the removal of it from the body.

13. List two factors that slow drug absorption and two factors that enhance it.

pp. 341 to 342

Factors that slow absorption are shock, acidosis, and peripheral vasoconstriction as caused by hypothermia.

Factors that enhance absorption include peripheral vasodilatation as caused by fever or hyperthermia which increase the blood supply at the injection site.

14. Define "blood brain barrier."

p. 342

The blood brain barrier is a mechanism that isolates the brain tissue from the blood stream and selectively allows a limited number of compounds into the brain.

15. Describe the theory of drug receptors, and give an example of one such receptor.

p. 343

Drug receptors are proteins on the surface of cells which receive drugs and initiate the desired biochemical response. Epinephrine contains alpha and beta agonists. They will bind to receptors in the lungs and heart and cause the intended response. If a Beta blocker such as Inderal is administered, it will bind to the sites and prevent Epinephrine from causing its desired effects.

16. Describe the principles of "therapeutic threshold," "therapeutic index," and "minimum effective concentration."

pp. 343 to 344

Therapeutic threshold is the point at which the drug begins to have the desired effect. A concentration of drug below this level will not produce the desired effect.

Therapeutic index is the difference between the therapeutic threshold and toxic concentrations. The higher the therapeutic index, the greater the latitude in drug administration. If a drug has a small therapeutic index it must be carefully titrated to ensure the therapeutic effect is obtained without toxic effects.

Minimum effective concentration is essentially the same as the therapeutic threshold. It is the minimum dose of a drug which will produce the desired effects, and hence, is the safest dose.

17. Define the following terms.

pp. 349 to 352

Agonist is a drug which binds to a receptor and causes an action.

Antagonist is a drug which binds to a receptor, causes no action, and prevents an agonist from affixing to the receptor.

Sympathomimetic drugs are those which stimulate the sympathetic nervous system. An example is Epinephrine.

Sympatholytic drugs are those that inhibit the sympathetic nervous system. An example is Propranolol.

Parasympathomimetic drugs stimulate the parasympathetic nervous system.

Parasympatholytic drugs block the actions of the parasympathetic nervous system.

CASE STUDY REVIEW

Reread the case study in **PARAMEDIC EMERGENCY CARE** and then read the discussion below.

This case study highlights the sophistication of pharmacology and the importance it plays in advanced prehospital care. It identifies only some of the drug considerations which the paramedic needs to keep in mind as he or she administers medications in the care of patients.

Chapter 13 Case Study

The paramedics in this case study are presented with a patient who displays the classic signs and symptoms of a heart attack. The patient has substernal chest pain, is pale and sweating, and has some cyanosis. He is assessed and found to have a rapid pulse and an EKG consistent with the myocardial infarction. The chest should be evaluated to determine if there is any evidence of pulmonary edema, which frequently accompanies heart failure. The presence of pulmonary edema is also important in determining the medication regimen for this patient.

Assessment also reveals a great deal of information which must be considered when using drugs in prehospital care. The blood pressure of this patient (150/90) is an important sign because many of the drugs used to treat the myocardial infarction may lower the blood pressure. The drugs which may be contraindicated in the hypovolemic patient include nitroglycerin and morphine sulfate. While nitroglycerin will reduce cardiac preload and after-load, and the cardiac workload, it will also reduce the blood pressure. A patient with a blood pressure of 80 mm Hg, for example, cannot afford a reduction in the blood pressure for it may adversely affect vital organ perfusion.

Morphine sulfate has a similar action, though its major use is to relieve pain and in some cases reduce the edema secondary to congestive heart failure. The paramedics in the hypotension scenario would be better advised to administer dopamine to increase the blood pressure and follow it with morphine if the pressure rises significantly and the pain persists. Dopamine is a potent vasoconstrictor and will increase the myocardial workload so its administration must be carefully regulated (titrated).

In this case study the paramedics are reasonably safe in employing the lidocaine and morphine. The lidocaine reduces the myocardial irritability and should diminish the number of premature ventricular contractions and the chance of one causing ventricular fibrillation. The morphine sulfate will lower the cardiac workload as well as reduce the patient's pain. In the face of the myocardial infarction these drugs are helpful in reducing the damage done to the heart and in reducing the possibility of cardiac arrest. In many cases and with this patient, arrest may still occur.

The patient becomes unconscious, is assessed and the arrest protocol is used. The patient receives defibrillation at 200, 300, and 360 joules and basic cardiac life support is begun. The patient is then given 1 mg of epinephrine. The 360 joule defibrillation is repeated and is successful, possibly because the epinephrine has increased the likelihood that counter shock will be effective. It is followed by a lidocaine bolus and drip, and careful monitoring of the vital signs and of the ECG.

New advances in the treatment of the myocardial infarction are employed at the hospital. The TPA is a drug which works on dissolving the clot obstructing the patient's coronary artery. While his pain subsides he must be monitored carefully over the next few days to ensure no further complications occur. He is taken to the CCU.

READING COMPREHENSION SELF-EXAM

1. Drugs are chemical agents which are used in the ....

   A. diagnosis of disease.
   B. treatment of disease.
   C. prevention of disease.
   D. all of the above.
   E. A and B.

   Answer D

2. Most of the drugs used by the paramedic are for ....

   A. cardiovascular emergencies.
   B. hemodynamic emergencies.
   C. allergic reactions.
   D. unconscious states.
   E. none of the above.

   Answer A

3. Which of the following are common sources of drugs?
   1. plants
   2. minerals
   3. animals
   4. synthetics

   Select the proper grouping.

   A. 1, 2
   B. 1, 3
   C. 2, 4
   D. 1, 3, 4
   E. 1, 2, 3, 4

   Answer E

4. Which of the following is the origin of the drug lidocaine?

   A. plant
   B. mineral
   C. synthetic
   D. animal
   E. none of the above

   Answer C

5. Under which schedule of medications do Demerol (meperidine) and morphine fall?

   A. schedule I
   B. schedule II
   C. schedule III
   D. schedule IV
   E. schedule V

   Answer B

6. The federal agency which bears primary responsibility for enforcement of the Controlled Substances Act is the ....

   A. Federal Bureau of Investigation.
   B. Division of Narcotic Enforcement.
   C. Drug Enforcement Agency.
   D. Harrison Narcotic and Controlled Substance Commission.
   E. Food and Drug Administration.

   Answer C

7. The name "naloxone" is an example of which of the following?

   A. chemical name
   B. official name
   C. generic name
   D. trade name
   E. schedule name

   Answer C

8. Narcan is an example of which of the following?

   A. chemical name
   B. generic name
   C. trade name
   D. official name
   E. schedule name

   Answer C

9. In which of the following references for drugs might the paramedic find photographs of drugs to assist in identification?

A. AMA Drug Evaluations
B. Physicians' Desk Reference
C. Manufacturer's drug inserts
D. Prehospital Emergency Pharmacology
E. B and D

Answer B

10. Dextrose 5% in water (D5W) is an example of which of the following drug forms?

A. solution
B. tincture
C. suspension
D. spirit
E. elixir

Answer A

11. Parenteral drugs are ....

A. low viscosity fluids.
B. administered other than via the digestive track.
C. administered from one person to another.
D. given by various routes yet must be isotonic in composition.
E. none of the above.

Answer B

12. In prehospital emergency medicine, most drugs are supplied in what type of packaging?

A. ampules
B. single-dose vials
C. prefilled syringes
D. multi-dose vials
E. suspended and bagged solutions

Answer C

13. The characteristic action of a drug which is unique to an individual is ....

A. idiosyncracy.
B. cumulative.
C. refractory.
D. synergism.
E. untoward.

Answer A

14. When two drugs, administered in combination, produce a greater effect than the sum of their isolated effects, this characteristic is called ....

A. idiosyncrasy.
B. synergism.
C. hypersensitivity.
D. untoward reaction.
E. potentiation.

Answer B

15. The expected and intended action of a drug is referred to as its ....

A. cumulative action.
B. indication.
C. therapeutic action.
D. tolerance.
E. design factor.

Answer C

16. Which of the following are elements of drug pharmacokinetics?
1. absorption
2. distribution
3. elimination
4. biotransformation
Select the proper grouping.

A. 1, 3
B. 2, 4
C. 1, 2, 4
D. 2, 3, 4
E. 1, 2, 3, 4

Answer E

17. The study of a drug's actions upon the body is called ....

A. pharmacokinetics.
B. pharmacodynamics.
C. pharmacology.
D. synergism
E. none of the above.

Answer B

18. The process of the blood or target tissue converting a drug into its useful form is called ....

A. active transport.
B. biotransportation
C. biotransformation.
D. facilitation.
E. glycolysis.

Answer C

19. Drugs are removed from the vascular system by ....

A. the kidneys.
B. the liver.
C. the lungs.
D. the intestinal tract.
E. all of the above.

Answer E

20. Medications that are relatively safe to administer have a ....

A. a low therapeutic threshold.
B. a high therapeutic threshold.
C. a high minimum effective dose.
D. a high therapeutic index.
E. a low therapeutic index.

Answer D

EMERGENCY DRUG CARDS

In the appendix of this workbook you will find perforated index cards for each of the commonly used emergency medications. Detach them from the book and use them as a study guide for pharmacology and for the remaining chapters of PARAMEDIC EMERGENCY CARE. Practice being able to identify the general description, indications, contraindications, precautions, dosage, and route for each of the cards. As you prepare for each unit and division test offered in your course, practice with the drugs which are covered within that chapter as well as those which have been already covered in a chapter. Notice that most of the emergency pharmacology comes with the cardiology chapter; it might be a good idea to work on some of those drugs before those classes begin.

You will notice that the cards leave enough space to add notes of your own. Often each system uses drugs slightly differently from another. Use the space provided to identify any modifications or special situations identified by your instructor, medical director or protocols.

EMERGENCY MEDICATIONS

The following are the drugs discussed within PARAMEDIC EMERGENCY CARE as possible choices for administration by the paramedic.

oxygen
epinephrine
norepinephrine (Levophed)
isoproterenol (Isuprel)
dopamine (Intropin)
dobutamine (Dobutrex)
labetalol (Trandate) (Normodyne)
lidocaine (Xylocaine)
bretylium tosylate (Bretylol)
procainamide (Pronestyl)
verapamil (Isoptin) (Calan)
atropine sulfate
sodium bicarbonate
morphine sulfate
nitrous oxide (Nitronox)
furosemide (Lasix)
nitroglycerin (Nitro Stat)
nifedipine (Procardia)
calcium chloride
aminophylline
racemic epinephrine
(microNEFRIN) (Vaponefrin)
terbutaline (Brethine)
albuterol (Proventil) (Ventolin)
50% dextrose in water
thiamine
methylprednisolone (Solu-Medrol)
diazepam (Valium)
oxytocin (Pitocin)
magnesium sulfate
diphenhydramine (Benadryl)
syrup of ipecac
activated charcoal
naloxone (Narcan)
haloperidol (Haldol)
promethazine (Phenergan)
adenosine (Adenocard)

13

EMERGENCY PHARMACOLOGY

Part II - *(pages 344 to 398)*

Review of the Objectives for Chapter 13

After reading this chapter, you should be able to:

18. Describe the autonomic nervous system and its role in pharmacology.

pp. 344 to 352

The autonomic nervous system is divided into two opposing systems: the sympathetic and the parasympathetic. The sympathetic system is responsible for the "fight-or-flight" aspects of nervous function and, in general, increased metabolism. The parasympathetic system is the "feed-or-breed" system and slows metabolism. They are generally balanced in a cycle of rest and activity. They are mediated by several chemical mediators and receptor sites and can be controlled by pharmacological intervention. The receptors of the sympathetic system are the alpha, beta, and dopaminergic receptors. Blocking or stimulating these sites can cause various actions within the body.

19. Describe the location and action of Alpha and Beta adrenergic receptors.

p. 349

Alpha receptor sites are found in the vascular system and the lungs. Stimulation of these sites will cause peripheral vasoconstriction and possibly mild bronchoconstriction.

Beta receptors are located in the heart (B_1) and cause increased heart rate, contractile force and electrical conduction. They are also located in the lungs and vascular system (B_2) and will cause dilatation.

20. Define the metric system.

p. 352

The metric system is a system of measurement for mass, length, and volume. It uses the decimal system (each unit is 10 times larger or smaller than the next). Its basic units are grams, meters, and liters.

21. Demonstrate the ability to do routine calculations and conversions using the metric system.

pp. 352 to 356

See the medication math guide and work sheets found later in this workbook chapter

22. Be able to calculate any given drug dose for all medications used in your EMS system.

pp. 352 to 356

See the medication math guide and work sheets found later in this workbook chapter

23. List ten routes of medication administration, and give the advantages and disadvantages of each.

pp. 356 to 364

Intradermal is the injection of a medication into the skin. It is a superficial route which is limited in its use due to slow absorption and small volumes of drug which can be administered. The administration site can be easily viewed and is used for diagnostic tests.

Sublingual administration allows absorption of the drug through the capillary bed under the tongue. Nitroglycerin and nifedipine are administered via this route.

Oral administration is the most common route of medication administration, however, it is too slow and unpredictable for emergency medications.

Transdermal is a route of absorption through the skin. It is a slow and unpredictable route, though nitroglycerin and hormone preparations are administered via this route.

Subcutaneous injection places the drug under the dermis. The route is slow and limited in the volume of medication which can be given.

Intramuscular injection has a slow but predictable rate of absorption and will allow administration of more drug.

Intravenous injection is the most common route for the administration of emergency drugs because it is a rapid route for distribution and will accept large volumes of medication either by bolus or drip. The rapid administration of drugs carries the danger of severe reaction.

Transtracheal administration of medications is rapid (as rapid as intravenous), though limited to a few drugs.

Sublingual injection is more rapid than normal intramuscular injection because of the vast capillary network of the tongue. The drugs available for administration via this route are limited.

Intracardiac injection places the drug directly in the heart and while this places the medication in the central circulation, it is accompanied by many complications.

24. Describe and list the indications, contraindications, and dosages for the emergency drugs used in your system.

pp. 356 to 398

(See the drug cards found at the end of this workbook)

READING COMPREHENSION SELF-EXAM

21. The type of drug which binds to a receptor and causes the expected response is called an antagonist.

A. True
B. False

Answer B

22. A drug which blocks the action of the sympathetic nervous system is called a ....

A. vagalytic.
B. sympatholytic.
C. parasympathomimetic.
D. parasympatholytic.
E. dopaminerolytic.

Answer B

23. Which of the following are true regarding the sympathetic nervous system?
   1. it is the "fight-or-flight" nervous system
   2. it is the "feed-or-breed" nervous system
   3. it releases norepinephrine
   4. it effects the dopamine receptors
   5. its chief neurotransmitter is acetylcholine

Select the proper grouping.

A. 2, 5
B. 1, 5
C. 2, 4, 5
D. 1, 3, 4
E. 1, 3, 4, 5

Answer D

24. Atropine is classified as a ....

A. parasympatholytic.
B. sympatholytic.
C. sympathomimetic.
D. parasympathomimetic.
E. neurotransmitter.

Answer A

25. Which of the following do you as a paramedic need to know about the drugs you are able to administer?
   1. incompatibilities with other drugs
   2. common side effects
   3. common indications
   4. the contraindications
   5. the recommended dosage range

Select the proper grouping.

A. 1, 3
B. 2, 4, 5
C. 1, 3, 5
D. 2, 3, 4, 5
E. 1, 2, 3, 4, 5

Answer E

26. Arrange the following metric prefixes in order from smallest to largest.
   1. deci
   2. milli
   3. micro
   4. kilo
   5. centi

Select the proper grouping.

A. 3, 2, 5, 1, 4
B. 2, 3, 5, 1, 4
C. 2, 5, 3, 4, 1
D. 5, 3, 4, 2, 1
E. 4, 5, 2, 1, 3

Answer A

27. The metric units for mass, length, and volume are which of the following, respectively?

A. meter, liter, gram
B. liter, meter, gram
C. meter, gram, liter
D. gram, meter, liter
E. gram, liter, meter

Answer D

28. The route of administration which permits a medication to be absorbed through the skin is ....

A. intradermal.
B. subcutaneous.
C. intramuscular.
D. oral.
E. none of the above.

Answer E

29. Which drug listed below can be administered via the endotracheal tube?

A. naloxone
B. atropine
C. epinephrine
D. lidocaine
E. all of the above

Answer E

30. The most common route for the administration of drugs for emergency medical service is via the ....

A. intramuscular route.
B. intravenous route.
C. subcutaneous route.
D. oral route.
E. sublingual route.

Answer B

PHARMACOLOGY MATH

Guide to easier drug calculations

While there might be more rapid systems to calculate drip rates and concentrations, the following step-wise approach is designed to help you understand the math so you are able to solve almost any problem. While math is an essential skill for the paramedic, most drip calculations are simple, standard, and easy to use once you become familiar with the drugs and drips used in your system.

Step I **Identify all known elements**

Elements for most drip calculations

R Rate (either in gtts/min., mcgtts*/min. or mL/min.)
V Volume (convert to mL)
T Time (convert to minutes)
D Drip conversion (gtts or mcgtts per mL)

Elements for most drug dose calculations

- C Concentration (g, mg or mcg per mL)
- W Weight (g, mg, or mcg)
- V Volume (convert to mL)

* mcgtts refers to microdrops

Step II **Select the proper formula**

The element which you don't know (and need to find) should be equal to the remainder of the formula.

Rate = Volume / Time (R = V / T)
Volume = Rate x Time (V = R x T)
Time = Volume / Rate (T = V / R)

Concentration = Weight / Volume (C= W / V)
Weight = Volume x Concentration (W = V x C)
Volume = Weight / Concentration (V = W / C)

Step III **Convert all variables into common terms**

Use the drip conversion figure or other conversion formula to convert all values to metric and standard values

Rate - into milliliters or milligrams / minute
Volume - into milliliters
Concentration - into milligrams / milliliter

Time - into minutes
Weight - into milligrams

Step IV **Plug in the known values**

Complete the formula, inserting the values identified in step I.

Step V **Cancel out labels**

Cross multiply labels to cancel them out. The result should leave you with the resulting label in terms of the unknown value.

$$\text{Volume} = \text{Rate x time} = \frac{X\text{ mL}}{\text{min.}} \text{ x } Y\text{ min.} = \frac{X\text{ mL x }Y\text{ min.}}{\text{min.}} = X * Y\text{ mL}$$

Step VI **Do the mathematical operations**

Multiply, divide, add, or subtract as necessary.

3 x 7 = 21 3 / 7 = 0.43 7 - 3 = 4 7 + 3 = 10

Step VII **Apply any needed conversions**

Use the mathematical conversions needed, such as the drip conversion to give you the final answer. Ensure that your answer is provided in the form and label which the question asks for.

$$X\text{ mL / min. using a }Y\text{ mcgtts / mL} = \frac{X\text{ mL}}{\text{min.}} \text{ x } \frac{Y\text{ mcgtts}}{\text{mL}}$$

$$= \frac{X\text{ x }Y\text{ mcgtts}}{\text{min.}} = X\text{ x }Y\text{ mcgtts / min.}$$

DRIP MATH WORKSHEET

Formulas

Rate = Volume/Time	mL/min = gtts per min/gtts per mL
Volume = Rate x Time	gtts / min = mL per min x gtts per mL
Time = Volume/Rate	mL = gtts/gtts per mL

Please complete the following drug and drip math problems:

[1] You are running a D5W drip (60 mcgtts/mL) into a patient at 15 mcgtts / min. During a 25-minute trip to the hospital, how much fluid would you infuse?

[2] Medical Command requests that you infuse 250 mL of a solution during a one hour transport. What rate do you need to set for a 60 mcgtts/mL infusion set?

for a 10 gtts/mL infusion set?

[3] If a 50 mL bag of normal saline is hung and running through a 45 mcgtts/mL administration set at 32 drops per minute, how long will the fluid last?

[4] If you are running a macro drip (10 gtts/mL) at 4 drops per second, how much fluid could you infuse in 45 minutes?

[5] Medical Command orders you to infuse 1.5 mL of a solution every minute. What drip rate would you set with a 60 mcgtts/mL set?

with a 45 mcgtts/mL set?

with a 10 gtts/mL set?

DIVISION REVIEW

PREPARATORY INFORMATION

Chapters 8 to 13

The following scenario based questions are designed to help you review the previous six chapters of **PARAMEDIC EMERGENCY CARE.** *They combine the knowledge gained thus far through your reading and course work.*

Scenario I

You arrive on the scene of a cardiac arrest with basic life support being performed by first responders. Your partner is a senior paramedic who assigns you to airway. You prepare to intubate while he readies the defibrillator. The patient is a rather large sized male with a short thick neck. The airway is well suctioned and the basic life support providers have been effective in ventilating the patient.

1. Just prior to intubation, assure the ventilator ....

   A. suctions the airway again.
   B. depresses the epigastric area.
   C. hyperventilates the patient.
   D. inserts an oral airway.
   E. all of the above.

   Answer C

2. You prefer to lift the epiglottis with the laryngoscope blade to visualize the glottis. Which laryngoscope blade should you select for this patient?

   A. a number 4 straight blade
   B. a number 2 straight blade
   C. a number 2 curved blade
   D. a number 4 curved blade
   E. any of the above

   Answer A

You quickly place the laryngoscope blade in the patients mouth and displace the tongue to the right. Even with great lifting pressure you are still unable to visualize the vocal cords.

3. Which of the following techniques would you employ if presented with the situation described above?

   A. nasotracheal intubation
   B. blind intubation
   C. digital intubation
   D. rapid sequence intubation
   E. A or C

   Answer E

You intubate the trachea and then auscultate for sounds at the epigastrium.

4. How would you describe the location of your stethoscope disc in relation to the xiphoid process?

   A. inferior
   B. superior
   C. proximal
   D. distal
   E. medial

Answer A

5. You hear gurgling sounds with each ventilation. You should do which of the following?
   1. leave the endotracheal tube in place
   2. withdraw the endotracheal tube, immediately
   3. hyperventilate the patient with a bag-valve-mask
   4. re-attempt intubation

   Select the proper grouping.

   A. 1, 3
   B. 1, 3, 4
   C. 2, 3
   D. 2, 4
   E. 2, 3, 4

Answer B

Bilateral breath sounds are clear and the patient's chest rises symmetrically. Your partner has given three countershocks with the defibrillator and asks you to initiate an IV line. Meanwhile he is preparing to administer twice the normal IV dose of epinephrine down the endotracheal tube.

6. The administration of twice the IV dose via ET tube is considered ....

   A. an inappropriately high dose.
   B. high but still within an acceptable dosage range.
   C. an inappropriate route for administration.
   D. appropriate.
   E. epinephrine is not indicated for arrest.

Answer D

7. As you insert the requested intravenous catheter you notice a good flashback of blood. You advance the catheter, withdraw the needle and connect the administration set. You open the drip valve and the fluid doesn't flow. Which of the following might be the cause of the problem?
   1. the IV bag needs to be higher
   2. the IV tubing is kinked
   3. the patient's blood pressure is too high
   4. the venous tourniquet needs to be released
   5. the catheter may be up against a valve

   Select the proper grouping.

   A. 1, 3, 4
   B. 2, 3, 5
   C. 1, 2, 5
   D. 1, 2, 4, 5
   E. 1, 2, 3, 4, 5

Answer D

8. As you begin the infusion of fluid, you notice an area of tissue swelling around the IV site. You should ...

A. securely tape the catheter and tubing to the patient's arm.
B. lower the IV to decrease the infusion pressure.
C. close the drip valve, apply pressure to the infusion site.
D. discontinue the IV and attempt at another location.
E. do none of the above.

Answer E

9. The drug epinephrine stimulates the sympathetic nervous system and is hence called a ....

A. parasympatholytic.
B. sympatholytic.
C. parasympathomimetic.
D. sympathomimetic.
E. sympathetic agonist.

Answer A

Scenario II

Your rescue unit has been called to the scene of a one car accident with a single patient with serious injuries. You arrive on the scene two minutes after dispatch and about four minutes after the actual accident. Your initial evaluation of the patient reveals a conscious, alert male with a blood pressure of 124/86, pulse of 72, and respirations of 26. You employ spinal precautions including a cervical collar, an extrication device, prepare a long spine board, and take a second set of vital signs. The blood pressure is 122/94, the pulse rate is now 88, respirations are 32 and shallow, and the patient appears agitated.

10. What is accounting for the changing patient vital signs?

A. post-accident anxiety
B. the confinement of the spine board
C. hypovolemic shock (compensated)
D. hypovolemic shock (decompensated)
E. hyperventilation

Answer D

11. Which of the following care steps would you provide for this patient?
1. PASG
2. Rapid IV fluid infusion
3. high-flow oxygen
4. rapid transport

Select the proper grouping.

A. 1, 3
B. 1, 2
C. 2, 3, 4
D. 3, 4
E. 1, 2, 3, 4

Answer E

You quickly load the patient into the ambulance and are underway. You begin the physical assessment and note a crackling sensation while palpating the left chest. Auscultation reveals diminished breath sound on the left and a gentle crackling sound heard during inspiration. The patient's left flank is tender and the belly reveals rebound tenderness.

12. The crackling upon palpation of the chest area is called ....

    A. subcutaneous emphysema.
    B. spontaneous pneumothorax.
    C. rhonchi or rales.
    D. tension pneumothorax.
    E. none of the above.

    Answer A

13. The sound heard during inspiration is best described as which of the following?

    A. normal
    B. rhonchi
    C. rales
    D. stridorous
    E. incipient

    Answer C

14. The left flank pain is most likely related to an injury to which of the following organs? Is lower and in back.

    A. kidney
    B. large bowel
    C. stomach
    D. liver
    E. none of the above

    Answer A E C.

Scenario III

You are administering a lidocaine drip to a patient with cardiac irritability. The drip was mixed by adding 2 gm of lidocaine to a 250 ml bag of D_5W and is run in at 60 microdrops per minute. Suddenly the patient complains of yellow vision, numbness "all over" and his level of consciousness is dropping.

15. Given the patient response to the drip, you should do which of the following?

    A. increase the drip rate
    B. decrease the drip rate
    C. re-mix the drug and run at the same rate
    D. discontinue the drip
    E. leave the drip as it is

    Answer D

16. The reaction to the drip displayed by this patient is best described as ....

    A. untoward.
    B. synergistic.
    C. expected.
    D. therapeutic.
    E. allergic.

    Answer A

17. The concentration of the drip of lidocaine is ....

A. 1 mg/ml.
B. 2 mg/ml.
C. 3 mg/ml.
D. 4 mg/ml.
E. 8 mg/ml.

Answer E

18. The rate of administration of the drip is ....

A. 0.25 ml/min.
B. 0.50 ml/min.
C. 0.75 ml/min.
D. 1.0 ml/min.
E. 1.5 ml/min.

Answer D

19. The dosage of lidocaine you are giving in this scenario is within the normal therapeutic range.

A. True
B. False

Answer B

The patient in this scenario begins to seize. It is followed by seizure after seizure without the patient regaining consciousness.

20. Which drug would be indicated to control these seizures?

A. lidocaine
B. morphine sulfate
C. nitrous oxide
D. meperidine
E. diazepam

Answer E

21. What dose of the above drug would you administer?

A. 2 mg IV
B. 4 mg IV
C. 10 mg IV
D. 25 mg IV
E. 100 mg IV

Answer C

22. If the airway became a problem and you could not open the clenched teeth what method might you still use to establish an airway?

A. nasal intubation
B. PTL airway
C. EOA or EGTA
D. combi-tube
E. digital intubation

Answer A

14

THE KINETICS OF TRAUMA

Review of the Objectives for Chapter 14

After reading this chapter, you should be able to:

1. Describe the prevalence and significance of trauma.

p. 402

Prevalence

Third most common cause of death in the United States
140,000 lives lost to trauma per year
44,000 lives lost in auto accidents each year

Significance

Obvious injury not necessarily life threatening
Subtle injuries often life endangering

2. Explain the "Golden Hour" concept and describe how it applies to prehospital emergency medical service.

p. 404

Time from accident to surgery, ideally one hour maximum
Observation of the "Golden Hour" reduces trauma mortality
Prehospital scene care is alloted 10 minutes of the "Golden Hour"
10 percent of trauma patients fall into this need category

3. Identify, and explain by example, Newton's Laws of Inertia and Conservation of Energy.

p. 406

A body in motion or at rest will remain so unless acted upon by an outside force.

Example: two autos, slowing from 55 to 0 mph., one by braking (friction) and the other by impact with a stationary object such as a tree or another auto.

Energy can neither be created nor destroyed.

Example: when an auto collides with a tree, the kinetic energy is released as the noise of the crash, the bending and heating of metal, and the injuries suffered by the patient.

4. Apply the principles of kinetic energy and force to various types of trauma.

pp. 406 to 407

$$KE = \frac{M * V^2}{2} \qquad F = M * A$$

Kinetic energy is the energy any object or vehicle has while in motion. It increases directly as the mass of an object increases and/or as the sum of the square of the velocity increases.

Kinetic energy becomes very important in understanding the tremendous energy associated with a gunshot wound. The projectile, though very small and light. has a very great amount of energy because of its speed.

Force is the strength of the impact and is directly related to the increase (acceleration), or decrease (deceleration) in velocity. Force is a very important consideration when looking at the devastation caused by the auto accident or fall. The rate of deceleration (or acceleration) plays an important role in how much damage will be done to the car and passengers inside.

5. Compare and contrast the types of impact associated with auto and motorcycle accidents.

pp. 408 to 420

In **frontal** impact two pathways are identified: the down and under, and the up and over. The down and under path impacts the knee with the fire wall or dash and transmits the energy along the thigh. The up and over pathway impacts the chest with the steering wheel or dash, and the head with the windshield or dash.

Rear end impact pushes the automobile forward with rapid acceleration. The patient's body is forced forward with tremendous energy while the head remains stationary.

Lateral impact does not benefit from the large expanse of auto body metal between the impacting object and the patient. The deceleration is more extreme than either the frontal or rear end impact.

Rotational impact benefits from the transfer and exchange of forces rather than complete dissipation. The auto is deflected from its path rather than being stopped abruptly. The mechanism of injury is a mixture of lateral, frontal and rear end forces.

The **roll-over** accident, as with the rotational impact, combines mechanisms of injury. The energy needed to rollover an auto is great and the patient injuries may be severe. Ejection is a commonly associated outcome.

Motorcycle accidents are generally more severe than the auto because of limited protection afforded the rider. Frontal impact produces ejection and entrapment of the femurs while angular impact will crush the lower extremity between the bike and object. Helmets reduce head injuries but do not affect the incidence of neck injuries.

6. Predict the injuries expected from the various types of auto impacts and other blunt and penetrating trauma.

pp. 411 to 418

Frontal - the down and under pathway is likely to produce knee, femur and pelvic fractures, while the up and over pathway will cause anterior chest, neck and head injuries.

Rear end - the most common pathology related to rear impact is the neck injury. The patient is well protected unless unrestrained and thrown about during secondary impacts.

Lateral - this impact induces extremity fractures but reduces the incidence of rib fractures. There is also an increase in the incidence of great vessel, head and neck trauma.

Rotational - the incidence and severity of injury is somewhat reduced; however, the injuries found may be any of those expected from the lateral, frontal or rear end impact.

Roll-over - as with the rotational impact, the injuries expected are related to the actual point or points of impact. The incidence of ejection is increased and, with that, the chances of serious injury or patient mortality.

Blunt trauma occurs from falls, blasts, physical assaults, etc. The spectrum of injury is similar to those injuries expected from auto accidents.

Penetrating injuries result in low and high energy trauma. Low energy usually affects only the area of tissue contacted. High energy projectiles, bullets, have the ability to transmit energy and damage to surrounding tissue.

7. Discuss the benefits and disadvantages of auto restraint and motorcycle helmet use.

pp. 410 to 420

Lap belts greatly reduce injury and the chances of ejection. However, they may result in abdominal, lower spine or pelvic injury.

Shoulder belts add to the effectiveness of the lap belt, though when used alone may cause neck injury or decapitation.

Air bags are effective for initial frontal impact only.

Helmets reduce the incidence of head injury yet do not affect the incidence of neck injury.

8. Describe the significance and meaning of the terms velocity, cavitation, and profile, as they relate to penetrating trauma.

pp. 426 to 429

Velocity is the speed at which a projectile travels. As the velocity changes, the kinetic energy changes by the square of the change in velocity.

Cavitation is the energy wave transferred to the patient as the projectile passes through the body tissue.

Profile is the surface of the projectile, which actually contacts the tissue and transfers energy. The greater the profile, the more rapid the energy transfer.

9. Associate various types of penetrating trauma with the extent of injury they can involve.

pp. 429 to 431

The extent of internal injury is dependent on the pathway and amount of energy transmitted to the tissue. The low velocity injuries (knife, arrow, etc.) are limited to the object pathway. Higher velocity injuries (handgun, shotgun and rifle) are dependent upon the amount of energy transferred to and through the tissue.

10. Describe how the environment and mechanism of injury can alert you to specific types of injury.

pp. 402 to 431

Analysis of the circumstances which caused injury and the injury process can lead to an anticipation of the nature and severity of the patient's injuries. This is called the index of suspicion.

CASE STUDY REVIEW

Reread the case study in **PARAMEDIC EMERGENCY CARE** and then read the discussion below.

This case review applies the kinetics of trauma to an accident scene. The result is an orderly and controlled scene in which the patients are quickly assessed, prioritized, immediately stabilized and transported. The accident is analyzed to anticipate both the nature and severity of patient injuries. This information is used in combination with the data gathered through the patient assessments to develop a clear picture of what happened to the auto passengers and to determine what resources will be distributed to each patient.

Chapter I4 Case Study

The information given by the dispatcher allows the paramedic to begin planning for arrival at the scene. The information describes a severe accident with the potential for several injured persons. Trauma equipment should be located in the ambulance and set out on the stretcher for quick transport to the patient's side. 1000 ml. bags of lactated Ringer's solution might be readied in the ambulance with trauma tubing, pressure infusers, and large bore catheters, just in case the decision is made to rapidly transport. The paramedic may also use this time to review the responsibilities, which begin with arrival at the scene.

Given the police update, the paramedic should begin thinking about the kinetic energies of the accident and the injuries that are likely to result. One auto was stopped and hit from behind by a vehicle at "highway speed." The injuries suspected should include potential neck injury, with the rest of the body well protected except for secondary impact. The paramedic should also anticipate the need for spinal precautions.

The auto traveling at highway speed most likely impacted the other, frontally. The occupants may have traveled either through the down and under, or up and over, pathway, or they may have been protected by lap, lap and shoulder or airbag restraint systems (remember that the air bag restraint system is beneficial only for the initial head-on impact). Internal head injuries, respiratory embarrassment and shock are the leading trauma killers. The paramedic should ensure that these have not occurred or are not occurring.

The paramedic can gain a great deal of information quickly during the survey of the scene. Hazards, the number of patients, the resources available and the mechanism of injury can all be identified. From this analysis of the mechanism of injury, the paramedic can anticipate the nature and extent of injuries. By examining what happened, how badly the auto is damaged, from what direction, etc., the paramedic can garner enough information to anticipate who is the most seriously injured patient.

In this case the red car was struck from behind by the green car. The red car sustained severe rearend damage, reflecting a strong impact. The passenger would have been pushed forward with great acceleration by the auto seat while the unsupported head remained in position. A helpful observation was that the head rest was in the "up" position. This may have limited the forceful hyperextension of the head and neck and limited injury. The seat belt would also limit the danger of secondary impact as the car came to a rest.

The second car (the green one) sustained front end damage and two spider webs in the windshield. This suggests an unrestrained driver and passenger, the up and over pathway, and a potential for severe head and internal injuries. The deformity of the steering wheel also suggests that the driver may have sustained a chest injury.

Assessment confirms the injuries anticipated by review of the impact and the degree of auto damage. The driver of the red car appears only shaken up. His vitals are within normal limits, given the circumstances. The choice was made to leave him with a first responder while care was provided to the patients within the green car. While it would be ideal to have a paramedic by the side of each patient, this decision is justified based upon the first responder assessment and the analysis of the mechanism of injury.

The occupants of the green auto are in a much different situation. The driver has sustained chest trauma and is experiencing dyspnea, though her breath sounds are clear at this time. She is stable for now. However, she has the potential to deteriorate rapidly at any time. Her passenger is moving rapidly into hypovolemic shock, presumably due to pelvic and femur fractures, and internal hemorrhage. She is also unconscious either due to the hypovolemia or the head impact. The passenger is a candidate for immediate transport. The driver, though more stable, is a candidate for immediate transport also.

This case study demonstrates the value a good scene analysis can have in triaging, in anticipating the findings of assessment, and in determining the care needed by the patient. While the analysis of the kinetics of trauma does not give absolute information on the nature and extent of patient injuries, it can complement the overall assessment of both the scene and each individual patient.

READING COMPREHENSION SELF-EXAM

1. Highway accidents are responsible for approximately how many deaths each year?

   A. 22,000
   B. 44,000
   C. 75,000
   D. 100,000
   E. 150,000

   Answer B

2. The paramedic is given how much of the "Golden Hour?"

   A. 1 minute
   B. 10 minutes
   C. 20 minutes
   D. 30 minutes
   E. the whole hour, but no more

   Answer B

3. The study of motion is called ....

   A. kinetics.
   B. physics.
   C. ballistics.
   D. inertia.
   E. none of the above

   Answer A

4. Two autos accelerate from a stop sign to a speed of 30 mph., the first one by normal acceleration and the second when it was struck from behind by another vehicle. Assuming that both vehicles have the same weight, which vehicle gained the most kinetic energy?

   A. the vehicle in normal acceleration
   B. the vehicle struck from behind
   C. both vehicles gained the same kinetic energy
   D. neither vehicle since the kinetic energy is not known
   E. neither vehicle, since the force is not known

   Answer C

5. Which of the following is an example of energy dissipation from the auto accident?

   A. sound of the impact
   B. bending of the structural steel
   C. heating of the compressed steel
   D. internal injury to the occupant
   E. all of the above

   Answer E

6. The type of auto impact that occurs most frequently is the ....

   A. lateral.
   B. rotational.
   C. frontal.
   D. rear end.
   E. roll-over.

   Answer C

7. The anatomical region most commonly injured in the rear end collision is the ....

A. head.
B. neck.
C. chest.
D. extremities.
E. pelvis.

Answer B

8. In motorcycle accidents, the highest index of suspicion for injury should be directed at the ....

A. neck area.
B. head area.
C. extremities.
D. pelvic area.
E. femurs.

Answer B

9. In the auto/pedestrian (child) auto accident, you would expect the victim to turn into the impact.

A. True
B. False

Answer A

10. Place the following injuries in order of frequency in which they cause death in the auto accident:
   1. internal injuries
   2. head injuries
   3. spinal and chest injuries
   4. extremity fractures

   Select the proper grouping.

A. 1, 2, 3, 4
B. 3, 2, 4, 1
C. 2, 1, 3, 4
D. 4, 2, 3, 1
E. 4, 3, 2, 1

Answer C

11. The mechanism that causes patient injury in the blast is (are) ....

A. a pressure wave.
B. flying debris.
C. the patient being thrown into objects.
D. all of the above.
E. A and B.

Answer D

12. The extent of damage that results from penetrating trauma is most related to which of the following?

A. speed
B. weight
C. kinetic energy
D. mass
E. acceleration

Answer C

13. The pressure wave that accompanies a bullet as it travels through human tissue is called .....

A. drag.
B. cavitation.
C. trajectory.
D. ballistics.
E. none of the above.

Answer B

14. A penetrating wound to the area of the rib margin should be suspected of involving the ....

A. spleen or liver.
B. kidneys.
C. abdominal and thoracic organs.
D. left, right or both lung fields.
E. diaphragm.

Answer C

15. Generally, powder burns and tattooing around the entrance wound suggests ....

A. a gun used at close range
B. a high powered rifle
C. a handgun
D. the use of a black powder
E. none of the above

Answer A

SPECIAL PROJECTS

Turn to each of the pages in Paramedic Emergency Care listed below. There you will find a photograph of an accident scene. Identify the type of impact that has occurred and list at least three injuries that you would expect have occurred.

Page 468 Mechanism of injury Auto Accident – frontal Impact.

Anticipated injuries

Down & under pathway — Knee Fracture, femur fracture, Hip dislocation

Up & over pathway — Head injurys Neck injurys – chest injurys

Page 419 Mechanism of injury motorcycle – Auto Accident

Anticipated injuries

Bilaterial femur fractures — Spine injurys

Abdominal injurys — upper extremity Fractures

head injury's (note Helmet)

15

HEAD, NECK, AND SPINE INJURY

Review of the Objectives for Chapter 15

After reading this chapter, you should be able to:

1. List the structures that protect the central nervous system from trauma, and describe how they accomplish this function.

pp. 435 to 439

The **scalp/soft tissue** of the back will absorb a great deal of energy from blunt and penetrating trauma.

The **skull and vertebral bodies** provide rigid skeletal protection for the brain and spinal cord. The skull forms a rigid vault for the brain which will not expand should the pressure within increase.

The **meninges** are three layers of tissue: the pia mater, the arachnoid, and the dura mater. The dura is a tough fibrous layer which lines the interior of the skull and spinal foramen. The pia mater is a delicate membrane covering the convolutions of the brain and spinal cord. The arachnoid is a web-like structure under which the cerebral spinal fluid is found. The cerebral spinal fluid "floats" the brain and cord to help absorb the energy of trauma.

2. List the components of the central nervous system and explain how they help control the human body.

pp. 439 to 442

The **brain** consists of the cerebrum, cerebellum, pons and brainstem. It is an electrochemical computer which stores and processes information necessary for body function.

The **spinal cord** is the major communications conduit which distributes the brain's commands to the body's organs and directs information back to the brain.

3. List the signs and symptoms for the following conditions.

pp. 444 to 453

Soft tissue injuries (of the scalp, face and neck) - swelling, ecchymosis (late sign), deformity, instability, hemorrhage, pain

Skull fracture - mechanism of injury, fluid drainage from the ears or nose, deformity, Battle's sign or periorbital ecchymosis (late signs), pain

Central nervous system injury

Brain injury - mechanism of injury, altered level of consciousness, personality change, pupillary inequality, increased B.P., decreased pulse rate, deep gasping respirations, headache

Increasing intracranial pressure mechanism of injury, diminishing level of consciousness, personality changes, headache

Spinal cord injury mechanism of injury, local pain, swelling, paresthesia or paralysis distal to injury

Special sense organ injury mechanism of injury, eye - painless loss of vision, curtain in front of vision. ear - vertigo, hearing loss

4. Identify the various head, neck, and spine injuries and explain the progression of their respective injuries.

pp. 444 to 453

Scalp injury can lead to severe hemorrhage, though it is usually easy to control.

Skull fracture is a skeletal injury which, alone, is not serious. It has the potential for injury beneath, which is of concern to the paramedic.

Vertebral fracture may occur at several points. Again, it is the reduced stability and the potential for spinal cord injury which is the greatest concern.

Facial injury (both soft tissue and skeletal injury to the facial region) will present with deformity, instability and possibly severe hemorrhage. The major concern, however, is the protection of the airway and hemorrhage control.

Neck injury can endanger the airway and some of the body's major blood vessels. Attention must be directed at reducing hemorrhage and the chance of air aspiration, as well as maintaining an open airway.

Brain injury presents with problems of two types: physical injury and increasing intracranial pressure. Physical injury will cause immediate manifestations that will normally improve with time. Increasing intracranial pressure may be caused by hemorrhage or cerebral edema and will progressively reduce blood flow to the brain.

5. Explain the significance of the primary assessment as it relates to CNS injury.

pp. 453 to 456

Survey of the scene - if the survey of the scene suggests a possibility of CNS injury, the patient should be treated as though one exists, throughout prehospital care.

Level of consciousness - the level of consciousness should be determined initially and evaluated periodically to determine if any changes are occurring. Any altered level of consciousness indicates brain injury until proven otherwise.

Breathing - any irregular or exaggerated respiratory pattern suggests head injury. Abdominal breathing suggests spinal injury below the C-3 level.

Circulation - any pulse rate below 60 in the trauma patient increases suspicion of increased intracranial pressure. Any cool and dry region of the skin may suggest CNS loss and spinal injury.

Disability - any disability or loss of sensation which cannot be linked to other injury should be suspected to be of CNS origin.

6. Identify the proper care steps for the following conditions.

pp. 460 to 467

Central nervous system injury

Brain injury - ensure airway, respirations and utilize high-flow oxygen. Do not halt fluid flow from ears or nose. Transport quickly to a neurocenter. Treat as a spinal cord injury also. Monitor level of consciousness.

Spinal cord injury - immobilize spine in a neutral position. Maintain positioning throughout care (including manual stabilization, cervical collar and rigid fixation) and transport.

Soft tissue injury (of the scalp, face, neck) - stop hemorrhage with direct pressure except in unstable skull fracture. Ensure the airway is clear and dress the wound as prioritized in assessment.

Skull fracture - care for as brain injury. Do not apply direct pressure over a depressed skull fracture or cranial instability.

Special sense organ injury - protect from further harm.

7. Describe the assessment of a patient with a head, neck, or spinal injury, and list the care steps required for each finding named.

pp. 453 to 467

The assessment of the head, neck, and spine injured patient must concentrate on the mechanism of injury to determine if one of these injuries could have occurred. Any evidence from the primary assessment, secondary assessment, vital signs, or patient history which suggests the possibility of one of these injuries should be a cause for immediate care and transportation.

Head injury - a possible head injury patient should receive high flow oxygen, serial evaluation of vital signs and level of consciousness, spinal immobilization and possible pharmacological therapy.

Neck injury - soft tissue injury to the neck should receive assessment that observes for possible threat to the airway, severe hemorrhage, and possible air embolism. Any bleeding wound should be covered with an occlusive dressing and the hemorrhage controlled.

Spine injury - any suggestion of spine injury should be met with immediate and continued manual spinal immobilization (including a cervical collar), followed by fixation to a spinal immobilization device.

CASE STUDY REVIEW

Reread the case study in **PARAMEDIC EMERGENCY CARE** and then read the discussion below.

This case study presentation addresses the considerations of CNS injury in the auto accident. It looks at the elements of scene survey, patient assessment, care, and transport, all with regard to the patient with potential head and spine injury.

Chapter I5 Case Study

The medics of unit 765 are dispatched to a typical auto accident with one patient. The scene is secure, and the survey finds a broken windshield corresponding to the driver's head. The auto and the history of the patient's unconsciousness both support the probability of head injury. The patient, from this information, will be assessed and transported quickly.

The history of the patient's unconsciousness causes the paramedics to monitor the level of consciousness frequently during care. The initial evaluation will be noted in subjective terms which can be compared against patient responses later on. Any change will be noted and will call for immediate transport if not already underway.

The physical assessment reveals a patient who cannot remember the events of the accident. This is a relatively common response, called retrograde amnesia. It is normal and alone reflects a psychological response rather than a physiologic injury. Questioning later on may find the patient beginning to remember the accident.

The chest injury is of concern and raises the index of suspicion for lung, great vessel or heart injury. These are cared for with oxygen, cardiac monitoring (to recognize any signs of myocardial contusion) and close observation of the vital signs. The chest is auscultated and evaluated frequently to watch for development of pneumothorax, edema or chest pain.

Monitoring of the vital signs and level of consciousness may give evidence of progressing intracranial hemorrhage. An increase in blood pressure, reduction in pulse rate and erratic respirations would support the diagnosis. These signs and any other neurologic deficits will be documented and related to medical command to help identify the location of the injury and its progression.

As the assessment continues, the patient becomes less alert and the left pupil becomes dilated. Finally unconsciousness ensues and the patient responds only to painful stimuli. These findings indicate that the patient has developing intracranial pressure. The only effective care is to release that pressure, a surgical process which can be accomplished only at a neurocenter. The patient is spine-boarded quickly and transported. Time is of primary importance. Oxygen therapy is aggressive and guided by oximetry. Airway protection is accomplished by oral intubation with the head maintained in a neutral position. The paramedics place the tube quickly to reduce the increase in intracranial pressure which occurs during intubation attempts.

READING COMPREHENSION SELF-EXAM

1. Which of the following bones is not a part of the cranium?

   A. frontal
   B. zygoma
   C. occipital
   D. sphenoid
   E. temporal

   Answer B

2. The protrusion of the axis that allows the large degree of motion of the head and yet ensures that the first and second vertebra remain in alignment is called the ....

   A. atlas.
   B. cauda equina.
   C. spinal foramen.
   D. odontoid process.
   E. foramen magnum.

   Answer D

3. If intracranial pressure affects the tentorium, the third cranial nerve may be compressed. This would most likely cause which of the following?

   A. Kussmaul respirations
   B. pupillary disturbances
   C. decreased pulse rate
   D. increased blood pressure
   E. none of the above

   Answer B

4. It is common for the paramedic to observe either Battle's sign or bilateral periorbital ecchymosis in the patient who has just sustained a basilar skull fracture.

   A. True
   B. False

   Answer B

5. Which of the following head injuries generally get worse in the first few hours after the accident?
   1. cerebral concussion
   2. cerebral edema
   3. brainstem contusion
   4. intracranial hemorrhage

   Select the proper grouping.

   A. 1, 3
   B. 1, 4
   C. 2, 4
   D. 1, 3, 4
   E. 1, 2, 4

   Answer C

6. The injury which causes the brain to be damaged on the side opposite of the impact is called ....

A. reversed affect.
B. subdural hematoma.
C. subluxation.
D. contrecoup.
E. a concussion.

Answer D

7. The injury which classically presents with unconsciousness immediately after the accident followed by a lucid interval and then a decreasing level of consciousness is most likely a(n) ....

A. concussion.
B. epidural hematoma.
C. subdural hematoma.
D. cerebral hemorrhage.
E. a brainstem contusion.

Answer B

8. Which of the following are signs of pressure on the medulla oblongata?
   1. vomiting without nausea
   2. lowering level of consciousness
   3. increasing blood pressure
   4. slowing heart rate
   5. pupillary dilatation

Select the proper grouping.

A. 1, 2, 3
B. 2, 4, 5
C. 1, 3, 4, 5
D. 1, 2, 3, 4
E. 1, 2, 3, 4, 5

Answer E

9. The collection of blood in front of a patient's pupil and iris due to blunt trauma is called ....

A. hyphema.
B. retinal detachment.
C. icterus.
D. anterior chamber hematoma.
E. none of the above.

Answer A

10. Blood vessel injury in the neck region carries with it the hazard of ....
   1. severe venous hemorrhage.
   2. severe arterial hemorrhage.
   3. development of subcutaneous emphysema.
   4. air aspiration.

Select the proper grouping.

A. 1, 2
B. 1, 3
C. 1, 2, 4
D. 2, 3, 4
E. 1, 2, 3, 4

Answer C

11. Which of the following respiratory patterns would be indicative of brain injury?
    1. eupnea
    2. Biot's respirations
    3. central neurogenic hyperventilation
    4. Cheyne-Stokes respirations
    5. agonal respirations

    Select the proper grouping.

    A. 1, 2, 5
    B. 2, 3, 5
    C. 1, 3, 4, 5
    D. 2, 3, 4, 5
    E. 1, 2, 3, 4, 5

    Answer D

12. The elements of the Glasgow Coma Scale include ....
    1. level of orientation.
    2. motor response.
    3. verbal response.
    4. AVPU.
    5. eye opening.

    Select the proper grouping.

    A. 1, 2, 4
    B. 2, 3, 5
    C. 1, 3, 5
    D. 2, 3, 4, 5
    E. 1, 2, 3, 4, 5

    Answer B

13. "Belly breathing" would normally suggest which of the injuries below?

    A. cerebral concussion
    B. cerebral contusion
    C. brainstem injury
    D. increasing intracranial pressure
    E. none of the above

    Answer E

14. The major reason for allowing fluid to drain from the nose or ear is that ....

    A. it may slow the rise of intracranial pressure.
    B. its flow will prevent pathogens from entering the meninges.
    C. it is impossible to stop the flow anyway.
    D. regeneration of CSF is beneficial to the healing process.
    E. none of the above.

    Answer A

15. The paramedic should move the head and neck of a patient with a suspected spine injury into the neutral position unless ....

    A. it can be immobilized in the position found.
    B. resistance is noted during the attempt.
    C. the patient experiences pain during the movement.
    D. the patient has no noticeable deficit.
    E. B and C.

    Answer E

16. Which endotracheal intubation techniques are recommended for the patient with a suspected spine injury?
    1. standard oral intubation
    2. digital intubation
    3. nasal intubation
    Select the proper grouping.

    A. 1
    B. 2
    C. 3
    D. 1, 2
    E. 2, 3

Answer E

17. Repeated or prolonged intubation attempts should be avoided because they may induce dysrhythmias and increase intracranial pressure in the head injury patient.

    A. True
    B. False

Answer A

18. The patient with head or spine injury should be watched for the development of, and protected against, hypothermia or hyperthermia.

    A. True
    B. False

Answer A

19. Which of the following pharmacologic agents might be given to the patient with a head or spine injury?
    1. oxygen
    2. methylprednisolone
    3. diazepam
    4. furosemide
    Select the proper grouping.

    A. 1, 3
    B. 2, 4
    C. 1, 2, 3
    D. 2, 3, 4
    E. 1, 2, 3, 4

Answer E

20. If methylpredisolone is ordered for a patient with suspected cerebral edema, it should be administered at which of the following dosages?

    A. 30 mg/Kg
    B. 45 mg/Kg
    C. 3 g/Kg
    D. 5 g/Kg
    E. 10 g/Kg

Answer A

SPECIAL PROJECTS

The authoring of both the radio message to the receiving hospital and the written run report are two of the most important tasks you will perform as a paramedic. Read the following information, reread the case study in your textbook, and then compose a radio message and complete the run report for this call.

The Call:

Dispatch to the call comes from the 911 Center at 2:15 a.m. You are called to an auto accident at the junction of highway 127 and county trunk H, in Wilbur Township. You and your team, Mary Greapt (Paramedic) and Tom Klien (EMT) arrive at the scene at 2:32.

The initial care of the patient includes cervical collar (2:34), vitals (2:36) and oxygen @ 6 L via nasal cannula (2:36). A second set of vitals is taken just after the patient becomes unconscious. They reveal a pulse of 52, respirations of 22 deep and labored, blood pressure of 136/92, and a pulseox reading of 98%. The patient is responsive to painful stimuli only (2:40). The patient is immobilized to a long spine board (2:41), loaded on the stretcher and moved to the ambulance at 2:42 with transport begun immediately.

The en route IV is initiated in the left forearm with a 16 ga. angiocath to run normal saline T.K.O. You are headed to Community Hospital, the closest facility and the base of your medical command.

Medical command is contacted and you call in the following:

Unit 765 to medical command, we are enroute to community hospital with a victim of a one car auto accident - frontal impact. The patient was reported as initially unconscious, but was conscious alert through somewhat disoriented upon, our arrival. He is now unconscious and responsive only to painful stimuli. He did complain of chest pain which varied with breathing, breath sounds are clear. He has a small contusion on his forehead. Vitals are BP 136/92. Pulse 52 Resp 22 + deep and a SaO_2 98%. We have established an IV with 1,000 mL N.S. running TKO and have applied O_2 a cervical collar has been applied and spinal imobilization is underway.

The medical command physician directs your patient to the Medical Center and orders that an endotracheal tube be placed if possible. A 8.0 mm. tube is positioned orally via digital technique with good bilateral breath sounds auscultated (2:51). The vitals are repeated (pulse 50, B.P. 140/92, respirations: 15, deep and irregular, pulseox 97%).

You contact medical command and provide the following update:

Unit 765 to medical Center. Our Patient Remains unconscious And responsive only to deep painful stimuli. He is orally intubated with assisted Respirations via Bag-valve-mask @ 25 Current vitals BP 140/92 pulse 50 + SaO2 97% ETA 15 minutes

ETA - 15 minutes

The second enroute vital signs are as follows: B.P. 140/90, pulse 50 and bounding, respirations 25 (assisted by BVM) and pulse oximetry of 97% (3:01). The patient is delivered to the Medical Center at 3:15 and you report for service at 3:35.

Complete the run report on the following page from the information contained in the narrative of this call.

Compare the radio communication and run report form which you prepare against the example in the answer key section of this workbook. As you make this comparison, realize that there are many "correct" ways to communicate this body of information. Ensure that the information you have recorded contains the major points of your assessment and care, and enough other material to describe the patient and his condition to the receiving physician and anyone who might review the form. Remember that this document may be the only record of your assessment and care for this patient. When you are done, it should be a complete accounting of your actions.

DRUGS USED IN HEAD INJURY

Emergency management for head injury utilizes many of the pharmacologic agents which are available to the paramedic. Please review and memorize the various names, indications, therapeutic effects, contraindications, side effects, routes of administration and recommended dosages for the following.

furosemide (Lasix)

methylprednisolone (Solu-Medrol)

diazepam (Valium)

Date 5 / 10 / 94 — Emergency Medical Service Run Report — Run # 913

Patient Information

Name: John Doe
Address: 112233 South Street
City: GG CA 96813 St: CA Zip: 92641
Age: 31 Birth: / / Sex: [M][F] (M marked)

Service Information

Agency: Unit 765
Location: Hwy 127 + Cty tr. H.
Call Origin:
Type: Emrg[X] Non[ ] Trnsfr[ ]

Times

Rcvd 2 : 15
Enrt 2 : 15
Scne 2 : 32
LvSn 2 : 42
ArHsp 3 : 15
InSv 3 : 35

Nature of Call: 1 Auto Accident/frontal impact
Chief Complaint: Chest pain which varies with Resp/unconsciousness

Description of Current Problem: Pt is a 31 y/o male victum of an Auto Accident. He impacted the Steering wheel and wind-sheild. Though initially unconscious, the pt was consious Alert though disoriented upon our arrival and complaining of chest pain only. During extrication, his left pupil dilated, his level of consciousness began to drop and he became unresponsive. Physical assesment did reveal a small contusion on his forehead with limited swelling and no crepitation

Medical Problems

Past		Present
[ ]	Cardiac	[ ]
[ ]	Stroke	[ ]
[ ]	Acute Abdomen	[ ]
[ ]	Diabetes	[ ]
[ ]	Psychiatric	[ ]
[ ]	Epilepsy	[ ]
[ ]	Drug/Alcohol	[ ]
[ ]	Poisoning	[ ]
[ ]	Allergy/Asthma	[ ]
[ ]	Syncope	[ ]
[ ]	Obstetrical	[ ]
[ ]	GYN	[ ]

Other:

Trauma Scr: 16 Glascow: 15

On Scene Care: C-Collar, Spinal Imm. oxygen, IV 16ga (L) Forearm - NS. 8.0mm Et tube digital - ass Resp @ 25 by BVM 15 L O^2

First Aid: none. Police Report the patient was unconscious when they arrived
By Whom?

O2 @ 6 L 2 : 36 Via NC — C-Collar 02 : 34 — S-Immob. 02:41 — Stretcher 02 : 42

Allergies/Meds: None
Past Med Hx: None.

Time	Pulse	Resp.	BP S/D	LOC	EKG
2 : 36	R: 70 [r][i]	R: 20 [s][l]	130 / 88	[a][v][p][u]	NSR

Care/Comments: Concious & alert, CP on Resp; Clear breath sounds 16ga IV-NS.

Time	Pulse	Resp.	BP S/D	LOC	EKG
2 : 41	R: 52 [r][i]	R: 22 [s][l]	136 / 88	[a][v][p][u]	NSR SaO_2 98%

Care/Comments: Pt becomes unconcious, responds to painful stimuli, Left pupil Dilated.

Time	Pulse	Resp.	BP S/D	LOC	EKG
2 : 51	R: 50 [r][i]	R: 15 [s][l]	140 / 92	[a][v][p][u]	NSR SaO^2 97%

Care/Comments: Pt is unconcious 8.0 Et tube - BVM hyperventilating

Time	Pulse	Resp.	BP S/D	LOC	EKG
3 : 01	R: 50 [r][i]	R: 15 [s][l]	140 / 90	[a][v][p][u]	NSR SaO^2 97%

Care/Comments: Pt is unresponsive to all but painful stimuli

Destination: medical Center
Reason: [ ]pt [ ]Closest [X]M.D [ ]Other
Contacted: [X]Radio [ ]Tele [ ]Direct
Ar Status: [ ]Better [ ]UnC [X]Worse

Personnel:	Certification
1. Cindy Robertson	[P][E][O]
2. Mary Kreapt	[P][E][O]
3. Tom Klein	[P][E][O]

16

BODY CAVITY TRAUMA

Review of the Objectives for Chapter 16

After reading this chapter, you should be able to:

1. Describe the incidence, mortality, and morbidity of body cavity injury in the trauma patient.

p. 470

Chest and abdominal trauma account for the second highest cause of death in the auto accident. It is a common area for injury in all types of trauma which can then involve the respiratory, cardiovascular, digestive or urinary system. However, if the paramedic can quickly recognize the injury (either through analysis of the mechanism of injury or the signs and symptoms), then appropriate care and transport can improve mortality and morbidity.

2. Locate and explain the function of the organs and major structures found within the thorax and abdomen.

pp. 471 to 475

The **lungs** fill all but the central portion of the chest cavity and are found on either side of the mediastinum. They are the gas exchange structures which consist of the airways, the air sacs (alveoli) and the capillary beds.

The **heart** is located in the left central chest and is the major pumping element of the cardiovascular system.

The **mediastinum** is the central portion of the chest cavity containing the heart, trachea, esophagus and great vessels.

The **diaphragm** separates the chest and abdominal cavities. It is a major muscle of respiration, moving up and down to diminish and increase the volume of the thoracic chamber.

The **liver** is located in the right lower quadrant just under the diaphragm. The liver is responsible for detoxifying the blood, storing energy sources for the body, and producing plasma proteins.

The **gall bladder** is directly beneath the liver. Bile, a byproduct of the liver, is stored in the gall bladder.

The **kidneys** are located in their respective upper quadrants; left and right. They are posterior and filter the blood, removing excess water, body salts, and waste products.

The **pancreas** is located in the first curve of the small bowel and in the lower portions of the left and right upper quadrants. It produces insulin and digestive juices.

The **alimentary canal** is a hollow tube running through all of the abdominal quadrants. It contains the digesting food and absorbs the needed nutrients and water.

The **spleen** is found in the left upper quadrant just beneath the kidney. It is responsible for some of the immune system activities and the production of white blood cells.

The **bladder** is located in the lower pelvic cavity. It contains and stores urine, awaiting its removal from the human system.

3. Explain the process of respiration, including the function of the bellows system, the pleura, and the airway.

pp. 471 to 473

The **bellows system** is powered primarily by the intercostal muscles and the diaphragm. The diaphragm contracts downward while the intercostals contract and raise and expand the chest. The increase in the size of the thorax causes the pressure to drop and the air rushes through the airway to equalize. Expiration occurs as the diaphragm and costals settle.

The **pleura** is a two-layer lining of the interior of the thoracic cage. It is designed to ensure that the lungs move with the expanding and contracting thorax.

The **airway** is a tube from the mouth and nose to the alveoli deep within the lungs. The airway must be open and unobstructed to ensure effective respiration.

4. Identify various injuries associated with chest and abdominal trauma.

pp. 476 to 482

Rib fracture, atelectasis, pulmonary contusion, flail chest, traumatic asphyxia, closed pneumothorax, open pneumothorax, tension pneumothorax, pericardial tamponade, aortic aneurysm, mediastinum injury, blunt abdominal trauma, penetrating abdominal trauma, and evisceration.

5. Describe the signs and symptoms most commonly found in cases of chest and abdominal trauma, noting the cause and/or effects of each condition.

pp. 476 to 482

Rib fracture presents with pain and crepitation on palpation. It induces severe pain during breathing and will cause the patient to reduce the pain by reducing respiratory excursion.

Atelectasis causes dyspnea which improves with time. Atelectasis reduces the surface area for gas exchange. In the traumatic instance, the patient may feel unable to catch his or her breath because the re-expansion of alveoli is a slow process.

Pulmonary contusion results in pulmonary edema, rales, rhonchi, dyspnea. Since the injury involves the lung tissue, the patient may experience progressive dyspnea, and pulmonary edema.

Flail chest displays with paradoxical respiration, dyspnea and results in the bellows system functioning inefficiently. The chest will appear to be moving paradoxically because the effort expended to exhale will push the flail segment out. The expanding of the chest to inhale, conversely, will draw the segment in. The patient will use great effort in breathing and move little air in and out of the respiratory system. The patient may experience severe pain from the motion of the numerous fracture sites.

Traumatic asphyxia can be recognized by the mechanism of injury, bulging blood shot eyes, distended neck veins, and dyspnea. It will cause the patient severe dyspnea and upper torso discoloration. The dyspnea is due to the compression of the chest cavity while the discoloration is due to an extreme reduction in venous return from the head and neck.

Closed pneumothorax will cause progressive dyspnea and diminished breath sounds on affected side. The pathology will generally present with dyspnea which may or may not be progressive. The trachea may tug toward the affected side with each inspiration due to the fixed volume of the pneumothorax. Breath sounds may be reduced on the affected side as a result of the lung displacement by the air.

Open pneumothorax is characterized by frothing blood at open wound and the signs and symptoms of closed pneumothorax. The open wound permits air to move through the opening instead of through the airway (hence called a sucking chest wound).

Tension pneumothorax has the signs and symptoms associated with closed pneumothorax and severe dyspnea, jugular vein distension, and tracheal deviation. The pneumothorax will begin to displace the uninjured lung and shift the trachea away from the injury site. The increased intrathoracic pressure will slow venous return and produce jugular vein distension.

Pericardial tamponade may induce shock, diminished heart sounds and a narrowing pulse pressure. The narrowing pulse pressure is due to the increasing peripheral resistance to maintain blood pressure in a low cardiac output state.

Aortic aneurysm may cause a tearing sensation in the chest as the vessel begins to tear apart. The delamination of the vessel may involve the branches to the left upper extremity causing diminished pulse and numbness. Rapid hypotension and death may follow if the vessel ruptures.

Mediastinum injury may be identifiable by mechanism of injury or central chest pain. It may involve any of the structures within, including the heart, great vessels, esophagus and trachea. The injuries will present with signs and symptoms reflective of the structure involved. Tracheal injury may present with subcutaneous emphysema and esophageal injury with a burning sensation, though it may only become apparent well after the trauma.

Blunt abdominal trauma may be recognized by abdominal tenderness, rebound tenderness, pain or pulsing mass. It may involve any of the abdominal or retroperitoneal organs. Signs will be superficial such as contusions or, more likely, erythema. Symptoms may result from the injury or from blood, body fluids or bacteria (a much later development) in the peritoneal cavity.

Penetrating abdominal trauma will present with an entrance wound and, possibly, an exit wound. It may also manifest with the signs and symptoms of blunt abdominal trauma due to the same mechanisms.

Evisceration will be evident by the protrusion of bowel from an open abdominal wound.

6. Describe how the elements of primary assessment relate to chest and abdominal injury.

pp. 482 to 485

Mechanism of injury is probably the most important body of information to use in the assessment and management of the patient. Use what information is available to suggest expected and possible injuries.

Airway assessment will identify the effectiveness of respiratory effort and may alert the examiner to the sounds of lower airway obstruction such as wheezes, gurgling, etc. These may suggest trauma and pulmonary contusion, bleeding into the respiratory tract or aspiration of vomitus due to loss of the gag reflex.

Breathing assessment - the evaluation of the depth, rate and regularity of respiration may suggest bellows system problems. Rib fractures, pneumothorax, flail chest, tension pneumothorax and traumatic asphyxia will generally display with dyspnea increasing with each, respectively. Deviations from symmetrical motion of the chest and any signs of trauma suggest injury as the chest is inspected and palpated. Flail chest and its paradoxical wall motion may be especially visible.

Circulation assessment - pulse rate and strength will reveal the first signs of shock and may suggest chest pathology. Examine for jugular vein distension reflective of pericardial tamponade, tension pneumothorax, or traumatic asphyxia in the trauma patient.

Disability assessment - a lowered level of consciousness may provide some of the first evidence of shock or respiratory inefficiency. Paralysis may also suggest the cause of diaphragmatic breathing.

Exposure of the chest and abdomen - observation of the chest and abdomen may be the best way to assess for injury. The regions should be quickly and completely observed and palpated. Contusions or reddening should lead the paramedic to suspect injury to the organs beneath. Any overt pulsing of the abdomen should increase the index of suspicion for abdominal aorta injury and aneurysm.

7. Describe a complete secondary assessment of the chest and abdomen, including the following tasks.

pp. 485 to 489

Inspection and examination - the entire chest and abdomen should be examined for any discoloration, asymmetrical motion, pulsing masses, hemorrhage, etc. It should also be palpated for any deformity, pain, tenderness, point tenderness, etc. Lastly, the chest should be auscultated for breath sounds, assuring they are bilaterally equal and without rales or rhonchi.

Vital signs - blood pressure, pulse rate and respiratory rate should be established and serially evaluated for trends. Signs of shock - rapid weak pulse, rapid shallow respiration or dropping blood pressure may indicate internal abdominal or chest hemorrhage.

Patient history - ask the patient to identify the mechanism of injury and report any symptoms of his or her injuries. Examine with care any report of dyspnea or pain in the chest or abdomen.

8. Identify, order and describe the care steps for chest and abdominal penetrating and blunt trauma.

pp. 489 to 496

Airway - the airway should be secured by head positioning, oral airway or endotracheal tube if the patient is unable to protect it on his or her own.

Respiratory assistance should be provided in the presence of dyspnea. It may also be of great value in the flail chest patient, even though a reasonable amount of air is being exchanged.

Oxygen should be administered with any dyspnea, shock or suspected chest injury. Observe caution if the patient has a history of chronic respiratory disease.

Positioning - in chest injury the patient should be placed on the affected side. The abdominally injured patient may be placed on the left side with the legs drawn up or in some other comfortable position.

Splinting and bandaging should be specific to the injury. Rib fractures are not splinted in the field setting, with the exception of the flail chest. Flail chest is stabilized with a pillow or other bulky dressing to limit paradoxical chest wall movement. Any open chest wound should be covered with an occlusive dressing, sealed on three sides to allow the release of any increasing intrathoracic pressure. Abdominal wounds should be bandaged in traditional ways with the evisceration covered with a non-adherent occlusive dressing to prevent tissue drying.

PASG - apply the PASG to any patient who may have significant internal injuries. It should be inflated when the patient is found to have the signs and symptoms of shock. Care should be employed if the patient has a chest injury with dyspnea to ensure it doesn't worsen with PASG inflation.

Fluid replacement - initiate fluid replacement to rapidly infuse crystalloids - two large-bore catheters connected to normal saline or lactated Ringer's solution with trauma tubing and run wide open with pressure infusers, if needed. Do not take time at the scene to initiate an IV except in cases of patient entrapment.

Transport - since chest and abdominal injuries account for a great number of trauma deaths, the patient should be considered for rapid transport if significant injury is suspected.

CASE STUDY REVIEW

Reread the case study in **PARAMEDIC EMERGENCY CARE** and then read the discussion below.

This case study presents many of the important elements of assessment and care for the patient who has suffered penetrating injury to the chest. It identifies the need to recognize and aggressively manage the patient. It also highlights the value of rapid transport, when called for.

Chapter 16 Case Study

The paramedics on Medic Rescue 3 use the time during their response to identify the necessary duties, equipment, and medical procedures. Of primary concern is scene safety for both the paramedics and the patient, especially when shots have been fired. The paramedics are also concerned about the severity of the injuries that may have resulted. They mentally review the steps of assessment and management of both chest and abdominal injuries. As the rescue unit arrives, it is obvious that the police have secured the scene and concern can be directed to the patient.

The primary assessment of the patient presents only minor signs of injury. The wounds are small and not bleeding severely. The patient does not appear to be in much pain. The paramedics do notice that the level of consciousness and the patient's color suggest shock, as does the labored, rapid and shallow breathing. The assessment also demonstrates that the wound was caused by a gun held at close range (the tattooing and powder burns) and that the projectile entered anteriorly and exited posteriorly, as shown by the wound characteristics. Even though the wounds are small in nature, the paramedics remember the severe injuries a bullet can produce.

The care is traditional, with the wounds covered and high flow oxygen administered. Careful and continued assessment, however, reveals a continuing degeneration in patient condition. The paramedics search for a possible cause. Breath sounds suggest a developing pneumothorax, possibly a tension pneumothorax. The team first tries to relieve the condition by unsealing the dressings at the wound sites, both front and back. Neither action is successful so medical control is contacted for orders. The paramedics are authorized to needle decompress the thorax using either the second intercostal space, mid-clavicular line or the fifth intercostal space, mid-axillary line locations. The attempt is successful, as noted by the escaping air. The dressings are re-applied and a valve assembly is applied to the needle hub. The paramedic's will watch this patient very carefully for the redevelopment of the tension pneumothorax.

READING COMPREHENSION SELF-EXAM

1. Chest and abdominal trauma accounts for ....

   A. the greatest cause of mortality in auto accidents.
   B. the second greatest cause of mortality in auto accidents.
   C. the third greatest cause of mortality in auto accidents.
   D. a minor incidence of mortality in auto accidents.
   E. none of the above.

   Answer B

2. The structure which divides the chest cavity from the abdominal cavity is the ....

   A. mediastinum.
   B. peritoneum.
   C. perineum.
   D. diaphragm.
   E. vena cava.

   Answer D

3. The structures found within the mediastinum include ....
   1. heart.
   2. trachea.
   3. lungs.
   4. esophagus.
   5. great vessels.

   Select the proper grouping.

   A. 1, 3, 4
   B. 1, 2, 3
   C. 1, 2, 4, 5
   D. 1, 3, 4, 5
   E. 1, 2, 3, 4, 5

   Answer C

4. The sac surrounding the heart is called the ....

   A. myocardium.
   B. endocardium.
   C. pericardium.
   D. parietal cardiac sheath.
   E. ligamentum arteriosum.

   Answer C

5. The structure which ensures that the lung expands with the thoracic cage wall and diaphragm is the ....

   A. pleura.
   B. hilum.
   C. ligamentum arteriosum.
   D. lobular attachment.
   E. none of the above.

   Answer A

6. Which of the organs listed below are found (at least partially) in the right upper quadrant?
   1. spleen
   2. kidney
   3. liver
   4. stomach
   5. pancreas

   Select the proper grouping.

   A. 1, 3, 4
   B. 2, 3, 5
   C. 2, 4, 5
   D. 1, 2, 4, 5
   E. 1, 3, 4, 5

   Answer b

7. The condition in which a part of the chest wall moves in opposition to the rest of the chest due to numerous rib fractures is called ....

   A. pneumothorax.
   B. tension pneumothorax.
   C. hemothorax.
   D. atelectasis.
   E. none of the above.

   Answer e

8. The organs found in the retroperitoneal space include ....
   1. the stomach
   2. the liver
   3. part of the pancreas
   4. the kidneys
   5. part of the duodenum

   Select the proper grouping.

   A. 1, 2, 5
   B. 2, 3, 5
   C. 2, 4, 5
   D. 3, 4, 5
   E. 1, 2, 3, 4, 5

   Answer D

9. The patient who is experiencing increasing dyspnea due to an open or closed pneumothorax which has a valve-like function and allows intrathoracic pressure to increase is referred to as ....

   A. subcutaneous emphysema.
   B. traumatic asphyxia.
   C. hyperbaric mediastinal displacement.
   D. tension pneumothorax.
   E. none of the above.

   Answer D

10. Traumatic asphyxia classically presents with which of the following?
    1. bulging blue tongue
    2. flat neck veins
    3. pale upper body
    4. hyperventilation
    5. bloodshot eyes

    Select the proper grouping.

    A. 1, 3
    B. 1, 5
    C. 2, 3, 4
    D. 1, 3, 5
    E. 1, 2, 3, 4, 5

    Answer B

11. A patient presents with the signs of shock, jugular vein distension, distant heart sounds, and a narrowing pulse pressure. The lung fields are clear. Which condition is most likely the cause?

    A. tension pneumothorax
    B. hemothorax
    C. traumatic asphyxia
    D. pericardial tamponade
    E. atelectasis

    Answer D

12. Signs and symptoms of abdominal injury are generally less noticeable than those of thoracic trauma.

    A. True
    B. False

    Answer A

13. Your patient was involved in a lateral impact auto accident. The car is greatly deformed, though the patient does not have many signs of injury. During your assessment he complains of a tearing sensation in his central chest and numbness in his left upper extremity. Your highest index of suspicion of injury is for which of the following?

A. traumatic asphyxia
B. pulmonary contusion
C. dissecting aortic aneurysm
D. myocardial contusion
E. none of the above

Answer C

14. Your patient presents with a rapid pulse, cool clammy skin, slow capillary refill, shallow breathing and no external signs of injury, though there is a history of trauma. You should suspect hemorrhage in which of the following areas?

A. cranial cavity
B. thoracic cavity
C. abdominal cavity
D. B and C
E. A, B and C

Answer D

15. While assessing a supine patient the jugular veins are found to be distended. This finding alone suggests ....

A. a normal patient.
B. pericardial tamponade.
C. tension pneumothorax.
D. traumatic asphyxia.
E. B, C and D.

Answer A

16. A patient who displays subcutaneous emphysema is most likely to have which of the conditions listed below?

A. traumatic asphyxia
B. tension pneumothorax
C. the paper bag syndrome
D. pulmonary contusion
E. none of the above

Answer B

17. The paramedic should examine the thorax for ....
   1. erythema.
   2. abrasions.
   3. tenderness.
   4. deformity.
   5. crepitation.

Select the proper grouping.

A. 1, 3, 5
B. 2, 4, 5
C. 1, 2, 3, 5
D. 2, 3, 4, 5
E. 1, 2, 3, 4, 5

Answer E

18. By the conclusion of the primary assessment, which of the following care steps should be applied?
    1. administration of oxygen
    2. stabilization of any flail chest
    3. sealing any open pneumothorax
    4. airway protection as needed
    5. decompression of any noted tension pneumothorax

    Select the proper grouping.

    A. 1, 2, 3
    B. 1, 2, 4
    C. 2, 4, 5
    D. 1, 3, 4, 5
    E. 1, 2, 3, 4, 5

    Answer e

19. Your patient has received chest trauma yet did not initially present with rales or rhonchi. However, as the assessment continues, they are heard in both the lower lung fields. This condition is most likely a result of which of the following?

    A. pulmonary contusion
    B. hemothorax
    C. pneumothorax
    D. aortic aneurysm
    E. pericardial tamponade

    Answer A

20. Which of the following patients merit immediate transport?
    1. traumatic asphyxia
    2. tension pneumothorax
    3. rapid pulse, slow capillary refill
    4. dissecting aortic aneurysm
    5. patient disorientation
    6. isolated humerus fracture

    Select the proper grouping.

    A. 1, 3, 4, 6
    B. 2, 3, 4, 6
    C. 1, 2, 3, 5
    D. 1, 2, 3, 4, 5
    E. 1, 2, 3, 4, 5, 6

    Answer D

21. Which of the following problems would most likely result in a chest area which was dull to percussion?

    A. pneumothorax
    B. tension pneumothorax
    C. hemothorax
    D. subcutaneous pneumothorax
    E. pericardial tamponade

    Answer C

22. The injury associated with either blood or bowel contents released into the abdominal cavity will result in a rapidly developing presentation of severe discomfort and pain.

    A. True
    B. False

    Answer B

23. Pulsus paradoxus is a condition where the strength of the pulse is greater during inspiration than expiration. It is opposite of the normal trend and may reflect pericardial tamponade.

A. True
B. False

Answer A

24. In which of the following traumatic chest injuries would you expect the patient's dyspnea to improve with time?

A. traumatic asphyxia
B. tension pneumothorax
C. atelectasis
D. pericardial tamponade
E. pulmonary contusion

Answer C

25. The patient who is suspected of a significant chest injury should be placed ....

A. on the uninjured side.
B. on the injured side.
C. supine with legs elevated.
D. on the left lateral side.
E. none of the above.

Answer B

26. The drug Nitronox is administered via which of the following routes?

A. intravenous
B. intramuscular
C. subcutaneous
D. inhalation
E. orally

Answer D

27. Nitronox (nitrous oxide) is contraindicated in which of the following conditions?

A. head injury
B. chest injury
C. abdominal injury
D. suspected shock
E. all of the above

Answer e

28. In the patient who is trapped in a wrecked auto and suspected of having traumatic asphyxia care, should include which of the following?

A. two large bore IVs
B. normal saline or lactated Ringer's solution
C. fluids run via pressure infusion as available
D. PASG prepared for rapid application
E. all of the above

Answer e

29. Which of the following drugs would be considered for the patient who has experienced traumatic asphyxia for more than 10 minutes?

A. decadron
B. sodium bicarbonate
C. morphine sulfate
D. demerol
E. dopamine

Answer B

30. Which locations are recommended for pleural decompression?
1. 2nd or 3rd intercostal space, mid-clavicular line
2. 5th intercostal space, mid-clavicular line
3. 5th intercostal space, mid-axillary line
4. just beneath the breast

Select the proper group.

A. 1
B. 2
C. 3
D. 1, 3
E. 1, 2, 4

Answer D

SPECIAL PROJECTS

Problem Solving - Chest Injury

One of the more serious respiratory-related emergencies is the tension pneumothorax. On the next few lines, identify the signs and symptoms you would expect to find in a patient with this pathology and its increasing intrathoracic pressure.

mechanism of Injury — TRAchial deveation away from Injury
progressive dyspnea — Subcutenous emphysema
diminished Breath Sounds (Injured) Side — hyper-resonant precussion injured Side.
Jugular Vein distension — Signs & Symptoms of Shock

Give a patient report to medical command based upon the signs and symptoms identified above. Use only that information you feel important for the medical control physician. (You are attempting to receive permission to provide pleural decompression.)

Chest trauma Patient — progressive dyspnea
unequal Breath Sounds. — Jugular Vein distension
Side involved

Identify the exact location of your decompression attempt.

mid-CLAVICULAR line 2nd or 3rd Intercostal Space.
mid-AXILLARY line - 5th or 6th intercostal Space (nipple line)

17

MUSCULOSKELETAL INJURIES

Review of the Objectives for Chapter 17

After reading this chapter, you should be able to:

1. Identify the long bones of the extremities, and describe their general structure.

pp. 501 to 505

Upper extremity	Lower extremity
Humerus	Femur
Radius	Tibia
Ulna	Fibula
Carpals	Talus
Metacarpals	Calcaneus
Phalanges	Tarsals
	Metatarsals
	Phalanges

The **diaphysis** is the hollow skeletal shaft of the long bone and contains the yellow bone marrow. It is covered by the periosteum which contains sensory nerve fibers and initiates the bone repair cycle.

The **metaphysis** is the transitional region between the diaphysis and the epiphysis. In this region the thin layer of compact bone of the diaphysis shaft becomes the honeycomb of the weight-bearing epiphyseal region.

The **epiphysis** is the weight-bearing end of the bone. Through the widening of the metaphysis, and the cancellous bone underneath, the weight-bearing, articular surface distributes support over a large area.

Articular cartilage is a smooth, shock-absorbing surface which allows free movement between the two articular ends of the adjoining bones. It is the actual joint surface.

Ligaments are bands of connective tissue that attach bones to each other. These bands encapsulate the joint and allow some stretch, while holding the articulating bones firmly together.

2. Describe the structure, attachment, and general action of the muscles of the extremities.

pp. 505 to 506

The muscles of the extremities are skeletal muscles under conscious nervous control. They consist of a muscle body and are secured to the skeleton at one or both ends by tendons. The muscle body consists of individual muscle fibers which can only contract. Hence most muscles are opposed by other muscles which will stretch when the latter contract. The attachment which remains stationary when the muscle moves is its origin, and the moving point of muscle attachment is its insertion.

3. Compare and contrast strains, sprains, subluxations, dislocations, and fractures.

pp. 506 to 510

Strain is an overstretching of a muscle body which produces pain. The muscle fibers have been damaged; however, there is usually no internal hemorrhage or associated discoloration.

Sprain is the tearing of the ligaments of a joint. The injury will produce pain, swelling and discoloration with time. Since the injury has damaged the joint integrity, further exertion may cause joint failure.

Subluxation is a transitional injury between the sprain and dislocation. The ligaments have been stretched and do not provide a stable joint. The range of motion may be limited and the region is very painful.

Dislocation is a displacement of one of the bones of a joint from the joint capsule. The area is noticeably deformed, the limb is fixed in position and the injury is very painful. Due to the proximity of blood vessels and nerves, there is a concern for involvement of these structures and loss of distal circulation and sensation.

Fracture is a break in the continuity of the bone. It may present with pain, false motion, angulation and possibly an open wound.

4. List the signs and symptoms normally associated with musculoskeletal injury, and describe their relative importance to the assessment process.

pp. 513 to 515

The signs and symptoms of musculoskeletal injury include pain, tenderness, deformity, discomfort, crepitation, inability to move, false motion, loss of distal pulse, loss of distal sensation, and/or a cool, clammy distal extremity.

Musculoskeletal injuries are not a high priority in the assessment and care of the trauma patient. With the exception of severe bleeding, extremity injuries are not assessed until the primary assessment is complete and problems found are then corrected. Note that pelvic or bilateral femur fracture may account for significant hemorrhage and possibly shock.

5. Order and describe the steps of assessment for trauma patients as they apply to extremity injury.

pp. 513 to 515

A complete trauma assessment includes the primary assessment, secondary assessment, and vital sign and history determination. During the primary assessment deformity of the skeletal injury may be evident. An absent distal pulse or loss of distal feeling, strength or control may be noticed. The secondary assessment will focus more specifically on the extremities and should identify the significant signs of fracture or disocation. History may reveal the mechanism of injury and other causative factors.

6. Describe the signs and symptoms of circulatory or nervous loss to a distal extremity, and the steps taken to correct this deficit.

pp. 515 to 517

Circulatory impairment due to a fracture or dislocation will present with the signs and symptoms of the injury as well as loss of distal pulses, slow capillary refill, cool, clammy skin, distal discoloration, and numbness and/or tingling. Nervous loss may present with the classic signs and symptoms of the fracture and, additionally, numbness, tingling, loss of motor function, loss of sensation - all distal to the injury site.

Should the signs and symptoms of nervous or circulatory deficit be evident, the limb may be manipulated slightly (towards alignment) in an attempt to restore the loss.

If resistance is met, or more than limited manipulation is needed, the limb should be splinted and the patient immediately transported.

7. Explain fracture or dislocation immobilization techniques for the following locations: **pp. 517 to 519**

The objective of splinting is to prevent further injury during transport to the emergency department. A splint should be chosen for ease in application, ability to immobilize the fracture or dislocation site (and the joint above and below), and patient comfort. The devices below should be utilized only as they can accomplish these goals effectively.

pelvis - PASG, long spine board with additional support.
hip - PASG, long spine board, orthopedic stretcher
femur - PASG, traction splint
knee - padded board splints
tibia and fibula - padded board splints, air splint
ankle - pillow splint, padded board splint, air splint
foot - pillow splint, padded board splint, air splint, conforming splint
shoulder - sling and swath
humerus - cuff and collar sling and swath
elbow - padded board splint
radius and ulna - padded board splint
wrist - padded board splint
hand - padded board splint, conforming splint
finger - conforming splint, padded board splint

CASE STUDY REVIEW

Reread the case study in **PARAMEDIC EMERGENCY CARE** and then read the discussion below.

This case presentation describes a typical skeletal injury in an elderly patient. It identifies some of the important aspects of skeletal injury assessment and care. It also presents the elderly patient who is a common victim of skeletal injury due to degeneration of strength in the aging bone.

Chapter I7 Case Study

The description of the events surrounding the fracture of this 85-year-old patient are typical of the geriatric hip fracture. Weakened with age, the femur can no longer withstand the stress of walking and will fracture. (It usually occurs on steps, where the stress is somewhat increased.) As the bone gives way the patient feels it snap and then falls. Since the injury is not of traumatic origin, the internal soft tissue damage is generally reduced and the patient may be relatively comfortable with the injury.

The primary assessment of Mrs. Jones reveals a hemodynamically stable patient with less pain than expected from a femur fracture. The extremity is angulated, unstable, and moderately painful. Further assessment reveals a cold extremity and diminished distal pulse. Both signs suggest circulatory compromise. The patient is considered a candidate for immediate transport based upon these findings.

Due to the past history of diabetes and a diuretic medication, the paramedics take precautionary measures of determining a blood sugar level by dextrose stick and auscultating the lung fields to rule out any pulmonary edema. The lungs are also evaluated because emboli from the fracture may travel there. All assessment points to a rather isolated skeletal injury, though the team initiates an IV for venous access and rapid infusion should the signs and symptoms of shock begin.

In the field of emergency care this call might seem routine and anything but exciting. Care of minor "emergencies," especially those dealing with the elderly, are common. While to the paramedic there may be the desire to consider this call a "taxi ride," to the patient it threatens lifestyle and is an important life event. The paramedics in this case realize their responsibility to make Mrs. Jones as comfortable as possible, to provide the appropriate assessment and care, and to place emphasis on an empathetic communication with her during care, packaging and transport. She is treated with respect and consideration.

READING COMPREHENSION SELF-EXAM

1. Which of the following positions is ideal for the immobilization of most extremity injuries?

   A. extended
   B. flexed
   C. hyperextended
   D. hyperflexed
   E. neutral

   Answer E

2. The covering of the shaft of the long bones that initiates the bone repair cycle is the ....

   A. periosteum.
   B. peritoneum.
   C. haversian canal.
   D. osteocyte.
   E. none of the above.

   Answer A

3. The tissue that is normally damaged in the sprain is the ....

   A. tendon.
   B. ligament.
   C. muscle.
   D. articular cartilage.
   E. all of the above.

   Answer B

4. The muscle attachment to the bone that moves when the muscle mass contracts is the ....

   A. flexor.
   B. extensor.
   C. origin.
   D. insertion.
   E. none of the above.

   Answer D

5. The overstretching of a muscle that presents with pain is the ....

   A. strain.
   B. sprain.
   C. cramp.
   D. spasm.
   E. none of the above.

   Answer A

6. The patient who has suffered a fracture due to degeneration secondary to aging is expected to experience what level of pain when compared to the traumatic fracture?

A. about the same
B. more pain
C. less pain
D. no pain at all
E. extreme pain

Answer C

7. Which of the fractures listed below are relatively stable?
   1. open fracture
   2. greenstick fracture
   3. hairline fracture
   4. impacted fracture
   5. closed fracture

   Select the proper grouping.

A. 2, 5
B. 3, 4
C. 1, 3, 5
D. 3, 4, 5
E. 1, 2, 3, 4, 5

Answer B

8. The greenstick fracture is an incomplete fracture which often must be completely broken to permit proper healing.

A. True
B. False

Answer A

9. The dislocation, or fracture in the area of a joint, is generally less significant than the long bone shaft fracture because it does not have as high an incidence of vascular and nervous injury.

A. True
B. False

Answer B

10. The energy and degree of manipulation needed to cause further injury after a bone has broken is much less than was initially needed to cause the fracture.

A. True
B. False

Answer A

11. The anterior hip dislocation will normally present with the ....
    1. foot turned outward.
    2. foot turned inward.
    3. knee flexed.
    4. knee turned outward.
    5. extremity shortened.

    Select the proper grouping.

A. 1, 4
B. 2, 4, 5
C. 2, 3
D. 1, 3, 5
E. 3, 5

Answer A

12. In general long bone shaft fractures should be splinted in which position?

A. aligned, except if resistance is experienced
B. as found
C. extended, except if resistance is experience
D. flexed, except if resistance is experienced
E. none of the above

Answer A

13. Any fracture within three inches of the joint should be treated as a dislocation.

A. True
B. False

Answer A

14. If a fracture of the pelvis, or of bilateral femurs, is suspected and patient vital signs are stable, the PASG should ....

A. be inflated to pop-off pressure.
B. be inflated until stabilization is achieved.
C. be applied but not inflated until vital signs begin to fall.
D. be withheld and the long spine board and traction splint used.
E. none of the above.

Answer B

15. Which of the fractures below should you consider for immediate transport because of possible internal blood loss?
1. humerus
2. femur
3. tibia
4. pelvic
5. clavicle
Select the proper grouping.

A. 1, 3
B. 2, 3
C. 2, 4
D. 2, 4, 5
E. 1, 2, 3, 4, 5

Answer C

16. Which of the following signs are reflective of a fracture?

A. distal pulse loss
B. crepitus
C. false motion
D. deformity
E. all of the above

Answer e

17. Due to the difficulty in differentiating the various muscular and skeletal injuries, one from another, it is best to "over-immobilize" rather than not properly splint a serious injury.

A. True
B. False

Answer A

18. The distal pulse should be checked at which times during the fracture and dislocation care process?
    1. during the secondary assessment
    2. before splinting
    3. during the splinting process
    4. at the conclusion of the splinting process
    5. during movement and transport

    Selecting the proper grouping.

    A. 1, 2, 4
    B. 2, 3, 5
    C. 1, 2, 4, 5
    D. 1, 2, 3, 5
    E. 1, 2, 3, 4, 5

    Answer e

19. In general, most fractures should be left in the position found because the splints of today are very effective in immobilizing the limb in the position found.

    A. True
    B. False

    Answer B

20. Dislocations of both the knee and elbow normally are found at what angle?

    A. 0 degrees
    B. 45 degrees
    C. 90 degrees
    D. 120 degrees
    E. 180 degrees

    Answer C

21. List the common signs and symptoms of dislocations.

Signs	Symptoms.
Angulation	loss of sensation
Pulse defecit	inability to move.
neurologic deficit	Pain
Joint deformity	
Pain	

22. List the common signs and symptoms of long bone fractures.

Signs	Symptoms.
false motion – limb Shortening	Pain
Angulation – Soft tissue wound.	loss of sensation
Crepitation	inability to move
Pulse defecit	
neurologic defecit	

18

SOFT-TISSUE TRAUMA AND BURNS

Review of the Objectives for Chapter 18

After reading this chapter, you should be able to:

1. Describe the structure and function of the skin.

pp. 522 to 525

The integumentary system provides the outer barrier of the body and protects it against environmental extremes and pathogens. It is a three-layer structure consisting of the:

The **epidermis** is a layer of dead or dying cells that provides a barrier to fluid loss, absorption and the entrance of pathogens.

The **dermis** is the true skin. It houses the sensory nerve endings, many of the specialized skin cells which produce sweat, oil, etc., and the upper level capillary beds which allow for the conduction of heat to the body's surface.

The **subcutaneous layer** is not a true part of the skin, but it works in concert with the skin to insulate the body from heat loss and the effects of trauma.

2. Identify the characteristics of contusion, abrasion, laceration, incision, avulsion, and amputation.

pp. 525 to 528

The **contusion** is a closed wound caused by blunt trauma which damages blood vessels. The blood vessels leak and the affected area becomes edematous. It is characterized by swelling, pain and, later on, discoloration. Since the wound is closed the danger of infection is remote.

An **abrasion** is a scraping away of the upper layers of the skin. It will normally present with capillary bleeding and, since the wound is open, can be associated with infection.

Laceration is the most common open wound. It is a tear into the layers of the skin and beneath and can involve blood vessels, muscles, connective tissue, and other underlying structures. Since it is an open wound it carries with it the danger of infection and external hemorrhage.

The **incision** is a very smooth laceration made by a surgical or other sharp instrument. It is otherwise a laceration.

Avulsion is a partial tearing away of the skin and soft tissues. It is commonly associated with blunt skull trauma, animal bites or machinery accidents. The degloving injury is a form of avulsion.

Amputation is a complete severance of a body part. The injury usually results in loss of the remaining extremity or digit; however, the severed tissue may be used for grafting to extend the length and usefulness of the remaining limb.

3. **Name the four types of burns**

pp. 529 to 533

Thermal - the most common of burns is the heat burn. It causes injury by increasing the rate of molecular movement thereby destroying the cell membrane.

Chemical - in the chemical burn the cell membrane is destroyed by the reaction between the chemical and the body's substance.

Electrical - burns caused by the passage of electrical current damage by the increased heat caused by the current. The electrical energy may also paralyze muscles.

Radiation - ionizing radiation causes internal damage by altering the genetic make up of the cell. Actual burns do not occur unless the exposure is very extreme.

4. **Explain the precautions to take when approaching a possible radiological incident, including the effect time, distance, and shielding upon exposure.**

p. 531

Radiation hazards cannot be seen, heard or felt yet they can cause both immediate and long-term health problems and death. The objective of rescue and care is to limit the exposure to both the patient and rescuer. The elements which affect the level of exposure are:

Time - radiation exposure is cumulative. The less time in an area of hazard, the less effect radiation will have on the human body.

Distance - the greater the distance from a radiation source, the less strength and potential to cause damage it has.

Shielding - radiation levels are diminished as the particles travel through dense objects. By placing more mass between the source and patient and rescuers, the exposure is reduced.

5. **Discuss the common causes of inhalation injuries.**

pp. 532 to 533

Toxic inhalation is caused when the patient inhales the toxic products of combustion. These substances include potassium cyanide, hydrogen sulfide, etc. They induce chemical burns of the lung tissue or systemic poisoning.

Thermal airway burns are caused most commonly by the inhalation of superheated steam during the fire process.

Carbon monoxide poisoning occurs when the combustion occurs in an enclosed space. The carbon monoxide displaces the oxygen-carrying power of the hemoglobin and the patient starves for oxygen at the cellular level.

6. **Explain the three degrees of thermal burns as well as the depth and effects these burns have on the human body.**

pp. 533 to 534

First degree burns involve only the upper layers of the epidermis and dermis. The effects are limited to an irritation of the upper sensory tissues with some swelling and erythema.

Second degree burns penetrate slightly deeper than first and will cause blistering, erythema, swelling, and pain. Since the cells which reproduce the skin's upper layers are still alive, complete regeneration is expected.

Third degree burns are full-thickness burns penetrating the layers of the skin and causing extensive destruction. The burned area can take on many colorations, the site is anesthetic and healing is prolonged. Third degree burns may involve not only the skin, but also underlying tissues and organs.

7. **Identify the two methods of approximating the burn surface area, and apply them to several burn patient descriptions.**

pp. 535 to 536

The **rule of nines** approximates the body surface area by assigning each of the following regions nine percent of the total: each upper extremity, the anterior of each lower extremity, the posterior of each lower extremity, the anterior of the abdomen, the anterior thorax, the upper back, the lower back, and the entire head. The remaining percent is assigned to the genitalia.

The **Palmar surface** method approximates burn surface area by assuming the victim's surface of the palm is equivalent to percent of the total body surface area. The care provider then estimates the burn surface area by determining the number of palmar surfaces it would take to cover the wound.

8. **Describe difficulties in assessing and caring for soft tissue injuries.**

pp. 538 to 551

In the prehospital setting, the assessment of soft tissue injuries is complicated only because the discoloration normally associated with these injuries takes a few hours to develop. The care of a soft tissue wound is simply met by three objectives:

Immobilize the wound site - this will assist the clotting and healing processes.

Keep the wound sterile - the bandaging of a soft tissue injury should keep the wound sterile or at least as clean as possible.

Apply direct pressure - the bandage should apply direct pressure and control all hemorrhage from the wound site.

9. **List the anatomical areas that, if burned, will increase the overall severity of the burn.**

pp. 541 to 542

Inhalation injury
Face
Circumferential neck
Circumferential chest
Circumferential abdomen
Circumferential limb
Joint areas
Genitals
Hands
Feet

10. **List the advantages and the disadvantages of each of the following methods of bleeding control.**

pp. 544 to 545

Direct pressure is a very effective first-line technique for the control of hemorrhage. Since hemorrhage is powered by blood pressure, digital pressure at the site of blood loss should easily stop blood loss.

Elevation can be used to complement direct pressure. By elevating an extremity the blood pressure to the limb will be decreased and the hemorrhage may be easier to control. Elevation should be used only for wounds on otherwise uninjured limbs, and only after direct pressure has proved ineffective.

Pressure point is an adjunct to both direct pressure and elevation. A proximal artery is located and compressed, reducing the pressure of the hemorrhage. It can be very helpful in the crush wound where the exact location of blood loss is difficult to find.

Tourniquet is the last technique to be used in attempts to control hemorrhage. A limb is circumferentially compressed above the systolic pressure under a wide band, such as a blood pressure cuff. If a lower pressure is used, the wound will bleed more severely. The tourniquet carries with it the additional hazard of toxins accumulating in the isolated limb. These toxins endanger the future use of the limb and the patient's life.

11. Identify the circumstances in which each of the above techniques, or a combination, might be best.

p. 544

In most circumstances direct pressure will control hemorrhage. Occasionally both direct pressure and elevation of the limb will be necessary. In severe cases of hemorrhage, pressure points will be needed. In extreme cases, such as crush injuries, a tourniquet may be called for.

12. List and explain the care steps for chemical burns and the special considerations given to lime and phenol burns.

pp. 548 to 550

Remove contaminated clothing, and protect the rescuers and patient from further contamination during the entire chemical burn care process.

Remove the agent by flushing with large volumes of cool water or, if the agent is a powder, by brushing gently and then flushing with water.

Cleanse the wound by gently irrigating the wound and washing the contaminated area with soap and water.

Continue irrigation throughout transport to the hospital to ensure any remaining chemicals have been removed.

Dry lime reacts violently with water. It should first be gently brushed off and then rinsed continuously with large volumes of cool water.

Phenol is an industrial chemical that is not water soluble and will cause severe tissue burns. It should be carefully removed with alcohol and then rinsed with large volumes of cool water.

CASE STUDY REVIEW

Reread the case study in **PARAMEDIC EMERGENCY CARE** and then read the discussion below.

The scenario presented in this chapter of Paramedic Emergency Care illustrates the dangers of inhalation injury and the difficulty you might have in recognizing and treating the problem.

Chapter I8 Case Study

The firefighter involved in this incident experiences the classic evolution of the burn and inhalation injury. He was initially found to be stable with signs, symptoms, and vital signs suggestive of minor injury. The major concern for this patient might well be the fractured forearm. The paramedics are cautious because of the history, hoarseness and the sooty sputum.

The belt, which is still smoldering, draws attention to an important concern regarding the assessment and management of the thermal burn patient. The paramedic must be careful regarding any articles of clothing or jewelry that could continue to burn or provide a constrictive band to the swelling that often accompanies burn injury. The paramedic's initial action should be to stop any further burning. This calls for complete inspection of the burn area and the surrounding clothing. Once the burn area is exposed, the depth and area involved can be assessed. In this case the patient has a fracture, possible inhalation injury and a burn. The combination of traumatic injury, burn, and inhalation injury are reasons to consider the burn serious.

The paramedics initiate an IV with a large-bore catheter and begin running normal saline. A 1,000 mL bag is hung with a trauma tubing administration set just in case the signs of shock appear. Fluids are run rapidly to get ahead of the loss normally associated with severe burns. If this were a 125 Kg. man with the burns identified (27% by the rule of nines) the needed fluid would be 4 mL. per 27% of 125 Kg. or a total of 13,500 mL in the first 24 hours. Half of this is needed in the first eight hours. That's more than 1,500 mL per hour.

The signs of respiratory involvement are even more significant than the burn or fracture. Inhalation injury is likely due either to the chemical burning caused by the products of combustion reacting with the soft tissue of the respiratory tract or thermal burns caused by superheated steam created when the water extinguished the flames. In either case respiratory damage can be extensive. Respiratory burns usually display progressive dyspnea, as in this case, developing before the paramedic's eyes. The only effective way to treat these problems is to anticipate the progression and be aggressive in airway care. Intubation equipment should be readied and used when signs of developing airway compromise appear. The patient should also be transported immediately because airway maintenance skills are difficult and, as with this case, may result in the need for surgical intervention.

The paramedics in this scenario must also be prepared for the worst. If the firefighter had experienced the dyspnea and airway restriction while twenty to thirty minutes from the hospital a needle cricothyrotomy would have been performed in the ambulance. Likewise, had they waited on the scene to bandage and care for the patient, they would also have had to perform the needle cricothyrotomy. This case study clearly identifies the need for rapid recognition and transportation of the patient with developing airway compromise.

READING COMPREHENSION SELF-EXAM

1. The layer of skin which is made up of mostly dead cells and provides the waterproof envelope which contains the body is the ....

A. dermis.
B. subcutaneous layer.
C. epidermis.
D. sebum.
E. corium.

Answer ____

2. Which of the following wounds are considered open?
   1. laceration
   2. abrasion
   3. contusion
   4. first degree burn
   5. avulsion

   Select the proper grouping.

A. 1, 2, 5
B. 2, 3, 5
C. 1, 2, 4, 5
D. 1, 3, 4, 5
E. 1, 2, 3, 4, 5

Answer ____

3. The injury in which the skin is pulled off a finger, hand or extremity by farm or industrial machinery is the ....

A. amputation.
B. avulsion.
C. complete laceration.
D. degloving injury.
E. none of the above.

Answer ____

4. Which of the following are important aspects of assessment and management of external hemorrhage?
   1. type of bleeding
   2. rate of hemorrhage
   3. volume of blood lost
   4. stopping further hemorrhage

   Select the proper grouping

   A. 2, 3
   B. 1, 4
   C. 1, 3, 4
   D. 2, 3, 4
   E. 1, 2, 3, 4

   Answer e

5. It is generally most difficult to locate the source and to control blood loss in the ....

   A. amputation.
   B. abrasion.
   C. puncture.
   D. electrical burn.
   E. crush wound.

   Answer e

6. The burn characterized by erythema, pain, and small blisters is the ....

   A. first degree burn
   B. second degree burn
   C. third degree burn
   D. electrical burn
   E. none of the above

   Answer B

7. The burn characterized by discoloration and lack of pain is the ....

   A. first degree burn.
   B. second degree burn.
   C. third degree burn.
   D. chemical burn.
   E. electrical burn.

   Answer C

8. Which of the following burns would be considered severe?
   1. a circumferential third degree burn to the chest
   2. first degree facial burns with sooty residue
   3. 10 percent first and second degree burns
   4. third degree burns to the elbow and hand
   5. 25 percent second degree burns in the geriatric patient

   Select the proper grouping.

   A. 1, 3
   B. 2, 5
   C. 1, 2, 4
   D. 2, 3, 4, 5
   E. 1, 2, 4, 5

   Answer e

9. A patient has received burns to the entire anterior chest and to the left upper extremity, circumferentially. Using the rule of nines, determine the percentage of body surface area involved.

A. 9%
B. 18%
C. 27%
D. 36%
E. 48%

Answer B

10. A patient has received burns to the entire left lower extremity and the genitals. Using the rules of nine, determine the percentage of the body surface area involved.

A. 9%
B. 10%
C. 18%
D. 19%
E. 21%

Answer D

11. An adult patient has first and second degree burns to her entire left thigh, leg and foot circumferentially. There appear to be no other complications. What severity of burn would you assign?

A. minor
B. moderate
C. severe
D. critical
E. none of the above

Answer B

12. In documenting the exposure of a patient to a chemical agent which caused a burn, the paramedic should note which of the following?
1. duration of contact
2. exact chemical name
3. precise areas initially affected
4. type of agent
Select the proper grouping

A. 1, 3
B. 1, 4
C. 1, 2, 3
D. 2, 3, 4
E. 1, 2, 3, 4

Answer e

13. In addition to the entrance and exit wounds normally expected with the passage of electrical current through the human body, the paramedic should expect ....

A. ventricular fibrillation.
B. cardiac irritability.
C. internal damage.
D. respiratory arrest.
E. all of the above.

Answer E

14. The paramedic can only presume a high tension electrical line is not energized when it no longer sparks or gives off a blue glow. Failure to observe these precautions can result in severe injury to the paramedic and patient.

A. True
B. False

Answer B

15. If the source of radiation cannot be contained or moved away from the patient ....

A. the patient should be brought to the paramedics.
B. care should be offered by paramedics in protective gear.
C. care should be offered by specialists in protective gear.
D. care should be offered by the highest ranking officer.
E. A or C.

Answer A

16. Which of the following is not one of the primary objectives of bandaging?

A. neat appearance
B. hemorrhage control
C. wound immobilization
D. maintaining wound sterility (cleanliness)
E. all of the above are primary objectives of bandaging

Answer A

17. The dangers of a tourniquet include ....

A. increased hemorrhage if pressure is not sufficient.
B. possible loss of limb.
C. accumulation of toxins in the limb.
D. tissue damage beneath the tourniquet.
E. all of the above.

Answer e

18. If after bandaging a forearm wound with severe hemorrhage you notice that the limb is cool, capillary refill is slowed, and the radial pulse cannot be found, you should ....

A. apply more dressing material and increase the pressure.
B. leave the bandage as it is.
C. loosen the bandage.
D. elevate the extremity and assess circulation again.
E. none of the above.

Answer C

19. If you find a patient who has suffered a finger amputation. Keep the amputated part ....

A. warm and dry.
B. warm and moist.
C. cool and dry.
D. cool and moist.
E. packed in ice.

Answer C

20. Local and minor burns (first and second degree) may be cared for by ....

A. direct pressure.
B. cool water immersion.
C. prolonged application of ice.
D. warm water immersion.
E. A and D.

Answer B

21. In general, moderate to severe burns should be cared for by ....

A. moist occlusive dressings.
B. dry sterile dressings.
C. cool water immersion.
D. plastic wrap covered by a soft dressing.
E. none of the above.

Answer B

22. In general, chemical contact and the resulting burns should be cared for by ....

A. dry sterile dressings.
B. chemical antidotes.
C. rigorous scrubbing.
D. cool water irrigation.
E. rapid transport.

Answer D

23. The chemical phenol is soluble in ....

A. water.
B. dry lime.
C. normal saline.
D. ammonia.
E. none of the above.

Answer E

24. Which element of patient rescue should be employed to reduce the exposure of the rescuer to a radiation source?

A. increase the distance from the source
B. decrease the time exposed to the source
C. increase the shielding between the rescuer and source
D. protect against inhalation of contaminated dust
E. all of the above

Answer E

25. Once exposed to a significant radiation source, the patient will become a source of radiation the rescuer must protect him- or herself against. No amount of decontamination will reduce this danger.

A. True
B. False

Answer B

DRIP MATH WORKSHEET II

Formulas

Rate = Volume/Time	mL/min = gtts per min/gtts per mL
Volume = Rate x Time	gtts / min = mL per min x gtts per mL
Time = Volume/Rate	mL = gtts/gtts per mL

Please complete the following drug and drip math problems:

[1] Upon arriving at the emergency department the physician asks how much fluid you infused into your trauma patient. Your on scene and transport time was 35 minutes and you ran normal saline at a rate of 120 gtts/minute through a 10 gtts/mL administration set. What would you report?

V = R×t = 120gtts/min × 35min

R = 120gtts/min

V =

T = 35min

D = 10gtts/ml

V = 120 gtts × 35min / min = 4200 gtts

V = 4200gtts/D = 4200gtts × ml / 10

= 420 ml

[2] Protocol calls for a drug to be hung and administered by drip at 45 ucgtts per minute based upon a 60 ucgtts/mL administration set. You find that the set you have administers 45 ucgtts/mL. How many drops per second should you set your chamber for?

R = 45mcgtts/min

D = 60mcgtts/ml

D = 45gtts/ml

R(ml) = R(min)/D = 45mcgtts/min / 60mcgtts/ml

R(ml) = 45mcgtts × ml / 60mcgtts × 60 min = 45ml = 0.75ml/min

R(min) = R(ml) × D = 0.75ml/min × 45gtts.

= 0.56 mcgtts/sec

[3] The transferring physician requests that you infuse 100 mL of a drug during your transport. Anticipated transport time is 1 hour and 55 minutes. At what rate would you set a 60 ucgtts/mL administration set?

R = ?

V = 100ml

T = 115min

D = 60gtts/ml

= 52mcgtts/min

[4] You are allowed to administer a drug by IV drip at a rate of between 45 and 100 mL per hour. What drip rate range can you use with a 60 mcgtts/mL set?

= 45mcgtts/min

a 45 ucgtts/mL set?

= 100mcgtts/ml

a 10 gtts/mL set?

= 33.75mcgtts/min

[5] After a call you can't remember at what rate you ran a fluid. You do know that 350 mL are left in the 500 mL bag and that the IV was running for one hour and five minutes. What would you record?

R(60) 0.75ml/min × 60mcgtts/ml / min × ml = 0.75ml × 60mcgtts = 75 mcgtts/ml

R(60) 1.67ml/min × 60gtts/ml / min × ml = 1.67ml × 60mcgtts = 7.5 gtts/min

R(45) = 0.75 ml/min × 45mcgtts/ml / min × ml = 0.75ml × 45mcgtts = 16.7gtts/ml

= 2.3ml/min

19

SHOCK TRAUMA RESUSCITATION

Review of the Objectives for Chapter 19

After reading this chapter, you should be able to:

1. Identify the importance of rapid recognition and treatment of shock in the trauma patient.

p. 557

Shock is the transitional state between cardiovascular homeostasis and death. It develops rapidly in the presence of blood loss, respiratory compromise and other problem? If you are to be successful in combating this problem, you must employ aggressive and specific care.

2. Compare and contrast compensated, decompensated, and irreversible shock.

pp. 557 to 559

Compensated shock is a state where the body is effectively compensating for fluid loss, or other shock-inducing pathology, and is able to maintain blood pressure and critical organ perfusion. If the original problem is not corrected or reversed, compensated shock may progress to decompensated shock.

Decompensated shock is a state where the cardiovascular system cannot maintain critical circulation and begins to fail. Hypoxia affects the blood vessels and heart so they cannot maintain blood pressure and circulation.

Irreversible shock is a state of shock where the human system is so damaged that it cannot be resuscitated. Once this stage of shock sets in the patient will die.

3. List mechanisms that compensate for blood loss, and describe how they provide this function.

pp. 557 to 558

Increased peripheral resistance is caused by the constriction of the blood vessels and provides two mechanisms which combat shock. The arterioles constrict and maintain the blood pressure, and they divert blood to only the critical organs.

Increased preload occurs when the veins constrict and reduce their volume. Since they account for about 60 percent of the blood volume this is reasonably effective in modest to moderate blood loss.

Increased heart rate is a mechanism in response to lowering blood pressure. In the presence of low preload it may not be effective.

Peripheral vascular shunting directs the blood away from the skin, conserves body heat and reduces fluid loss through evaporation. It also redirects blood to more critical areas.

Fluid shifts are the results of drawing fluid from the interstitial and cellular spaces into the vascular space. While this is a slow mechanism, it can provide the vascular system with several liters of fluid.

4. Identify signs and symptoms of hypovolemic shock, and explain why they occur.

pp. 557 to 559

Tachycardia occurs in attempts to maintain blood pressure when preload is reduced.

Weak pulse is secondary to the lowered preload and the reduced efficiency of the heart's pumping function.

Cool, clammy skin is due to the redirection of blood to more critical organs than the skin.

Ashen, pale skin may present due to hypoxia and peripheral vasoconstriction.

Agitation, restlessness, and reduced LOC will occur as the brain begins to receive a reduced flow of oxygenated blood. The hypoxia causes the defense mechanisms of agitation and restlessness, followed by a noticeable reduction in the level of consciousness.

Dull, lackluster eyes occur secondary to low perfusion and hypoxic states.

Rapid, shallow respiration may occur as shock progresses and respiratory effort becomes less efficient.

Dropping oxygen saturation may also provide evidence to support developing shock. As the peripheral circulation slows, the readings may drop or become erratic.

Falling blood pressure heralds the progression from compensatory to decompensated shock. As a late sign, it should not be used to determine the presence of shock.

5. List findings related to hypovolemic shock for each of the elements of the primary assessment.

pp. 560 to 562

Airway - the airway may be clear. However, as the level of consciousness drops, either due to head injury or shock, it may be endangered by loss of protective reflexes.

Breathing - respiration may increase in rate and decrease in volume, making it less efficient.

Circulation - the pulse will increase in rate and decrease in strength: the classic thready pulse. The capillary refill time will increase due to reduced circulating volume and peripheral vasoconstriction.

Disability - the patient's level of consciousness may diminish as the circulating volume decreases and hypoxia begins. Frequently agitation and restlessness will precede the diminished LOC.

Expose - in cases of external hemorrhage, bleeding may be evident or hidden. The paramedic should examine any hidden areas where significant hemorrhage could otherwise go unnoticed. Examination of the chest, abdomen, and pelvis may also present the external signs of internal hemorrhage.

6. Identify and explain the various steps taken in the care of patients with differing degrees of blood loss.

pp. 563 to 567

The patient suspected of hypovolemic shock should be cared for with the standard primary A-B-C-D-E assessment and any problems cared for as found. All significant bleeding should be controlled and high-flow oxygen applied. The patient should be positioned with legs elevated, the PASG applied and inflated as needed, and two large-bore IV's begun with trauma tubing and pressure infusers in place. The PASG and infusion rate should be guided by the progressing shock.

7. Explain benefits of, and indications and contraindications for, using the pneumatic antishock garment (PASG).

pp. 565 to 566

Benefits include:

Autotransfusion - while this effect of the PASG is controversial, it is apparent that 200 to 300 mL of blood may be autotransfused from the legs and abdomen to the critical circulation.

Increased peripheral vascular resistance - the PASG compresses blood vessels within the garment, thereby increasing the pressure needed to circulate blood through the areas enclosed. This helps maintain blood pressure and critical organ perfusion.

Hemorrhage control - the PASG is able to control, through direct pressure, hemorrhage in the pelvis, and to some degree in the abdomen and lower extremities.

Indications

- Hypovolemic or relative hypovolemic shock
- Hip fractures or bilateral femur fractures (for stabilization)

Contraindications

- Head injury
- Penetrating trauma to the chest
- Relative contraindications
  - Pulmonary edema
  - Late pregnancy - leg sections only
  - Impaled object - inflate segments below and not involved

8. Explain how catheter length and diameter, and fluid pressure affect the rate of intravenous infusion.

pp. 566 to 567

Catheter length - the longer the catheter, the greater its resistance to the flow of fluid and the slower an IV fluid will run.

Catheter diameter - the larger the diameter of a catheter, the more fluid can be infused through it. The relation is related to the power of four. If you double the diameter the flow will increase by a factor of sixteen.

Fluid pressure - the greater the pressure of a fluid, the more rapidly it will infuse.

9. List the signs and symptoms of circulatory overload in a patient receiving rapid crystalloid infusion.

p. 567

The common signs and symptoms commonly associated with circulatory overload associated with rapid field fluid resuscitation include dyspnea, rales and rhonchi, or dropping oxygen saturation

10. Describe the preparation of a patient for air medical transport.

pp. 567

The use of air medical transport of the trauma patient from the scene to a trauma center can significantly reduce transport time and save critical minutes of the "Golden Hour." A patient who will be flown should have the airway secured, a large-bore IV route established and the patient completely immobilized. You should be prepared to give a rapid and thorough patient report when the flight crew arrives.

11. Identify the benefits of helicopter use, and list the criteria for establishing a landing zone.

pp. 568 to 570

The helicopter has the ability to transport the trauma patient from the scene to the trauma center at a speed roughly twice that of ground transport and "as the crow flies." Since the object of prehospital trauma care is to bring the patient to surgery, the helicopter offers a great service to the trauma patient.

Landing zone size

- 60 x 60 feet - small helicopter
- 75 x 75 feet - medium helicopter
- 120 x 120 feet - large helicopter

- Flat surface
- Debris free
- Obstructions free - trees, utility lines, etc.
- Free of ignition sources

CASE STUDY REVIEW

Reread the case study in **PARAMEDIC EMERGENCY CARE** and then read the discussion below.

The patient presented within this case study has the typical signs and symptoms of shock and is cared for with the aggressiveness required if shock resuscitation is to be successful.

Chapter I9 Case Study

The patient presents with the classical signs and symptoms of shock. The carotid pulse is rapid and weak, reflective of volume depletion, and the heart's attempt to compensate with a rapid rate. The patient has a reduced level of consciousness, is not able to remember what happened, and is both anxious and combative. These signs reflect cerebral hypoxia. Breathing is also affected. The breaths are shallow and rapid, thus less efficient than slower and deeper respirations. The absence of distal pulses suggests both reduced blood pressure and peripheral vasoconstriction. This is supported by the cool, clammy skin and capillary refill time of over 4 seconds (normal being less than 2 seconds). The pulse oximetry reading is low, reflecting poor oxygenation. It is surprising that a reading was obtained at all. In low flow states the oximeter often provides an erratic reading, if one can be obtained at all.

This patient is certainly a candidate for rapid transport and aggressive shock care en route. Because of the entrapment, the rapid transport is not an immediately available option and aggressive field care is employed. The aggressive care offered by the paramedics includes two IVs begun with 14- or 16-gauge short catheters. This will allow the greatest infusion rates. The catheters are connected to trauma tubing for the rapid infusion of crystalloids and, eventually, blood in the emergency department. Pressure infusers are applied to the fluids. The paramedics use one 1,000 mL bag of lactated Ringer's solution and one of normal saline. The normal saline is hung because there is an incompatibility between blood and lactated Ringer's solution. This arrangement will allow the hospital to infuse the blood through the saline line, if they wish to do so.

The PASG provides a double benefit in this patient scenario. The pressure of the garment over the dressings is an effective application of direct pressure and hemorrhage control. The garment also effectively supports the body's compensatory mechanisms against shock.

The only action on the part of the paramedic team which might have improved patient care would have been to draw blood at the scene and have a police officer transport it to the emergency department. This would allow the ED staff to type and crossmatch whole blood for the patient much earlier than was otherwise possible. Instead, type O negative blood was given, which might not be the ideal blood type for this patient.

READING COMPREHENSION SELF-EXAM

1. Shock/trauma resuscitation takes place during which of the steps of patient assessment/management?

   A. survey of the scene
   B. primary assessment
   C. secondary assessment
   D. management
   E. transport

   Answer B

2. The total blood volume in an average adult is about ....

   A. 2 to 3 liters.
   B. 3 to 4 liters.
   C. 4 to 5 liters.
   D. 5 to 6 liters.
   E. 7 to 8 liters.

   Answer D

3. Which blood vessels are most responsible for the regulation of blood pressure?

A. arteries
B. arterioles
C. capillaries
D. veins
E. venules

Answer B

4. Shock is a transitional state between normal body function, a hemodynamic balance, and death.

A. True
B. False

Answer A

5. The presentation of shock depends on ....

A. the patient's state of health.
B. the rate of blood or fluid loss.
C. the patient's system's response.
D. the volume of blood or fluid lost.
E. all of the above.

Answer E

6. At which point in the shock process would you expect the blood pressure to drop precipitously?

A. early compensated shock
B. late compensated shock
C. decompensated shock
D. irreversible shock
E. none of the above

Answer C

7. Which of the following CNS responses would be consistent with the development of shock?
   1. anger and hostility
   2. restlessness
   3. lowering level of consciousness
   4. anxiety

Select the proper grouping.

A. 1, 2
B. 2, 3
C. 1, 2, 4
D. 2, 3, 4
E. 1, 2, 3, 4

Answer D

8. Chest and abdominal injuries are notorious for silently causing shock and death.

A. True
B. False

Answer A

9. If all the blood lost due to hemorrhage was immediately returned to the patient in decompensated shock, the condition would be reversed and patient recovery would be likely.

A. True
B. False

Answer A

10. It is the responsibility of the paramedic to assess and anticipate shock. Further, he or she must aggressively treat shock early in its course to be successful in its treatment.

A. True
B. False

Answer A

11. Place the following results of the primary assessment in order as they would be found.
   1. shallow respirations
   2. patient unable to remember accident
   3. absent radial pulse, weak carotid pulse
   4. inguinal hemorrhage
   5. snoring

Select the proper grouping.

A. 1, 2, 3, 4, 5
B. 2, 4, 1, 3, 5
C. 4, 2, 3, 1, 5
D. 5, 1, 3, 2, 4
E. 5, 2, 3, 1, 4

Answer D

12. A patient is found to be dead at the scene. What trauma score would he receive?

A. 0
B. 1
C. 2
D. 3
E. 5

Answer A

13. A trauma patient is breathing at 24 times per minute, has normal respiratory expansion, a blood pressure of 80 systolic, delayed capillary refill of 4 seconds, and a Glasgow Coma Scale of 12. What should you report as the trauma score to medical control?

A. 7
B. 9
C. 11
D. 13
E. 15

Answer D

14. Care rendered at the scene for a critical patient who is a candidate for rapid transport should not exceed ....

A. 3 minutes.
B. 5 minutes.
C. 10 minutes.
D. 12 minutes.
E. one hour.

Answer C

15. The PASG is expected to autotransfuse about ....

A. 250 mL of blood.
B. 500 mL of blood.
C. 750 mL of blood.
D. 1,000 ml of blood.
E. 1,250 mL of blood.

Answer A

16. A patient has been injured in a severe auto accident and has a low blood pressure, a thready pulse, and cool, clammy skin. She is late-term pregnancy and is conscious and alert, though restless. The PASG should be inflated as follows:

A. all chambers until the valves pop off
B. all chambers until the blood pressure rises
C. leg chambers only until the blood pressure improves
D. leg chambers only until the valves pop off
E. the PASG is contraindicated

Answer C

17. After applying the PASG the patient's blood pressure and level of consciousness improve. The patient begins to complain of dyspnea and has rales in the lower lung lobes. As a paramedic you should ....

A. immediately release a small amount of the PASG pressure.
B. immediately release all the PASG pressure.
C. leave the current pressure but stop inflation.
D. continue the inflation as called for by vital signs.
E. administer morphine and continue inflation.

Answer C

18. Which of the following would be the most ideal catheter for fluid rapid administration to the hypovolemic shock patient?

A. a 14-gauge 3-inch catheter
B. a 14-gauge 2-inch catheter
C. a 16-gauge 3-inch catheter
D. a 16-gauge 2-inch catheter
E. a 22-gauge 3-inch catheter

Answer B

19. It takes what volume of lactated Ringer's solution or normal saline to replace one liter of blood lost through hemorrhage?

A. 500 mL
B. 750 mL
C. 1,000 mL
D. 1,500 mL
E. 3,000 mL

Answer e

20. Normally the prehospital infusion of crystalloids in the resuscitation of a shock patient should be limited to ....

A. 500 mL.
B. 1,000 mL.
C. 2,000 mL.
D. 3,000 mL.
E. 5,000 mL.

Answer D

SPECIAL PROJECTS

Trauma Crossword Puzzle

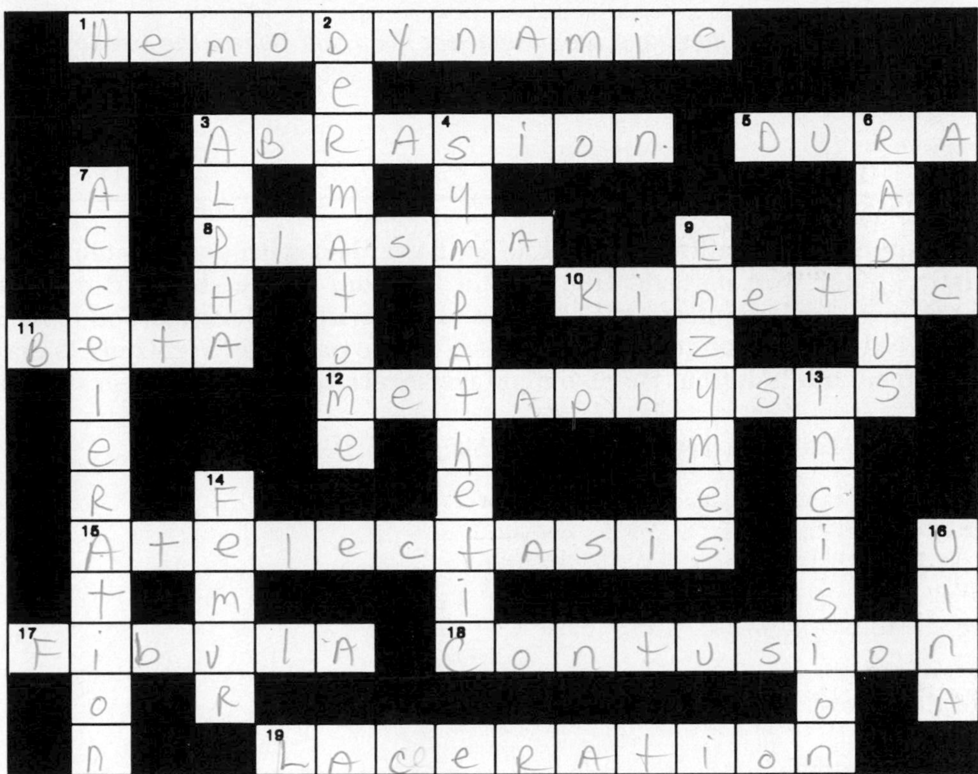

The crossword puzzle above addresses the vocabulary of chapters 14 through 19.

ACROSS

1. Referring to the regulation of the cardiovascular system.
3. An open wound caused by a scraping trauma.
5. The outermost layer of the meninges.
8. The fluid portion of the blood.
10. The type of energy related to motion.
11. Ionizing radiation which can penetrate only superficial layers of clothing or the skin.
12. The transitional region of the bone between the diaphysis and the epiphysis.
15. The collapse of the alveoli.
17. The smaller of the bones of the lower leg.
18. A closed soft tissue wound.
19. An open wound which may be gaping and jagged.

DOWN

2. A surface area of the body controlled by one peripheral nerve root.
3. The weakest form of ionizing radiation.
4. The "fight-or-flight" nervous system.
6. The lateral bone of the forearm.
7. Increase in velocity.
9. Biological catalysts which help break down food.
13. A smooth form of laceration.
14. The bone of the thigh.
16. The medial bone of the forearm.

DIVISION REVIEW

TRAUMA EMERGENCIES

The following scenario based questions are designed to help you review the previous six chapters of **PARAMEDIC EMERGENCY CARE.** *They combine the knowledge gained thus far through your reading and course work.*

Scenario I

Your rescue squad arrives at the scene of an auto accident with a wind shield broken in the characteristic spider web pattern. One patient is found inside slumped over the steering wheel. He has a severe laceration to the frontal region with moderate blood loss. He does not respond to verbal stimuli but does move ineffectively to pain. His breathing is erratic and he is snoring with each inhalation. He also displays severe hemorrhage from the left forearm.

1. What Glasgow Coma Score would you assign this patient?

   A. 0
   B. 3
   C. 5
   D. 9
   E. 12

Answer C

2. Which of the following head injuries do you suspect?

   A. epidural hematoma
   B. subdural hematoma
   C. intracerebral hemorrhage
   D. cerebral concussion
   E. any or all of the above

Answer E

Your partner quickly moves the patient to seated position and maintains the head in a neutral position. You affix a cervical collar and notice that the respirations remain erratic though the snoring has stopped. The patient is quickly lowered to a spine board and prepared for transport. During assessment you notice that the muscle tone on the left side of the patient's body is flaccid when compared to the patient's right side.

3. Which of the following care steps would you provide for this patient?
   1. high flow oxygen
   2. hyperventilation
   3. IV drug route
   4. endotracheal intubation

   Select the proper grouping.

   A. 1, 3
   B. 2, 4
   C. 1, 3, 4
   D. 1, 2, 3
   E. 1, 2, 3, 4

Answer E

4. If you chose to intubate this patient, which of the following techniques would you use?
   1. blind
   2. oral
   3. digital
   4. nasal

   Select the proper grouping.

   A. 1, 2
   B. 2, 3
   C. 1, 4
   D. 3, 4
   E. 2, 3, 4

   Answer E

5. The difference in the patient's muscle tone between right and left side is due to the head injury.

   A. True
   B. False

   Answer A

During transport to the hospital the patient begins to fight the restraints. He is now opening his eyes and is speaking clearly though he is disoriented to time and place.

6. Given the change in the patient's condition, the new Glasgow Coma Score would be about ....

   A. 4
   B. 8
   C. 12
   D. 14
   E. 16

   Answer D

Scenario II

Your rescue unit has been called to the scene of a two car accident with serious injuries. You arrive on the scene two minutes after dispatch and about four minutes after the actual accident. Your initial evaluation of the patient reveals a conscious, alert male with a blood pressure of 124/86, pulse of 72, and respirations of 26. You employ spinal precautions including a cervical collar, an extrication device, prepare a long spine board, and take a second set of vital signs. The blood pressure is 122/94, the pulse rate is now 88, respirations are 32 and shallow, and the patient appears agitated.

7. What is accounting for the changing patient vital signs?

   A. post accident anxiety
   B. the confinement of the spine board
   C. hypovolemic shock
   D. hyperventilation syndrome
   E. None of the above

   Answer C

8. Which of the following care steps would you provide for this patient?
   1. PASG
   2. Rapid IV fluid infusion
   3. high flow oxygen
   4. rapid transport

   Select the proper grouping.

A. 1, 3
B. 1, 2
C. 2, 3, 4
D. 3, 4
E. 1, 2, 3, 4

Answer E

9. The patient above would be considered in which type of shock?

A. stable
B. compensated
C. decompensated
D. irreversible
E. none of the above

Answer C

You quickly load the patient into the ambulance and are underway. You begin the physical assessment and note a crackling sensation while palpating the left chest. Auscultation reveals diminished breath sound on the left and a gentle crackling sound heard during inspiration. The patient's left flank is tender and the belly reveals rebound tenderness.

10. The crackling upon palpation of the chest area is called ....

A. subcutaneous emphysema
B. spontaneous pneumothorax
C. rhonchi or rales
D. tension pneumothorax
E. none of the above

Answer A

11. The sound heard during inspiration is best described as which of the following?

A. normal
B. rhonchi
C. rales
D. stridorous
E. incipient

Answer C

12. The left flank pain is most likely related to an injury to which of the following organs?

A. kidney
B. large bowel
C. stomach
D. liver
E. spleen

Answer e

Scenario III

A 23-year-old male has fallen from a ladder, a distance of about 12 feet. Upon your arrival, he is found seated, in moderate pain. Your assessment reveals a elbow which is fixed at about 90°, painful, and swollen. The patient has also sustained a deep laceration to the left interior thigh.

13 The most likely cause of the patient's problem is ....

A. muscle cramp.
B. wrist dislocation.
C. forearm fracture.
D. subluxation.
E. elbow dislocation.

Answer e

14. The best immobilization device for this fracture would be ....

A. an air splint.
B. a padded board splint.
C. PASG.
D. a traction splint.
E. pillow splint.

Answer B

15. The elbow would be best splinted in an extended position.

A. True
B. False

Answer B

16. Select the appropriate hemorrhage control steps for the thigh wound.
1. direct pressure
2. elevation
3. pressure points
4. PASG
5. Tourniquet

Select the proper grouping.

A. 1
B. 3
C. 2, 4, 5
D. 1, 3, 4, 5
E. 1, 2, 3, 4, 5

Answer D

The pulse distal to the elbow wound is absent and the capillary refill time is about 3 seconds.

17. The elbow should be cared for by ....

A. leaving it as is.
B. gently manipulating it once.
C. straightening the limb.
D. increasing the pressure of the splint.
E. applying the PASG.

Answer B

Scenario IV

A 16-year-old boy is burned while starting a lawn mower after filling it with gas. He has received burns to both lower extremities and is in severe pain. His clothing has burned away to reveal reddened skin which is already blistering. The entire left lower extremity, the genitalia, and the right lower extremity up to the knee are involved. The patient is conscious, alert, and oriented. Vitals are pulse 82, respirations 16 without any distress, and the blood pressure is 132/92.

18. Using the rule of nines, the boy burned what portion of his body?

A. 9%
B. 14%
C. 18%
D. 19%
E. 24%

Answer E

19. The type of burn described here would be classified as ....

A. first degree.
B. second degree.
C. third degree.
D. full thickness
E. eschar

Answer B

20. The severity of this burn would be classified as ....

A. minimal.
B. minor.
C. moderate.
D. severe.
E. critical.

Answer D

21. The best method of burn dressing for this patient would be ....

A. dry sterile dressing.
B. wet dressing.
C. petroleum impregnated gauze.
D. sterile plastic wrap.
E. none of the above.

Answer A

22. An inherent danger in a burn such as this is the development of an eschar and its threat to the distal circulation.

A. True
B. False

Answer B

20

RESPIRATORY EMERGENCIES

Review of the Objectives for Chapter 20

After reading this chapter, you should be able to:

1. Identify the historical factors to elicit when evaluating the respiratory system.

p. 575

How long has the dyspnea been present?
Was the onset gradual or abrupt?
Is the dyspnea affected by position?
Has the patient been coughing?
Is there pain associated with the dyspnea?
What is the patient's past medical history?
What medications are prescribed for the patient?
Does the patient have any allergies?

2. Identify specific observations and physical findings to evaluate in the patient with a respiratory complaint.

pp. 576 to 580

Symptoms

Anxiety may suggest respiratory problems. Dyspnea can induce extreme fear and anxiety.

Difficulty speaking - dyspnea can render the patient unable to speak in complete sentences without a break for air.

Distraction - a patient who is frequently distracted from questioning or conversation is experiencing significant symptoms especially if they are related to respiration.

Signs

Position may tell much about the patient's respiratory status. Most severely embarrassed respiratory patients will be found bolt upright.

Obesity can result in respiratory compromise.

Nasal flaring suggests difficult breathing and respiratory distress.

Tracheal tugging is reflective of dyspnea and the use of accessory muscles of respiration.

Intercostal retraction is also a sign of distress and commonly suggestive of airway restriction or obstruction.

Accessory muscle use is commonly reflective of respiratory distress. It suggests that normal respiratory muscles cannot inspire or expire the needed respiratory volume.

Cyanosis is a sign of hypoxemia and is usually related to inadequate respiratory volume.

Pursed lip breathing is used by the patient to maintain the smaller airways during exhalation. It is generally a sign of chronic respiratory disease.

3. **Describe the techniques of inspection, auscultation, and palpation of the chest.**

pp. 576 to 580

Inspection is the first and least invasive technique of patient assessment and possibly the most revealing. Observe for any signs of distress and watch the patient's breathing pattern, use of auxiliary muscles and general color. Visually examine the nose, mouth, neck, thorax and belly.

Auscultation - listen to the regions of the thorax distally, medially, posteriorly and anteriorly. Determine if sounds are clear and bilateral. Listen for rales, rhonchi, wheezes, stridor or other abnormal airway sound.

Palpation - feel for any crepitation or the crackling of subcutaneous emphysema. Also palpate the chest excursion to determine symmetry.

4. **Define the following terms:**

pp. 578 to 579

Snoring is the sound made as air passes the flaccid tongue or other similar soft mass. It is related to an upper airway partial obstruction.

Stridor is a harsh and high pitched sound occurring as air passes a restriction in the lower part of the upper airway. It is commonly associated with croup.

Wheezing is a whistling sound associated with narrowing of the lower airways. It may be caused by edema, bronchoconstriction or a foreign body.

Rhonchi are rattling sounds made by air passing mucous or other viscous fluids in the airway.

Rales are fine crackling sounds due to early pulmonary edema in the smaller air passages.

The **friction rub** is a sound made as inflamed parietal and visceral pleura rub against each other.

5. **Review the basic principles of respiratory management.**

pp. 581 to 599

The **airway** receives first priority in the management of any patient. It should be managed by obstruction removal, positioning, oro- or nasopharyngeal airway, or by endotracheal tube. In the potential spinal injury patient positioning should not extend the neck.

Oxygen should be given to any patient with respiratory distress. It should be administered to any patient with a disease or injury which suggests hypoxia. In suspected COPD it should be administered if hypoxia is suspected.

6. **Describe the difference between the normal respiratory drive and the respiratory drive of the patient with chronic obstructive pulmonary disease (COPD).**

pp. 583 to 586

Normal respiration is controlled by the level of carbon dioxide found in the blood and cerebrospinal fluid. As the level rises, the pH decreases, the fluid becomes more acidic and the respiratory centers are stimulated. The centers then send impulses to initiate respiration. This system offers fine control over the breathing process. Chronic obstructive pulmonary disease progressively increases the level of CO_2 retained in the alveoli. This high CO_2 state renders the normal mechanism of respiratory control ineffective. The system then relies on the level of oxygen and initiates a breath when the O_2 level drops; hence, called the hypoxic drive.

7. Review the pharmacology, action, dosage, side effects, contraindications, and routes of administration of the following drugs:

pp. 589 to 594

Please review the pertinent information regarding the following drugs as they apply to respiratory emergencies. (See the drug cards found at the end of this book.)

epinephrine
isoetharine
terbutaline
aminophylline
albuterol
metaproterenol
methylprednisolone

8. Discuss the pathophysiology, assessment, and management of the following conditions.

pp. 583 to 599

EMPHYSEMA

Pathophysiology - emphysema is a chronic obstructive pulmonary disease due to the destruction of the alveolar walls, most commonly due to smoking. The result is a less efficient respiratory system, elevated CO_2, and pulmonary hypertension.

Assessment - the patient will generally complain of dyspnea on exertion and progressive limitation of physical activity. The patient may present with a large barreled chest, decreased chest excursion, a thin frame, remain pink throughout most of the disease process and may breathe with pursed lips. Wheezes and rhonchi may be present, and respiratory sounds are diminished.

Management - establish an airway, apply supplemental oxygen at a low flow rate and monitor respirations carefully. Initiate an IV line with D_5W at a T.K.O. rate, and administer a bronchodilator as requested by medical control.

CHRONIC BRONCHITIS

Pathophysiology - chronic bronchitis is a chronic obstructive pulmonary disease. It is associated with an increase in the number of mucous secreting cells in the respiratory track due to long exposure to cigarette smoking or other toxic airborne material. The alveoli are not severely affected though the airways are narrowed and respiratory exchange is reduced. Hypoxia may result as may pulmonary hypertension.

Assessment - the patient is often heavy and cyanotic, hence referred to as the "blue bloater." There may be a history of frequent respiratory infection and auscultation may reveal rhonchi. Signs and symptoms of right heart failure may also be apparent.

Management - the chronic bronchitis patient is managed as is the emphysema patient.

ASTHMA

Pathophysiology - asthma is a common respiratory disease usually detected before age 10. It is an allergic reaction in which the bronchioles constrict and the mucous membranes lining the passageways swell. It may be triggered by inhaled irritants, respiratory infection, emotional distress or cold air.
As the attack progresses, the airways become increasingly narrowed, the lungs hyperinflate and exhalation becomes difficult.

Assessment - patients are most often aware of their disease and will understand what is happening. They will be experiencing severe dyspnea, anxiety and wheezing (unless the attack is extremely severe). Tachycardia frequently accompanies asthma.

Management - maintain the airway and administer high flow, humidified oxygen. Calm the patient and initiate an IV with D_5W T.K.O. Administer subcutaneous epinephrine and, with permission of medical control, aminophylline. In some systems, bronchodilators may be available. If epinephrine does not break the attack the paramedic may be required to intubate if the patient goes into respiratory arrest.

PNEUMONIA

Pathophysiology - pneumonia is a common respiratory problem usually of viral or bacterial origin.

Assessment - the patient will feel ill with fever, chills, malaise and generalized weakness. Frequently the patient will have a productive cough with rales, rhonchi and wheezes present.

Management - field care for suspected pneumonia is supportive, including oxygen and possibly beta agonists.

TOXIC INHALATION

Pathophysiology - toxic gases such as ammonia, nitric oxide, sulfur dioxide, or sulfur trioxide combine with the fluid found in the airway. They create corrosive agents that chemically burn the airway. Swelling and obstruction can occur. The pathology can also be initiated by inhalation of superheated steam and the toxic byproducts of combustion.

Assessment - the patient will have a history of inhalation and accompanying burning pain or progressive dyspnea. The patient will display the signs and symptoms of progressive respiratory obstruction including rhonchi, wheezes, stridor or hoarse cough.

Management - with consideration for rescuer safety, remove the patient from the exposure. Administer oxygen and closely monitor the airway. Endotracheal intubation may be required though it may be a difficult procedure to employ.

PULMONARY EMBOLISM

Pathophysiology - pulmonary emboli originate from some source in the venous system, travel to the right heart and finally lodge in the pulmonary circulation. The embolus prevents circulation through the capillaries of some alveoli. It causes increased resistance against which the right heart must pump and may induce congestive heart failure.

Assessment - the patient may complain of sudden, unexplained dyspnea that may be associated with chest pain and a history of recent surgery or immobilization. The patient may exhibit dyspnea, JVD, falling blood pressure and other signs of congestive heart failure.

Management - the airway must be kept clear, oxygen administered and an IV initiated to run T.K.O.

HYPERVENTILATION SYNDROME

Pathophysiology - hyperventilation syndrome is a common anxiety-produced rapid respiratory rate. Hyperventilation eliminates too much CO_2 and the body then finds respiration hard to control.

Assessment - the patient will be breathing rapidly and deeply in the presence of anxiety. The patient may also display carpal (finger) and pedal (feet) tingling or spasm due to the respiratory alkalosis.

Management - management for hyperventilation is focused on calming and reassurance. The condition should be treated as any case of dyspnea, with oxygen. It may be helpful to ask the patient to consciously breathe deeply and to slow the respiratory rate.

CENTRAL NERVOUS SYSTEM DYSFUNCTION

Pathophysiology - CNS dysfunction can cause many respiratory patterns, respiratory depression, and in some cases arrest. Causes include stroke, tumors, drugs and trauma.

Assessment of the CNS-injured or -impaired patient may reveal erratic breathing patterns. Note should be made of especially deep, irregular or belly breathing patterns.

Management - general support of the patient is required with special benefit of hyperventilation for the patient with possible intracranial pathology.

CASE STUDY REVIEW

Reread the case study in **PARAMEDIC EMERGENCY CARE** and then read the discussion below.

This narrative describes a respiratory emergency call that is relatively routine from start to finish. There are, however, many areas present where the patient, and the call in general, could deteriorate. While many respiratory distress patients present without complication, there is the potential for general dyspnea to move from an uncomfortable sensation to a dire medical emergency.

Chapter 20 Case Study

Many "medical emergency" calls are respiratory in nature. The presentation of the patient in this scenario is very common. It is important to understand that the patient with a chronic respiratory problem may ride a fine line between dyspnea and severe respiratory decompensation. As the chronic respiratory disease process develops, the patient adjusts to his or her malady and may lead a relatively normal life. If the patient is placed under abnormal stress, as on a very hot and humid day or is engaged in unusual exercise, the respiratory system may fail to move enough air to provide oxygen and remove carbon dioxide from the blood stream. The result may be a very life-threatening situation.

Smoking frequently plays an important role in chronic respiratory disease. The products of the combustion of tobacco are toxic and irritating. Eventually they damage the respiratory system. The risks associated with smoking are now well known and well publicized. However, many life-long smokers find it impossible to stop, even in the face of the known risks or terminal respiratory disease.

The presentation of this patient is typical of chronic obstructive pulmonary disease. He is sitting upright at the table and using accessory muscles to assist respirations. The paramedics use the venturi mask to administer the oxygen because it will accurately provide a modest level of oxygen. They are concerned that the patient may control breathing via hypoxic drive. If high-flow oxygen is administered the patient may stop breathing and leave them to intubate and ventilate by bag-valve-mask. The history of emphysema confirms their suspicions and underscores the correctness of their conservative approach.

The current medications used by the patient are important in planning the care for the patient. The patient's use of theophylline suggests that cardiac monitoring may reveal dysrhythmias due to sympathetic stimulation or hypoxia. It also may suggest the cautious use of albuteral, especially if the patient has recently taken high doses of theophylline.

In the future the patient described here may again call upon emergency medical service for help. The disease process of emphysema is progressive and will be fatal sooner if the patient continues to smoke. As time passes, his respiratory reserve (the difference between the vital capacity and tidal volume) will reduce. As it does, he will be less able to move about, communicate or experience physiologic stress. Eventually his respiratory volume will be unable to meet his body's needs and he will die.

READING COMPREHENSION SELF-EXAM

1. If the patient complains of pain associated with dyspnea, he or she should be questioned to determine the ....

   A. location of the pain.
   B. radiation of the pain, if any.
   C. duration of the pain.
   D. onset of the pain.
   E. all of the above.

   Answer E

2. The vibration felt over the central thorax while a patient is speaking is called ....

   A. pathologic tremors.
   B. raleous emphysema.
   C. tactile fremitus.
   D. thoracic bruit.
   E. laryngovibrious palpation.

   Answer C

3. The sound heard during auscultation that reflects friction between inflamed pleura is termed ....

   A. rales.
   B. rhonchi.
   C. tactile fremitus.
   D. friction rub.
   E. S-3 gallop.

   Answer D

4. Both emphysema and chronic bronchitis are progressive respiratory diseases that restrict air exchange and induce pulmonary hypertension.

   A. True
   B. False

   Answer A

5. During assessment the classic emphysema patient would be expected to display which of the following?
   1. cyanosis
   2. dyspnea
   3. obesity
   4. productive cough
   5. history of smoking

   Select the proper grouping.

   A. 1, 3
   B. 2, 5
   C. 1, 2, 3, 5
   D. 2, 3, 4, 5
   E. 1, 2, 3, 4, 5

   Answer B

6. Which of the following signs and symptoms would you expect to find in the chronic bronchitis patient?
   1. cyanosis
   2. dyspnea
   3. obesity
   4. history of smoking
   5. productive cough

   Select the proper grouping.

   A. 1, 3
   B. 2, 4
   C. 1, 2, 3, 4
   D. 2, 3, 4, 5
   E. 1, 2, 3, 4, 5

   Answer E

7. Care for both the chronic bronchitis and emphysema patients should include ....
   1. high-flow oxygen.
   2. establishing an airway.
   3. supine patient positioning.
   4. establishing an IV line.
   5. possible nebulized bronchodilator.

   Select the proper grouping.

   A. 1, 3
   B. 2, 4
   C. 1, 2, 3
   D. 2, 4, 5
   E. 1, 2, 3, 4, 5

   Answer D

8. Asthma ....
   1. is a common respiratory illness.
   2. is usually associated with allergies.
   3. may cause the patient to quickly deteriorate.
   4. results in occasional deaths, 50% of which occur before the hospital.
   5. is related to bronchospasm.

   Select the proper grouping.

   A. 1, 3, 4
   B. 2, 3, 5
   C. 1, 3, 4, 5
   D. 2, 3, 4, 5
   E. 1, 2, 3, 4, 5

   Answer E

9. Care of the asthma patient experiencing a severe attack may include ....
   1. oxygen therapy.
   2. solu-medrol.
   3. aminopylline.
   4. a nebulized bronchodilator.
   5. calming and reassurance.

   Select the proper grouping.

   A. 1, 3
   B. 2, 5
   C. 1, 2, 4
   D. 2, 3, 4, 5
   E. 1, 2, 3, 4, 5

   Answer E

10. The initials PEFR refer to the airflow rate during maximum expiratory flow and is a good indicator of air exchange.

A. True
B. False

Answer ____

11. Status asthmaticus is defined as a severe, prolonged asthma attack that cannot be broken by repeated doses of solu-medrol.

A. True
B. False

Answer ____

12. Pneumonia is generally treated in the field by ....
   1. supplemental oxygen.
   2. high-dose antibiotics.
   3. subcutaneous epinephrine.
   4. aminophylline drip.
   5. transport.

Select the proper grouping.

A. 1, 5
B. 1, 3, 5
C. 1, 3, 4, 5
D. 1, 2, 5
E. 1, 2, 3, 4, 5

Answer ____

13. Causes of inhalation injury usually include which of the following?

A. inhaled steam
B. chemical irritants
C. toxic products of combustion
D. superheated air
E. all of the above

Answer ____

14. The primary reason that carbon monoxide is poisonous is that it ....

A. causes chemical burns of the upper airway.
B. causes chemical burns of the lower airway.
C. induces severe metabolic acidosis.
D. replaces oxygen on the hemoglobin molecule.
E. congests the bronchioles, reducing effective air exchange.

Answer ____

15. The two most common sources of carbon monoxide poisoning are from automobiles and ....

A. camp fires.
B. chemical plant fires.
C. home heating devices.
D. used tire fires.
E. cutting torches.

Answer ____

16. The oxygen concentration provided to the patient who has suffered carbon monoxide poisoning should be in which percentage range?

A. 40 to 50%
B. 50 to 70%
C. 70 to 80%
D. 80 to 90%
E. 90 to 100%

Answer ____

17. A specialized treatment that will greatly benefit the patient suffering from carbon monoxide poisoning would be ....

A. neurosurgery.
B. hyperbaric oxygen therapy.
C. respiratory therapy.
D. thrombolytic therapy.
E. hemodialysis.

Answer ____

18. Which of the following would predispose a patient to pulmonary emboli?
1. coumadin use
2. prolonged immobilization
3. thrombophlebitis
4. cerebral edema
5. toxic inhalation
Select the proper grouping.

A. 1, 5
B. 2, 3
C. 1, 3, 4
D. 2, 3, 4, 5
E. 1, 2, 3, 4, 5

Answer ____

19. An otherwise healthy patient displays and complains of anxiety, rapid deep respirations, tingling, spasms of the feet and hands. Your first suspicion should be of ....

A. pulmonary edema.
B. pulmonary emboli.
C. carbon monoxide poisoning.
D. hyperventilation syndrome.
E. emphysema.

Answer ____

20. A patient who has a history of myasthenia gravis is experiencing dyspnea. Your care steps should include which of the following?
1. establishing an airway
2. providing respiratory assistance
3. oxygen
4. medications specific to the care of this disease
Select the proper grouping.

A. 1, 3
B. 2, 4
C. 2, 3, 4
D. 1, 2, 3
E. 1, 2, 3, 4

Answer ____

PHARMACOLOGY MATH WORKSHEET I

Formulas

Rate = Volume/Time
Volume = Rate x Time
Time = Volume/Rate

mL/min = gtts per min/gtts per mL
gtts / min = mL per min x gtts per mL
mL = gtts/gtts per mL

Concentration = Weight/Volume
Weight = Volume x Concentration1
Volume = Weight/Concentration

1 Kg = 2.2 lb.
gm = 1,000 mg
1 mg = 1,000 mcg

Please complete the following drug and drip math problems:

[1] You are asked to prepare a lidocaine IV add-mixture of 4 mg/mL. You will be adding the drug to a 250 mL bag of D_5W.

A) How much lidocaine will you add to the solution?

B) The request from Medical Command calls for 2mg/min. What drip rate would you set with a 60 mcgtts/mL drip set?

C) How long would you have to run this drip rate to infuse 300 mL?

[2] Aminophylline is ordered for an acute asthma attack.

A) What amount of the drug would you add to a 100 mL of D_5W to obtain a concentration of 2.5 mg/mL?

B) What drip rate (60 mcgtts/mL) would you set to obtain a 0.5 mg/min flow?

C) To obtain a 1.0 mg/min flow?

[3] A) In a patient with acute pulmonary edema, 250 mg of aminophylline should be added to what volume of solution to obtain a concentration of 12.5 mg/mL?

B) What flow of the drug are you administering at a drip rate of (60 mcgtts/mL set) 60 mcgtts/min?

Using a 45 mcgtts/mL administration set?

C) How much drug have you infused over a 30 minute transport at 30 mcgtts/min with a 60 mcgtts/mL administration set?

SPECIAL PROJECTS

Problem Solving - Asthma

One type of respiratory problem that can become a life threatening emergency is asthma. On the next few lines, identify the signs and symptoms you would expect to find in a 12-year-old patient who is experiencing an acute asthma attack. Please relate the signs and symptoms expected under each of the following aspects of your assessment.

Observation:

Dyspnea — accessory muscle use.
Tripoding — Speech broken by Respirations
Anxiety

Physical exam:

Dyspnea-Tachypnea — audible wheezes.
Tachycardia — Reduced title Volume.
Cyanosis or ashen color. — hyperextended Chest.

Patient history:

asthma & allergic Reactions, are they frequent, severe.
what medications - bronchodilators

Auscultation:

Rales — wheezes
Rhonchi — Quiet (Pathologic)

The medical control physician orders epinephrine.

What route would you use? SQ

What dose would you give? 0.3 - 0.5 1:1000

What other drugs might you consider? Albuterol
Beta 2 Specifics — Terbutaline Sulfate
Isotherine

21

CARDIOVASCULAR EMERGENCIES

Part I - *(pages 603 to 625)*

Review of the Objectives for Chapter 21

After reading this chapter, you should be able to:

1. Describe the size, shape, location, and orientation of the heart.

p. 603

The heart is a muscular organ, the size of a closed fist, located in the middle of the chest within the mediastinum. The upper portion of the heart is called the base and is centrally located in the central mediastinum. The apex is located just above the diaphragm and forms a blunt point, just to the left of center.

2. Describe the normal anatomy of the heart and peripheral circulatory system.

pp. 603 to 609

The **heart** is a four-chambered organ divided left to right by the cardiac septum and upper to lower by the cardiac skeleton (a cartilaginous structure). The upper chambers are the atria while the lower are the ventricles. The heart is a muscular organ with a wall somewhat thicker on the left side than the right.

Blood vessels are generally made up of three layers: the tunica intima, the tunica media, and the tunica adventitia. The tunica intima is the innermost lining of the vessel and provides a smooth interior lumen. The tunica media contains the muscle and elastic fibers that control the diameter of the vessel, the pressure within, and the flow through it. The tunica adventitia is the outer layer and is fibrous in nature. It is responsible for maintaining the maximum diameter of the vessel and, in the arteries, withstanding the strength of the cardiac contraction.

The **vascular system** is composed of five components: the arteries, the arterioles, the capillaries, the venules and the veins. The arteries distribute the cardiac output throughout the body. The arterioles control distribution from the arteries to the capillary beds found within the body organs. The capillary beds provide the exchange surface for gases, nutrients and waste products. The venules control the flow of blood back into the venous system. The veins collect the blood and return it to the heart.

3. Name and describe the location of the cardiac valves.

pp. 604 to 606

The **mitral valve** is located between the left atrium and the left ventricle.

The **pulmonic valve** is located between the right ventricle and the pulmonary arteries.

The **tricuspid valve** is located between the right atrium and the right ventricle.

The **aortic valve** is positioned between the left ventricle and the aorta.

4. Describe the anatomy of the coronary arteries and veins.

pp. 606 to 607

Coronary arteries are named such because they resemble a crown. They are a series of vessels which begin where the aorta leaves the heart. The left coronary artery supplies the left ventricle, the intraventricular septum and part of the right ventricle. The left coronary artery branches into the anterior descending and circumflex arteries. The right coronary artery supplies a portion of the right atrium and ventricle and part of the conduction system. It branches into the posterior descending and marginal arteries.

Coronary veins collect deoxygenated blood from the heart. The coronary sinus drains the left ventricle - otherwise coronary veins generally correspond to the coronary arteries.

5. Describe the differences between the structural and functional aspects of the arterial and venous systems.

pp. 607 to 609

Arterial structure - the arteries are high pressure vessels with thick adventitia. They are able to withstand the high pressure of the systolic blood pressure. The arterioles have greater tunica media mass, which allows them to constrict and control the flow of blood through them. The purpose of the arterial system is to distribute blood to the body organs and tissues, and to maintain blood pressure.

Venous structure - the venules are very similar to the arterioles in structure. The veins are large, low pressure vessels that collect and transport blood back to the heart. They have only limited tunica media though constriction of the veins vessels can return large volumes of blood to the heart. The purpose of the venous system is to return blood to the heart and to maintain preload.

6. Describe the structure and function of capillaries.

p. 608

Capillaries are the exchange vessels for oxygen, carbon dioxide, nutrients and waste products. Their walls are very thin and permit this exchange efficiently. They are so small as to only allow red blood cells to travel through in single file.

7. Describe the course of blood flow through the heart and lungs.

pp. 604 to 609

Blood enters the heart through the vena cavae and into the right atrium. The blood flows through the tricuspid valve into the right ventricle. From there it flows out through the pulmonic valve, into the pulmonary arteries and into the pulmonary circulation. Once oxygenated by passing through the pulmonary capillaries, the blood returns to the heart through the pulmonary veins. The oxygenated blood enters the left atrium and passes through the mitral valve into the left ventricle. The left ventricle contracts and sends the blood out through the aortic valve and into the systemic circulation via the aorta.

8. Describe the cardiac cycle.

pp. 609 to 610

The cardiac cycle is a series of electrically initiated events that result in contraction of the myocardium, blood being pumped through the heart and into the arterial system. The cardiac cycle begins with the contraction of the heart muscle, a stage called systole. During this stage, the ventricles are forcibly emptied and expel the blood through the pulmonary and systemic circulation. They then relax and are filled, in part, by the action of the atria contracting, in a stage called diastole. The cycle then repeats itself.

9. Define the following terms:

pp. 609 to 610

Stroke volume is the volume (usually between 60 and 100 mL) of blood pumped by the ventricles with each contraction.

Afterload is the pressure against which the heart must pump. It is the pressure found in the aorta as ventricular contraction begins - the diastolic pressure.

Preload is the pressure within the ventricle at the end of diastole.

Cardiac output is the volume of blood pumped by the heart in one minute. It is the stroke volume multiplied by the cardiac rate.

Starling's Law provides that the myocardium will contract more forcefully when stretched by atrial filling.

10. Describe the innervation of the heart.

pp. 610 to 612

Sympathetic - the heart is innervated through the cardiac plexus of the sympathetic nervous system. The nerves innervate both the atria and ventricles. The neurotransmitter for the sympathetic nervous system is norepinephrine. Stimulation is primarily beta and will result in increased heart rate and contractile force.

Parasympathetic - the parasympathetic nervous system controls the heart primarily through the vagus nerve. The nerve controls the atria and limited portions of the ventricles. The chief neurotransmitter is acetylcholine. Parasympathetic stimulation will slow the heart rate and electrical conduction.

11. Name the major electrolytes that affect cardiac function.

p. 612

Calcium is vital for depolarization and myocardial contraction. Increased calcium concentrations (hypercalcemia) may increase the contractility of the myocardium. Low calcium states may decrease contractility and cause electrical irritability.

Potassium plays an important role in repolarization.

Sodium plays a major role in the depolarization of the myocardium.

12. Describe the electrical properties of the heart.

pp. 612 to 616

Excitability is the ability to contract to a stimulus.

Conductivity is the ability to conduct an electrical impulse through the cell and to surrounding cells.

Automaticity is a special characteristic of the heart tissue which causes it to contract on its own. Also referred to as the property of self-excitation.

Syncytium is the property possessed by the heart tissue which permits the muscle to contract together, as one mass.

Chronotropy refers to the rate of the heart. It can be increased (positive chronotropic) or decreased (negative chronotropic) by various drugs.

Inotropy refers to the strength of the cardiac contraction. It can either be increased (positive inotropic) or decreased (negative chronotropic) by drugs.

13. Describe the normal sequence of electrical conduction through the heart.

p. 615

The electrical cycle of the heart begins with the release of an electrical impulse by the sino-atrial node. The impulse is carried through the internodal pathways to the atria. As the impulse reaches the atrio-ventricular junction, the impulse is slowed. The impulse is carried through the A-V node to the bundle of His. From the bundle of His the impulse is split to the left and right bundle branches. It finally reaches the Perkinje system and the myocardial cells of the ventricles.

14. Describe cardiac depolarization and repolarization.

pp. 613 to 614

Depolarization Cardiac depolarization is caused by the influx of sodium, and its positive charge, into the myocardial cell. This influx and changing charge causes the muscle to contract.

Repolarization Cardiac repolarization occurs as the cardiac cell membrane becomes impermeable to sodium ions and they are pumped out of the cell. Repolarization must occur before the myocardium is ready to contract again.

15. Name three areas of the heart with pacemaking capabilities, and list the intrinsic rate of each.

p. 616

Sino-atrial (SA) node	60 to 100
Atrio-ventricular (AV) node	40 to 60
Perkinje system	15 to 40

16. Describe the basic concepts of ECG monitoring.

pp. 616 to 619

The **Electrocardiogram (ECG)** is a graphic recording of the electrical activity of the heart against time. It does not tell the cardiac output or efficiency.

The **heart** is the largest producer of electrical activity in the body. It is monitored by the electrocardiogram to determine its rate and the characteristics of its electrical activity.

Monitoring is the sensing, amplification and display of the cardiac electrical activity. It reflects only the electrical activity and not the muscular activity of the myocardium, valve competency or blood flow.

ECG leads are placed on the surface of the body and allow the heart to be monitored through the use of electrical planes. The common leads used in prehospital care are leads I, II and III.

17. Describe the grids and markings on the ECG paper.

p. 619

ECG paper is subdivided by large and small grids to mark time intervals and the strength of the electrical signal. The larger squares are designed to reflect 0.20 seconds horizontally while they reflect 0.5 millivolts of energy vertically. The smaller boxes fit five per one large one in either the horizontal or vertical direction. Each small box accounts for 0.04 seconds. ECG paper also will have markings at the top and/or bottom that indicate three-second intervals.

18. Define the following terms or phrases.

pp. 619 to 620

The **P wave** is the first positive deflection of the baseline in the normal lead II ECG. It has a smooth rounded shape.

The **QRS complex** is the second deviation from the isoelectric in the normal lead II ECG. The first negative deflection is the Q wave. The first positive deflection is the R wave while the S wave is the first negative deflection after the R wave.

The **T wave** is a rounded deflection from the isoelectric following the QRS complex of the normal ECG. It is positive in its orientation in lead II.

The **U wave** is a seldom seen wave form which follows the T wave and is in the same orientation.

The **P-R interval** is the time, as measured in distance on the ECG paper, between the beginning of the P wave and the beginning of the QRS complex.

The **QRS duration** is the length of time between the first deflection of the QRS complex and the last.

The **Isoelectric line** is the baseline of electrical charge and is a horizontal line upon which the elements of the ECG are superimposed.

The **ST segment** is the region of the ECG between the end of the QRS complex and the beginning of the T wave. It is normally isoelectric.

19. Define refractory period, and describe the difference between the relative refractory period and the absolute refractory period.

p. 625

Refractory period is the period of time between the end of depolarization and complete repolarization.

Absolute refractory period is the portion of repolarization when no stimulus, no matter how strong, can initiate a contraction.

Relative refractory period is the later period of time during repolarization when an especially strong stimulus could initiate a contraction.

CASE STUDY REVIEW

Reread the case study in **PARAMEDIC EMERGENCY CARE** and then read the discussion below.

This narrative describes a relatively common cardiac emergency call. However, it also illustrates many important points regarding the response of the paramedic to the cardiac arrest. While most cases of cardiac arrest treated by the paramedic do not survive, despite proper and aggressive advanced life support, the outcome of this case study is patient survival and return of the patient to a relatively normal life.

Chapter 2I Case Study

This scenario is probably the most stressful for the paramedic. The patient is presented at the station with no warning. The team does not have the time to identify where the needed equipment is and to ready it, nor to mentally prepare for the response once at the scene. They are required to respond instantly without forewarning. Practicing the ACLS "mega-code" and local protocols pay off here because the response must be automatic, rapid, and exact. It is.

The first paramedic begins basic life support with ventilations and cardiac compressions. While CPR is a basic skill of emergency medical care and not emphasized in this chapter it is essential to the provision of the cardiac arrest protocols. Without it the oxygen given by bag-valve-mask and the endotracheal tube, and the drugs needed to enhance the defibrillation, would not circulate.

The second paramedic summons help, obtains the needed equipment, gathers some history from the patient's wife, and prepares for a quick look with the paddles. Ventricular fibrillation, which offers the best chance for successful resuscitation of the three arrest dysrhythmias, is observed. He responds with three defibrillations according to protocol and then initiates the advanced skills of intubation and IV initiation. The IV is successful so epinephrine is given by IV bolus. The IV in the arrest patient is difficult to start because of poor circulation. If it can not be started immediately, epinephrine can be given via the endotracheal tube.

The fourth shock converts the patient to a cardiac rhythm that stabilizes as sinus tachycardia. The paramedic is careful to confirm a pulse and watch for other signs of circulation. Lidocaine is given to prevent a reoccurrence of ventricular fibrillation and the patient is transported.

The patient will hopefully begin to breathe on his own. If he does, high flow oxygen will be administered. Otherwise, ventilation will continue via the bag-valve-mask with 100% oxygen. The level of consciousness will be monitored and serial vitals will be taken. The paramedics know that this patient may return to ventricular fibrillation at any time so they will carefully monitor him and the cardiac rhythm.

READING COMPREHENSION SELF-EXAM

1. List the layers of the heart from the outside to the inside.
   1. endocardium 4
   2. visceral pericardium 1
   3. myocardium 3
   4. epicardium 2

   Select the proper grouping.

   A. 2, 4, 3, 1
   B. 1, 3, 4, 2
   C. 3, 4, 1, 2
   D. 1, 4, 2, 3
   E. 4, 2, 3, 1

   Answer A

2. Which of the following statements regarding the heart is false?

   A. The apex is located against the diaphragm.
   B. The heart is a four chambered pump.
   C. The heart is approximately the size of a man's closed fist.
   D. Approximately two thirds of the heart is right of the midline.
   E. The heart is the most electrically active muscle in the body.

   Answer D

3. The right side of the heart is a low pressure pump because the pulmonary circulation does not offer much resistance to blood flow.

   A. True
   B. False

   Answer A

4. The valve which separates the right atrium from the right ventricle is the ....

   A. tricuspid valve.
   B. mitral valve.
   C. aortic valve.
   D. pulmonic valve.
   E. semilunar valve.

   Answer A

5. The major blood vessel which receives blood from the head and upper extremities and transports it to the heart is the ....

   A. aorta.
   B. superior vena cava.
   C. inferior vena cava.
   D. pulmonary artery.
   E. pulmonary vein.

   Answer B

6. The normal cardiac stroke volume is ....

   A. 20 to 50 mL.
   B. 40 to 60 mL.
   C. 50 to 75 mL.
   D. 60 to 100 mL.
   E. 75 to 150 mL.

   Answer D

7. The circumstance which allows blood to travel between arterial vessels through anastamoses and is a protective mechanism in the event of vascular occlusion is called ....

A. peripheral circulation.
B. tunica media.
C. collateral circulation.
D. chordae tendonae.
E. none of the above.

Answer C

8. The principle which states that the heart will pump more forcibly when it is filled and the ventricles are stretched is ....

A. Hering-Beuer reflex.
B. Starling's Law.
C. Poiseuille's Law.
D. stretch reaction principle.
E. none of the above.

Answer B

9. Cardiac output is a factor of which of the element(s) below ....

A. cardiac rate.
B. stroke volume.
C. systemic vascular resistance.
D. A and B.
E. A and C.

Answer D

10. The chief chemical neurotransmitter for the parasympathetic nervous system is ....

A. acetylcholine.
B. norepinephrine.
C. epinephrine.
D. atropine.
E. verapamil.

Answer A

11. The properties of the cardiac conduction system which make the cells different from other body cells includes which of the following?

- 1. automaticity
2. contractility
- 3. conductivity
- 4. excitability

Select the proper grouping.

A. 1, 2
B. 1, 3
C. 3, 4
D. 2, 4
E. 1, 3, 4

Answer E

12. The chief chemical neurotransmitter for the sympathetic nervous system is ....

A. acetylcholine.
B. norepinephrine.
C. epinephrine.
D. verapamil.
E. atropine.

Answer B

13. A positive chronotropic agent would ....

A. increase respiratory rate.
B. decrease respiratory rate.
C. increase heart rate.
D. decrease heart rate.
E. increase the strength of contraction.

Answer C

14. A negative inotropic agent would ....

A. increase the rate of respiration.
B. decrease the rate of respiration.
C. decrease the heart rate.
D. increase the heart rate.
E. decrease the strength of cardiac contraction.

Answer E

15. Place the following in order as the cardiac electrical impulse would travel through them.
1. bundle of His
2. Perkinje fibers
3. SA node
4. internodal pathways
5. AV junction

Select the proper grouping.

A. 3, 4, 5, 1, 2
B. 4, 3, 5, 2, 1
C. 1, 4, 3, 5, 2
D. 2, 3, 4, 5, 1
E. 3, 2, 4, 1, 5

Answer A

16. The intrinsic firing rate of the AV node is ....

A. 100 to 130 beats per minute.
B. 60 to 100 beat per minute.
C. 40 to 60 beats per minute.
D. 15 to 40 beats per minute.
E. none of the above.

Answer C

17. Lead II places the positive and negative electrodes ....

A. on the left leg and left arm, respectively.
B. on the right leg and right arm, respectively.
C. on the right leg and left arm, respectively.
D. on the left leg and right arm, respectively.
E. on the left arm and right arm, respectively.

Answer D

18. Which of the following can be determined from lead II monitoring of the heart?

A. presence of a myocardial infarction
B. chamber enlargement
C. presence of pumping action
D. location of a myocardial infarction
E. none of the above

Answer E

19. The large box of the ECG graph paper represents what time period in the cardiac cycle?

A. 0.01 sec.
B. 0.04 sec.
C. 0.10 sec.
D. 0.20 sec.
E. 0.25 sec.

Answer D

20. Which of the characteristics below are normal for the lead II P wave?
1. rounded
2. regular in rate
3. identical in shape, one to another
4. negative in deflection
5. following the QRS complex by 0.04 to 0.12 sec.

Select the proper grouping.

A. 1, 3, 5
B. 1, 2, 3
C. 2, 3, 5
D. 1, 2, 4, 5
E. 1, 2, 3, 5

Answer B

CARDIAC PHARMACOLOGY

Emergency management for cardiac emergencies utilizes many of the pharmacologic agents which are available to the paramedic. Since this represents a large number of the total drugs you will be using, it is recommended that you begin to review and memorize the various names, indications, therapeutic effects, contraindications, side effects, routes of administration and recommended dosages for the following:

oxygen
epinephrine
norepinephrine (Levophed)
isoproterenol (Isuprel)
dopamine (Intropin)
dobutamine (Dobutrex)
labetalol (Trandate) (Normodyne)
lidocaine (Xylocaine)
bretylium tosylate (Bretylol)
procainamide (Pronestyl)
verapamil (Isoptin) (Calan)
nitroglycerin spray (Nitrolingual Spray)
sodium bicarbonate
morphine sulfate
nitronox
furosemide (Lasix)
nitroglycerin (Nitro Stat)
atropine sulfate
nifedipine (Procardia)
diazoxide (Hyperstat)
calcium chloride
aminophylline
diazepam (Valium)

PHARMACOLOGY MATH WORKSHEET II

Formulas

Rate = Volume/Time
Volume = Rate x Time
Time = Volume/Rate

mL/min = gtts per min/gtts per mL
gtts / min = mL per min x gtts per mL
mL = gtts/gtts per mL

Concentration = Weight/Volume
Weight = Volume x Concentration
Volume = Weight/Concentration

1 Kg = 2.2 lb.
1 gm = 1,000 mg
1 mg = 1,000 mcg

Please complete the following drug and drip math problems:

[1] Medical Command asks you to administer isoproterenol via IV drip. 2 mg are added to a 250 mL bag of D_5W.

A) What is the resultant concentration?

B) While titrating to patient effect, you obtain a flow of 45 gtts/min using a 60 mcgtts/mL administration set. What weight of drug are you infusing per minute?

C) After 45 minutes, how much fluid have you given?

[2] Your protocol asks for 200 mg of dopamine to be added to a 250 mL bag of D_5W.

A) What is the resultant concentration?

B) If you are asked to administer 2 mcg/Kg/min. to a 220 lb. male, what drip rate would you use (60 mcgtts/mL)?

C) If your patient weights 100 lb. and you are requested to administer 8 mcg/Kg/min, what drip rate would you use (60 mcgtts/mL)?

D) After a 20 minute transport, how much drug have you administered in B ? in C ?

21

CARDIOVASCULAR EMERGENCIES

Part II - *(pages 618 to 683)*

Review of the Objectives for Chapter 21

After reading this chapter, you should be able to:

20. Explain what information can and cannot be obtained from the rhythm strip analysis.
p. 618

The single lead ECG can tell:

Heart rate - the ECG can tell the general rate of the heart.

Regularity - the ECG can tell if the heart is beating in a regular or irregular fashion.

Progression of the electrical impulse - the ECG can tell how the electrical impulse is traveling through the conduction system and identify any electrical disturbances in that system.

The single lead ECG cannot tell:

Presence of an infarction - the single lead ECG provides insufficient evidence to confirm or deny the presence of a myocardial infarction.

Axis deviation or chamber enlargement - the single lead ECG does not reflect cardiac enlargement or shifting of the axis of the heart.

Pumping action or efficiency - the ECG cannot relate the effectiveness of the heart regarding cardiac output.

21. Name twelve causes of dysrhythmias.
p. 627

Myocardial ischemia, necrosis, or infarction
Autonomic nervous system imbalance
Heart chamber distention
Blood gas abnormalities
Electrolyte disturbances
Myocardial trauma
Drug effects and toxicity
Electrocution
Hypothermia
CNS damage
Ideopathic occurrences
Normal events

22. Describe the etiology, ECG findings, clinical significance, and treatment for common dysrhythmias.

pp. 627 to 683

SINUS BRADYCARDIA

Etiology - sinus bradycardia may result from increased vagal tone, SA node disease, and drugs such as digitalis, propranolol and quinidine. It may also be found in a physically well-conditioned person.

ECG findings in lead II

Rate	less than 60
Rhythm	regular
Pacemaker site	SA node
P waves	upright and normal in shape
P-R interval	0.12 to 0.20 sec.
QRS complex	0.04 to 0.12 sec.

Clinical significance - can result in decreased cardiac output, hypotension angina, and CNS symptoms. A rate below 50 may induce atrial or ventricular ectopy.

Treatment - if the patient is significantly symptomatic, atropine may be considered, 0.5 mg every 5 minutes until 2.0 mg is given or the rate increases. Profound bradycardia may require pacing.

SINUS TACHYCARDIA

Etiology - exercise, fever, anxiety, hypovolemia, anemia, pump failure and increased sympathetic tone may cause sinus tachycardia.

ECG findings in lead II

Rate	more than 100
Rhythm	regular
Pacemaker site	SA node
P waves	upright and normal in shape
P-R interval	0.12 to 0.20 sec.
QRS complex	0.04 to 0.12 sec.

Clinical significance - sinus tachycardia may reflect decreased cardiac output, especially if the rate is greater than 140. Tachycardia can mean increased myocardial oxygen consumption and initiate and/or exacerbate an infarction.

Treatment - identify and treat the underlying cause.

SINUS DYSRHYTHMIA

Etiology It is a normal finding which corresponds to respiration. In some cases it may be caused by increased vagal tone.

ECG findings in lead II

Rate	60 to 100
Rhythm	irregular, increasing and decreasing with respiration
Pacemaker site	SA node
P waves	upright and normal in shape
P-R interval	0.12 to 0.20 sec.
QRS complex	0.04 to 0.12 sec.

Clinical significance - sinus dysrhythmia is a normal phenomenon.

Treatment - none is required.

SINUS ARREST

Etiology -sinus arrest is a failure of the sinus node to initiate an electrical impulse. It may lead to prolonged interruptions in the rhythm or atrial or ventricular escape beats.

ECG findings in lead II

Rate	normal to slow depending on frequency and duration of the arrest.

Rhythm irregular
Pacemaker site SA node
P waves upright and normal in shape when present
P-R interval 0.12 to 0.20 sec.
QRS complex 0.04 to 0.12 sec.

Clinical significance - frequent or prolonged arrest may reduce cardiac output or cause syncope. The SA node may fail altogether, which may result in asystole.

Treatment - observation for the asymptomatic patient. Associated bradycardia or a symptomatic patient may require atropine - 0.5 mg every 5 minutes until relief or until 2.0 mg has been given.

WANDERING PACEMAKER

Etiology - wandering atrial pacemaker occurs when other pacemaker sites in the atria initiate the cardiac contraction. It may be caused by ischemic heart disease, atrial dilatation or may be rather benign as with the young patient or if associated with sinus dysrhythmia.

ECG findings in lead II

Rate	usually 60 to 100
Rhythm	slightly irregular
Pacemaker site	SA node, atrium, and AV junction
P waves	shape changes with location of origin
P-R interval	may vary above or below the 0.12 to 0.20 sec range.
QRS complex	0.04 to 0.12 sec.

Clinical significance - wandering atrial pacemaker is rather benign.

Treatment - none is usually required.

PREMATURE ATRIAL CONTRACTIONS (PACs)

Etiology - premature atrial contractions (PACs) can occur due to stimulant ingestion, sympathomimetic drugs, ischemic heart disease, hypoxia, digitalis toxicity or for no identifiable reason.

ECG findings in lead II

Rate	dependent upon underlying rhythm
Rhythm	usually regular except for ectopy
Pacemaker site	ectopic site in the atria
P waves	P wave of the premature contraction will vary from the normal P wave. It will also occur earlier than the expected P wave.
P-R interval	usually normal but the PAC P-R interval may be less than 0.12 sec.
QRS complex	0.04 to 0.12 sec (at times it may be longer than 0.12 or completely absent if the ventricle is refractory)

Clinical significance - if PACs are not isolated but frequent, it may indicate underlying heart disease.

Treatment - none normally required

PAROXYSMAL ATRIAL TACHYCARDIA (PAT)

Etiology - is precipitated by stress, overexertion, smoking or caffeine. It may also be related to atherosclerotic or rheumatic heart disease.

ECG findings in lead II

Rate	150 to 250
Rhythm	regular except at initiation and termination
Pacemaker site	atria
P waves	abnormal shape but it is usually buried within the preceding T wave.

P-R interval	usually normal
QRS complex	0.04 to 0.12 sec.

Clinical significance - rapid rates may reduce cardiac output, inducing angina, hypotension, or congestive heart failure.

Treatment - vagal maneuvers, verapamil 5 mg, then 10 mg (if hypotension occurs following verapamil administer 0.5 to 1.0 gm of calcium chloride).

ATRIAL FLUTTER

Etiology - atrial flutter is usually associated with organic disease. It rarely is secondary to the MI but may be related to atrial dilatation as in CHF.

ECG findings in lead II

Rate	atrial - 250 to 350
Rhythm	regular, though conduction to the ventricles may be irregular
Pacemaker site	atria
P waves	flutter waves which are sawtooth in appearance
P-R interval	usually constant
QRS complex	0.04 to 0.12

Clinical significance - as the rate of ventricular response increases above 140, the cardiac output may drop and cardiac symptoms may develop.

Treatment - for symptomatic patients cardioversion, verapamil, or vagal maneuvers may be considered.

ATRIAL FIBRILLATION

Etiology - atrial fibrillation is commonly associated with underlying heart disease and with atrial dilation secondary to congestive heart disease.

ECG findings in lead II

Rate	atrial - indiscernible, ventricular - variable
Rhythm	irregularly irregular
Pacemaker site	numerous atrial pacemakers
P waves	none discernible
P-R interval	none
QRS complex	0.04 to 0.12 sec.

Clinical significance - atrial function is lost; hence, the cardiac output may be reduced by 20 to 25 percent. There may also be a pulse deficit. The pathology may result in hypotension, angina, infarct, CHF or shock.

Treatment - cardioversion @ 75 to 100 joules (preceded by 3 to 5 mg valium in the conscious patient), verapamil 5 mg repeated at 10 mg if ineffective except in the patient with a history of bradycardia, hypotension or congestive heart failure.

PREMATURE JUNCTIONAL CONTRACTIONS (PJCs)

Etiology - premature junctional contractions can result from tobacco, caffeine, alcohol, sympathomimetic drugs, ischemic heart disease, hypoxia or digitalis toxicity. It can also be found with no underlying cause.

ECG findings in lead II

Rate	rate is dependent on the underlying rhythm.
Rhythm	rhythm is regular except for the PJCs
Pacemaker site	the ectopic pacemaker is located in the junctional tissue.
P waves	the ectopic P waves are inverted and may be found closer than 0.12 sec. to within or just after the QRS complex.
P-R interval	the P-R interval will be normal except for the junctional beat. There it will be less than 0.12 sec. or found following the QRS complex.
QRS complex	usually the QRS remains normal unless there is aberrant conduction.

Clinical significance - frequent PJCs may suggest heart disease and may precede other junctional rhythms.

Treatment - unless symptomatic, the patient is only observed.

JUNCTIONAL ESCAPE COMPLEXES and RHYTHMS

Etiology - junctional escape complexes or a junctional rhythm may be due to increased vagal tone, A-V block or a pathology of the S-A node.

ECG findings in lead II

Rate	usually 40 to 60
Rhythm	irregular with escape beats, regular with junctional rhythm.
Pacemaker site	A-V junction
P waves	inverted either immediately preceding or following the QRS
P-R interval	less than 0.12 sec. if it can be determined
QRS complex	normal at 0.04 to 0.12 sec.

Clinical significance - the rhythm may be an escape rhythm overriding a profound bradycardia. It may not be rapid enough to maintain good perfusion and may lead to angina.

Treatment - normally no treatment is required. However, in some symptomatic cases atropine may be administered in boluses of 0.5 mg every 5 minutes until 2.0 mg has been given or the rate increases.

ACCELERATED JUNCTIONAL RHYTHM

Etiology - accelerated junctional tachycardia often results from ischemia of the A-V junctional tissue.

ECG findings in lead II

Rate	greater than 60
Rhythm	regular
Pacemaker site	A-V junction
P waves	inverted if found
P-R interval	less than 0.12 if before the QRS complex
QRS complex	normal unless aberrantly conducted

Clinical significance - alone, accelerated junctional rhythm is well tolerated, though it should be watched carefully due to possible underlying ischemia.

Treatment - usually not indicated

PAROXYSMAL JUNCTIONAL TACHYCARDIA

Etiology - paroxysmal junctional tachycardia is an abruptly occurring tachycardia due to caffeine, stress, overexertion, smoking, or rheumatic or atherosclerotic heart disease.

ECG findings in lead II

Rate	100 to 180
Rhythm	regular except at beginning or termination
Pacemaker site	A-V junction
P waves	inverted if found
P-R interval	less than 0.12 sec. if found
QRS complex	normal, 0.04 to 0.12

Clinical significance - in other than the young patient, rapid rates may reduce cardiac efficiency and induce angina, hypovolemia or CHF.

Treatment - if the patient is symptomatic: vagal maneuvers, verapamil, 5 mg then 10 mg and synchronized cardioversion at 75 to 100 joules.

VENTRICULAR ESCAPE COMPLEXES and IDIOVENTRICULAR RHYTHM

Etiology - may be caused by slowing of the supraventricular pacemaker sites or high degree blocks.

ECG findings in lead II

Rate	15 to 40
Rhythm	if isolated complexes, the rhythm will be irregular; otherwise the rhythm will be regular.
Pacemaker site	ventricle
P waves	none are usually found
P-R interval	unrelated to QRS if found
QRS complex	greater than 0.12

Clinical significance - as an escape phenomenon, this rhythm may provide circulation; however, it is usually not able to maintain life.

Treatment - 0.5 mg atropine every five minutes to increased rate or 2.0 mg. Isuprel 1 mg in 500 mL of D_2W run at 2 to 6 ug/min. Epinephrine may also be considered.

PREMATURE VENTRICULAR CONTRACTIONS (PVCs)

Etiology PVCs may be caused by ischemia, hypoxia, acid-base disturbances, electrolyte imbalances, increased sympathetic tone or unknown causes.

ECG findings in lead II

Rate	dependent upon underlying rhythm and PVC rate
Rhythm	irregular
Pacemaker site	ventricle
P waves	none
P-R interval	none
QRS complex	more than 0.12 and bizarre in nature

Clinical significance - in patients with heart disease, it may indicate irritability. Significant if more than six per minute, R on T phenomenon, couplets or runs, or multifocal in nature.

Treatment - if symptomatic, oxygen, lidocaine at 1 mg/Kg then 0.5 mg/Kg every 5 minutes until 5 mg/Kg and start drip at 2-4 mg/min. Procainamide or bretylium may also be considered.

VENTRICULAR TACHYCARDIA

Etiology May be caused by cardiac ischemia, hypoxia, electrolyte imbalances, increased vagal tone and unknown reasons.

ECG findings in lead II

Rate	100 to 250
Rhythm	regular or slightly irregular
Pacemaker site	ventricle
P waves	not related to QRS if present
P-R interval	none
QRS complex	greater than 0.12 and usually bizarre

Clinical significance - results in reduced stroke volume, reduced cardiac output and may or may not perfuse.

Treatment - if perfusing consider the administration of oxygen, lidocaine 1 mg/kg then 0.5 mg/kg until a total of 3.0 mg/kg, then consider procainamide. If the patient is unstable employ cardioversion; if nonperfusing, defibrillation.

VENTRICULAR FIBRILLATION

Etiology May occur secondary to advanced coronary artery disease, R on T, etc.

ECG findings in lead II

Rate	not determinable
Rhythm	not determinable
Pacemaker site	numerous within ventricles
P waves	not determinable

P-R interval not determinable
QRS complex not determinable

Clinical significance - lethal dysrhythmia

Treatment - defibrillation at 200, then 200 to 300, then 360 joules. Epinephrine, lidocaine, bretylium and then sodium bicarbonate.

ASYSTOLE

Etiology - massive myocardial infarction, ischemia or necrosis. May also present incomplete heart block.

ECG findings in lead II

Rate	none
Rhythm	none
Pacemaker site	none
P waves	none
P-R interval	none
QRS complex	none

Clinical significance - fatal dysrhythmia

Treatment - CPR, oxygen, epinephrine, atropine, sodium bicarbonate and possible defibrillation.

ARTIFICIAL PACEMAKER RHYTHM

Etiology Pacemakers are placed to correct a dysfunction of some part of the cardiac electrical system. They may respond to need (demand) or be preset (fixed).

ECG findings in lead II

Rate	pacemaker will be regular, underlying may not be.
Rhythm	regular if preset, irregular if demand.
Pacemaker site	dependent upon electrode placement.
P waves	there may or may not be normal P waves - you will notice pacemaker spikes.
P-R interval	the P waves may or may not be related to the ventricular complexes.
QRS complex	greater than 0.12 and bizarre, and preceded by a pacemaker spike.

Clinical significance - pacemakers can fail to function, leading to the patient's underlying rhythm returning or dysfunction leading to a competing or run-away rhythm.

Treatment - transport or care for underlying rhythm.

1st DEGREE AV BLOCK

Etiology - ischemia at the A-V junction is the most common cause.

ECG findings in lead II

Rate	dependent on the underlying rhythm
Rhythm	regular
Pacemaker site	S-A node or atria
P waves	normal
P-R interval	greater than 0.21 sec.
QRS complex	normal unless aberrantly conducted

Clinical significance - generally not significant except that it may lead to a more advanced block.

Treatment - usually none is indicated.

2nd DEGREE AV BLOCK (MOBITZ I)

Etiology - common causes include ischemia at the A-V junction, increased parasympathetic tone, and drugs.

ECG findings in lead II

Rate	atrial rate is more apid than the ventricular rate.
Rhythm	atrial rhythm is regular, ventricular is irregular.
Pacemaker site	atria, though some beats are blocked
P waves	normal
P-R interval	lengthens until a ventricular beat is missed
QRS complex	0.12 or less and normal unless aberrantly conducted.

Clinical significance - may reducc cardiac output and induce syncope and angina.

Treatment - if symptomatic, 0.5 mg atropine every five minutes until dysrhythmia abates or 2.0 mg have been given. Isuprel may be required.

2nd DEGREE AV BLOCK (MOBITZ II)

Etiology - usually associated with infarction or necrosis.

ECG findings in lead II

Rate	atrial rate more rapid than the ventricular rate
Rhythm	atrial rate regular, ventricular rate regularly irregular
Pacemaker site	atria or S-A node
P waves	normal
P-R interval	constant for conducted beats but may be more than 0.20 sec.
QRS complex	normal unless aberrantly conducted

Clinical significance - may compromise cardiac output and cause syncope and angina. Since it is related to necrosis the patient should be carefully monitored.

Treatment - if symptomatic, atropine at 0.5 mg every five minutes until increased ventricular rate or 2.0 mg. Isoproterenol drip or epinephrine may be required.

3rd DEGREE AV BLOCK

Etiology - may result from an acute MI, digitalis toxicity or degeneration of the conduction system.

ECG findings in lead II

Rate	atrial rate (60 to 100) and ventricular rate (15 to 40) are different
Rhythm	atrial and ventricular both regular but different
Pacemaker site	A-V junction or ventricles
P waves	normal but not related to QRS
P-R interval	no relationship between P wave and QRS
QRS complex	normal if pacemaker is at junction, longer than 0.12 if pacemaker is in the ventricles.

Clinical significance - can severely compromise the cardiac output because of slow rate and lack of coordination with the atria.

Treatment - if symptomatic, atropine 0.5 mg every five minutes until rate increases or 2.0 mg. Isoproterenol drip or epinephrine are usually required.

DISTURBANCES in VENTRICULAR CONDUCTION

Etiology - the ventricular response to electrical stimuli can be aberrantly conducted due to injury or defect in the bundle of His, bundle branches or the Perkinje system. These disturbances may be caused by ischemia, necrosis or a refractory pathway from a previous contraction.

ECG findings in lead II

Rate	based on the underlying rhythm
Rhythm	based on the underlying rhythm
Pacemaker site	based on the underlying rhythm

P waves	based on the underlying rhythm.
P-R interval	based on the underlying rhythm.
QRS complex	greater than 0.12 and bizarre

Clinical significance - the significance of aberrant conduction cannot be determined in the field.

Treatment - treat the underlying rhythm and patient symptoms.

PRE-EXCITATION SYNDROMES

Etiology - pre-excitation syndromes are caused by accessory pathways of conduction which induce a retrograde electrical path.

ECG findings in lead II

Rate	usually rapid
Rhythm	regularly irregular
Pacemaker site	S-A node or atria
P waves	usually normal
P-R interval	less than 0.12
QRS complex	greater than 0.12

Clinical significance - usually not significant unless underlying heart disease or pathology.

Treatment - treat any underlying rhythm and patient symptoms.

DYSRHYTHMIA RECOGNITION

It is helpful to apply a systematic analysis when evaluating dysrhythmias. The following order, and items of analysis, may help you consistently identify dysrhythmias.

Rate:	Determine the overall and underlying rate of the QRS complexes.
Rhythm:	Determine if the rate is regular, slightly irregular, regularly irregular or irregularly irregular.
P wave:	Determine if P waves are present and whether they are upright and rounded.
P-R interval:	Determine its length and if it is consistent.
QRS complex:	Determine the width of the QRS complex and its general shape.

Once the above items have been identified, they should be used to determine the dysrhythmia which is occurring. Compare each item to the criteria for the dysrhythmia you suspect. If all the criteria are met, then it is likely that it is that rhythm.

The next 24 rhythms are relatively classic ECG strips. They are uncomplicated and should be reasonably simple to analyze.

DYSRHYTHMIA RECOGNITION EXERCISE - A

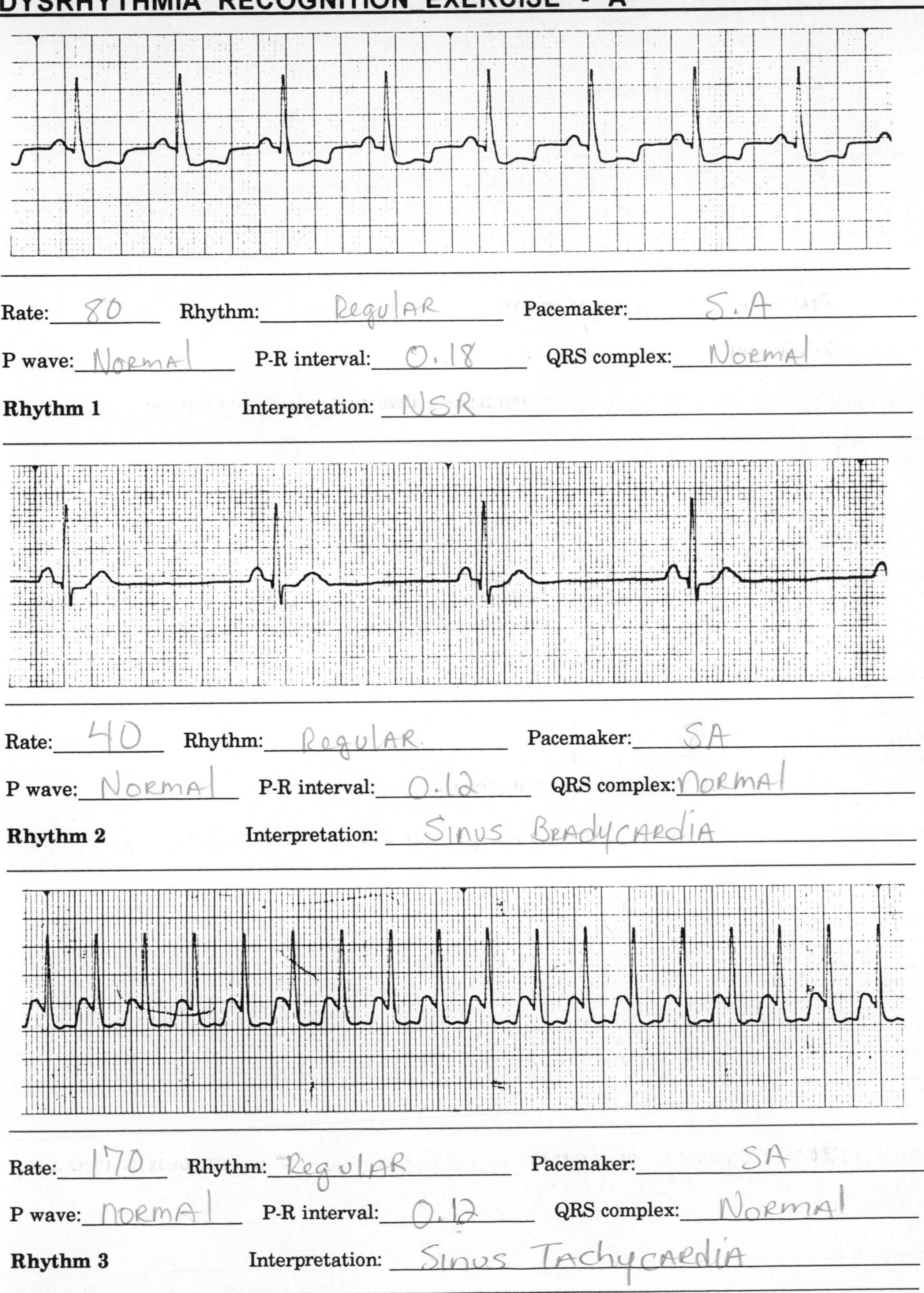

Rate: 80 Rhythm: Regular Pacemaker: S.A

P wave: Normal P-R interval: 0.18 QRS complex: Normal

Rhythm 1 Interpretation: NSR

Rate: 40 Rhythm: Regular Pacemaker: SA

P wave: Normal P-R interval: 0.12 QRS complex: Normal

Rhythm 2 Interpretation: Sinus Bradycardia

Rate: 170 Rhythm: Regular Pacemaker: SA

P wave: Normal P-R interval: 0.12 QRS complex: Normal

Rhythm 3 Interpretation: Sinus Tachycardia

DYSRHYTHMIA RECOGNITION EXERCISE - A (cont.)

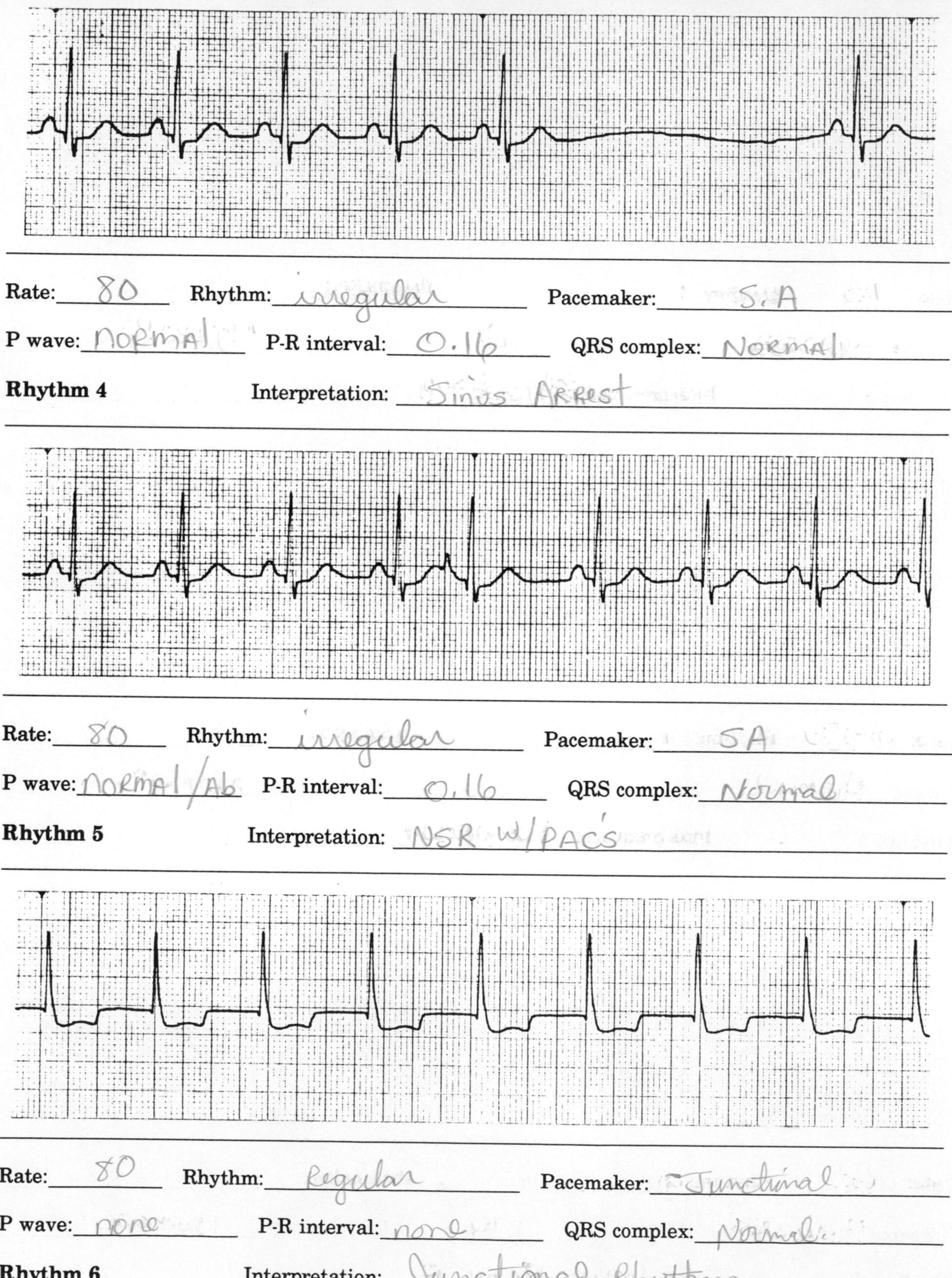

Rate: 80 Rhythm: irregular Pacemaker: S.A

P wave: normal P-R interval: 0.16 QRS complex: Normal

Rhythm 4 Interpretation: Sinus Arrest

Rate: 80 Rhythm: irregular Pacemaker: SA

P wave: normal/Ab P-R interval: 0.16 QRS complex: Normal

Rhythm 5 Interpretation: NSR w/PAC's

Rate: 80 Rhythm: Regular Pacemaker: Junctional

P wave: none P-R interval: none QRS complex: Normal

Rhythm 6 Interpretation: Junctional Rhythm

DYSRHYTHMIA RECOGNITION EXERCISE - A (cont.)

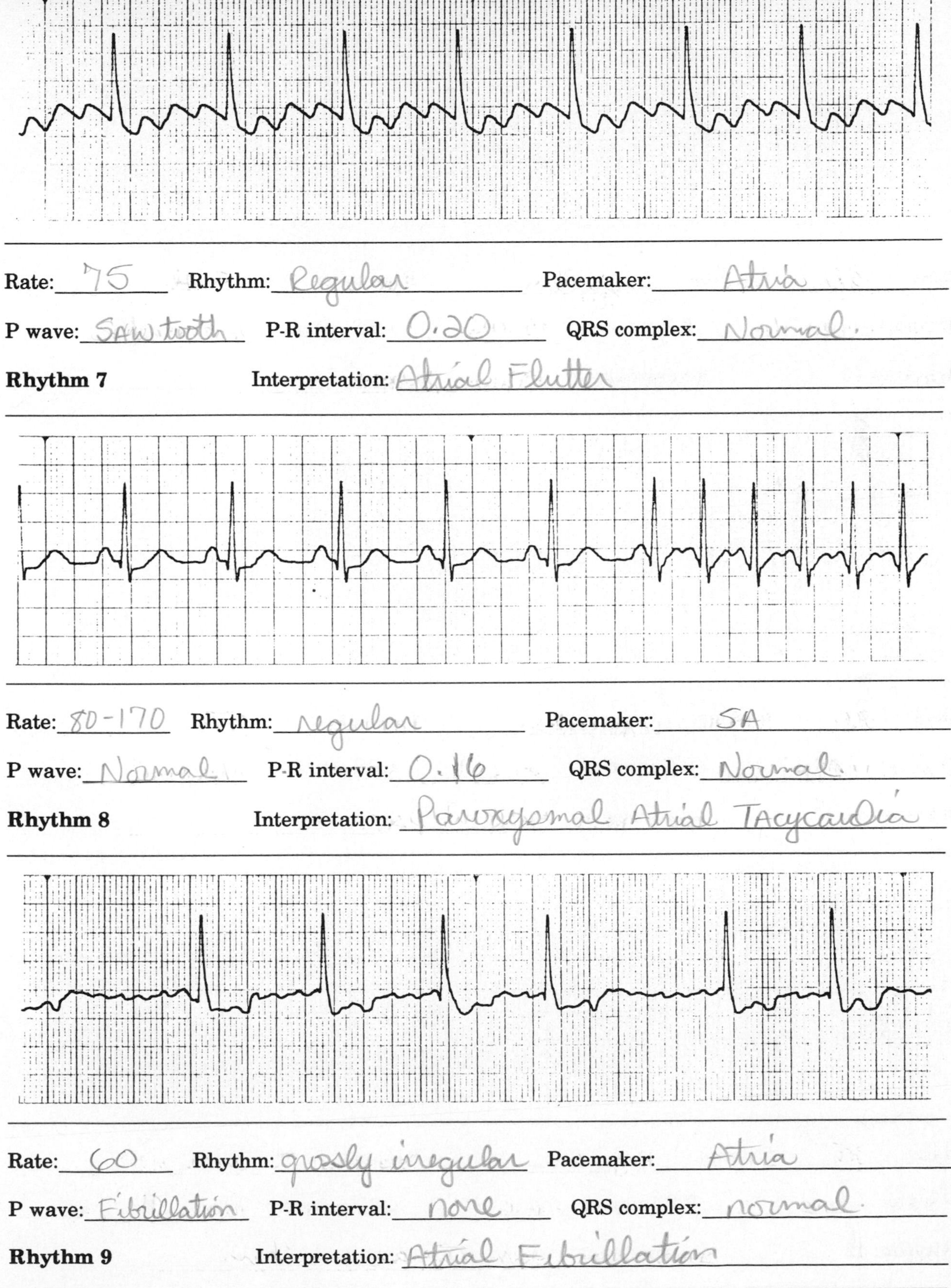

Rate: 75 Rhythm: Regular Pacemaker: Atria

P wave: SAW tooth P-R interval: 0.20 QRS complex: Normal.

Rhythm 7 Interpretation: Atrial Flutter

Rate: 80-170 Rhythm: regular Pacemaker: SA

P wave: Normal P-R interval: 0.16 QRS complex: Normal.

Rhythm 8 Interpretation: Paroxysmal Atrial TAcycardia

Rate: 60 Rhythm: grossly irregular Pacemaker: Atria

P wave: Fibrillation P-R interval: none QRS complex: normal.

Rhythm 9 Interpretation: Atrial Fibrillation

DYSRHYTHMIA RECOGNITION EXERCISE - A (cont.)

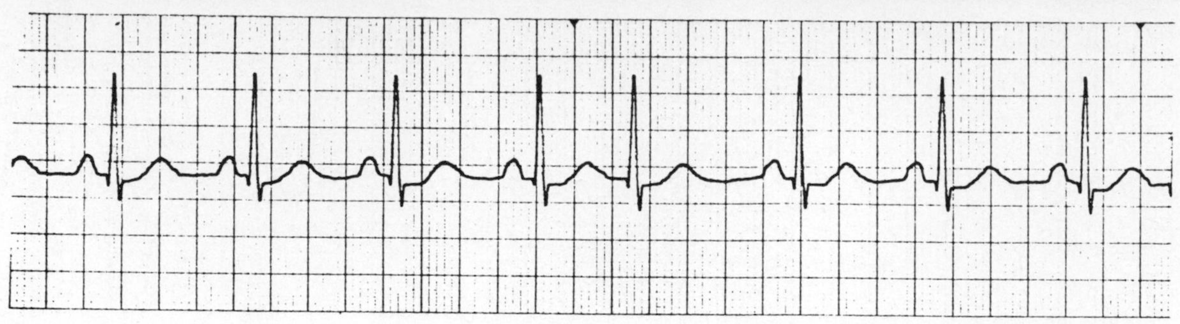

Rate: 80 Rhythm: irregular Pacemaker: SA-AV Junctions

P wave: normal/none P-R interval: 0.16 QRS complex: normal

Rhythm 10 Interpretation: NSR w/PACS

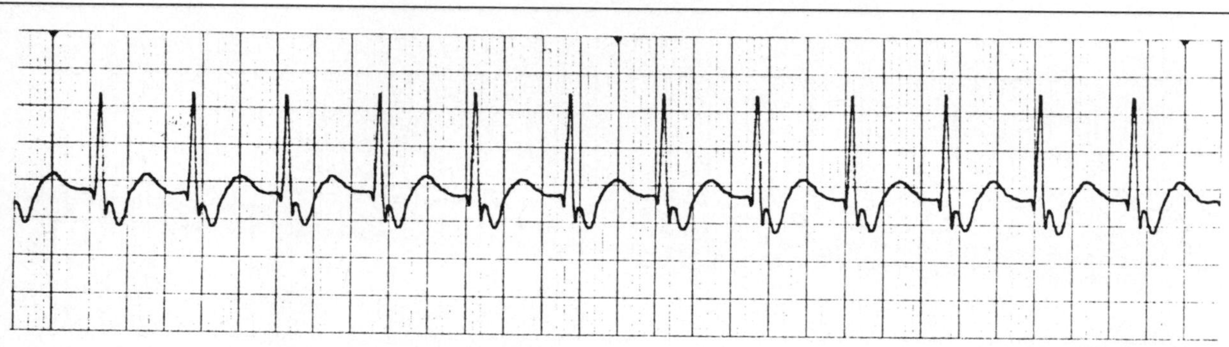

Rate: 120 Rhythm: regular Pacemaker: A-V Junction

P wave: none P-R interval: none QRS complex: normal

Rhythm 11 Interpretation: Accelerated Junctional Tachy.

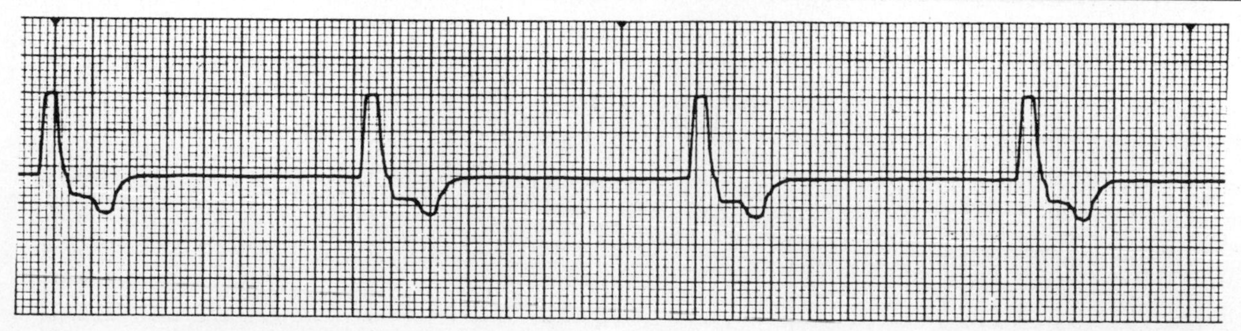

Rate: 35 Rhythm: regular Pacemaker: Pacemaker Ventricles

P wave: none P-R interval: none QRS complex: wide 0.14

Rhythm 12 Interpretation: Idioventricular Rhythm

DYSRHYTHMIA RECOGNITION EXERCISE - A (cont.)

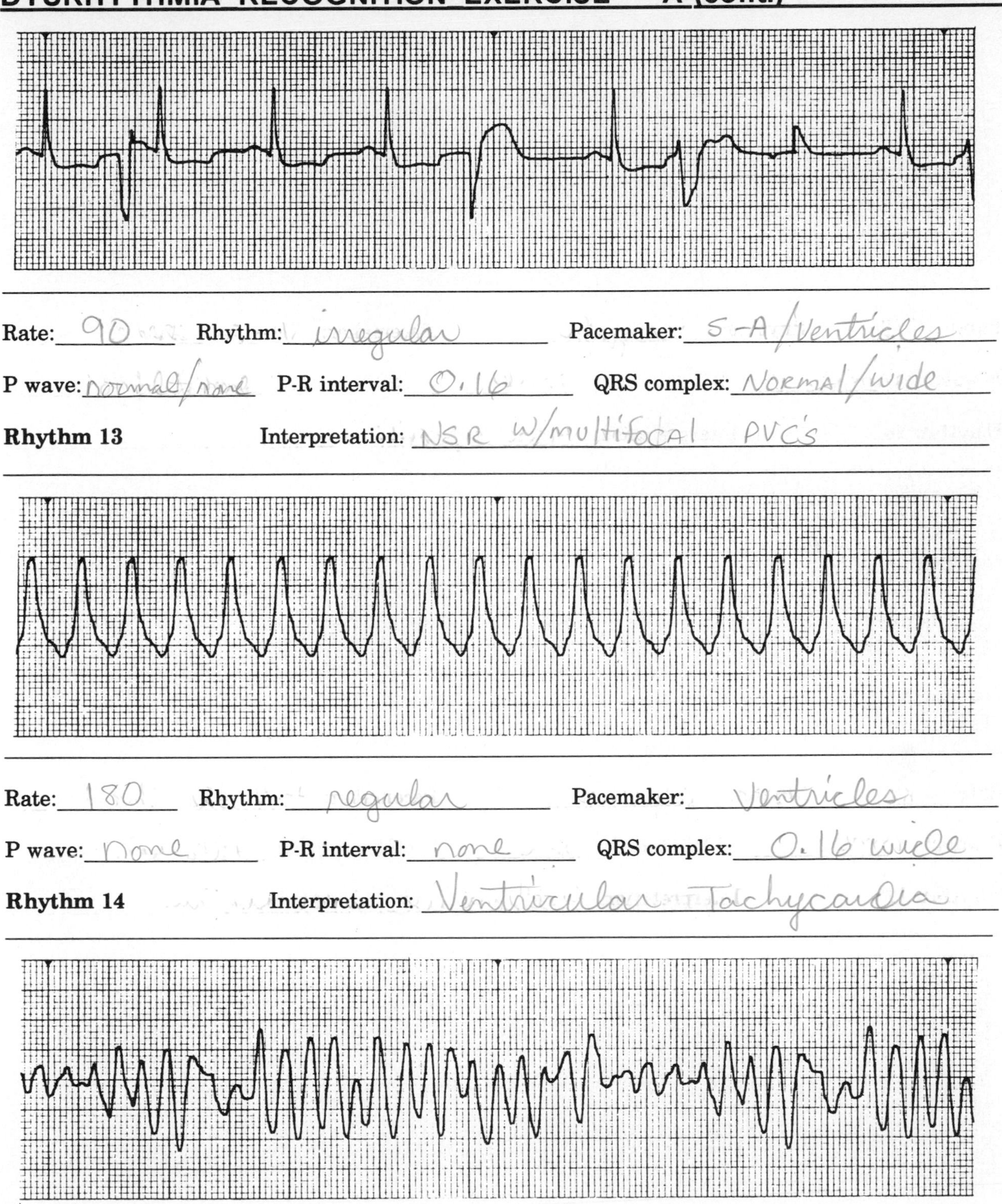

Rate: 90 Rhythm: irregular Pacemaker: S-A/Ventricles

P wave: normal/none P-R interval: 0.16 QRS complex: NORMAL/wide

Rhythm 13 Interpretation: NSR w/multifocal PVC's

Rate: 180 Rhythm: regular Pacemaker: Ventricles

P wave: none P-R interval: none QRS complex: 0.16 wide

Rhythm 14 Interpretation: Ventricular Tachycardia

Rate: none Rhythm: none Pacemaker: Ventricles

P wave: none P-R interval: none QRS complex: Fibrillation

Rhythm 15 Interpretation: Course Ventricular Fibrillation

DYSRHYTHMIA RECOGNITION EXERCISE - A (cont.)

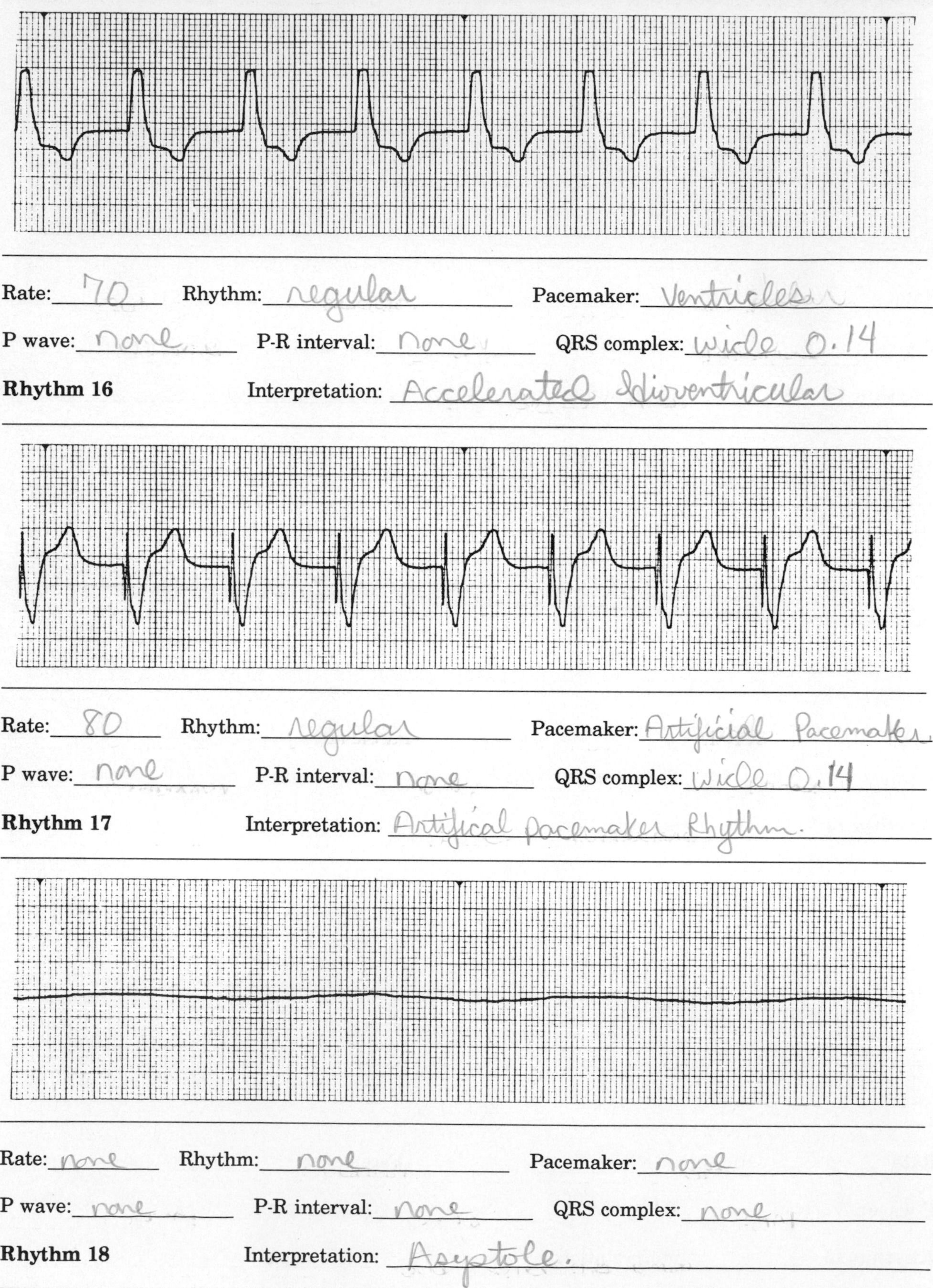

Rate: 70 Rhythm: regular Pacemaker: Ventricles

P wave: none P-R interval: none QRS complex: wide 0.14

Rhythm 16 Interpretation: Accelerated Idioventricular

Rate: 80 Rhythm: regular Pacemaker: Artificial Pacemaker

P wave: none P-R interval: none QRS complex: wide 0.14

Rhythm 17 Interpretation: Artifical pacemaker Rhythm.

Rate: none Rhythm: none Pacemaker: none

P wave: none P-R interval: none QRS complex: none

Rhythm 18 Interpretation: Asystole.

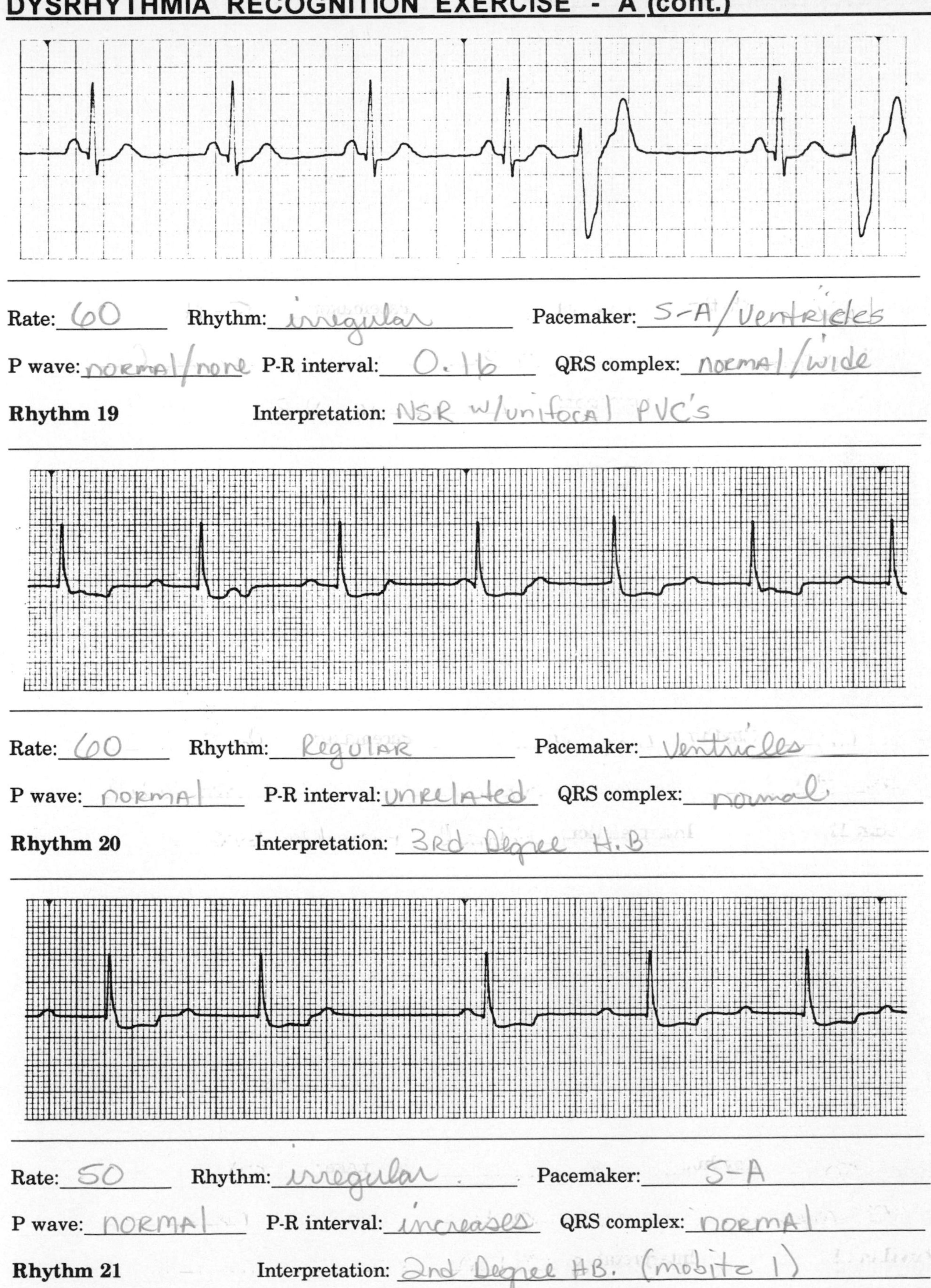

DYSRHYTHMIA RECOGNITION EXERCISE - A (cont.)

Rate: 60 Rhythm: irregular Pacemaker: S-A/Ventricles

P wave: normal/none P-R interval: 0.16 QRS complex: normal/wide

Rhythm 19 Interpretation: NSR w/unifocal PVC's

Rate: 60 Rhythm: Regular Pacemaker: Ventricles

P wave: normal P-R interval: unrelated QRS complex: normal

Rhythm 20 Interpretation: 3rd Degree H.B

Rate: 50 Rhythm: irregular Pacemaker: S-A

P wave: normal P-R interval: increases QRS complex: normal

Rhythm 21 Interpretation: 2nd Degree HB. (mobitz 1)

DYSRHYTHMIA RECOGNITION EXERCISE - A (cont.)

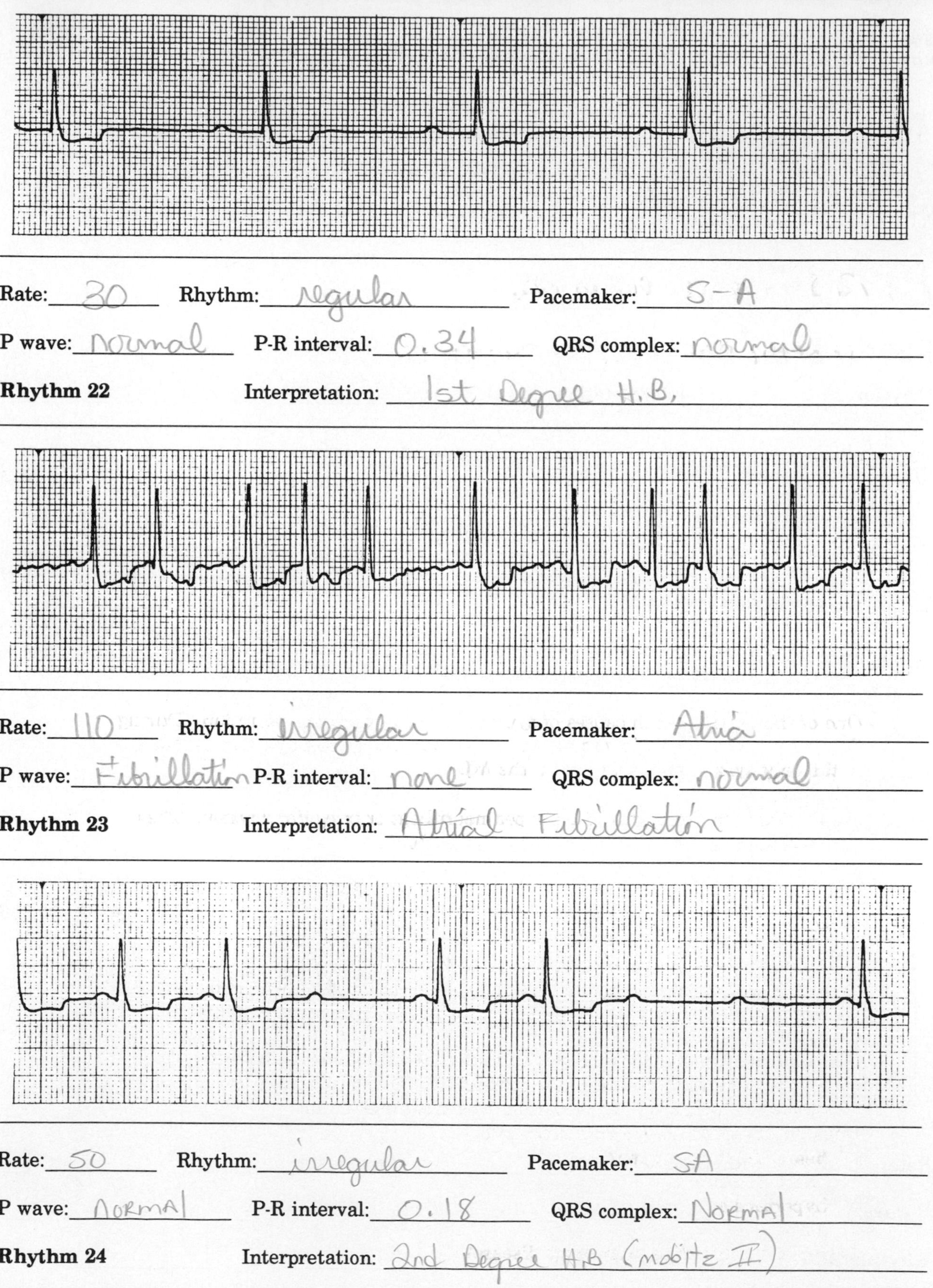

Rate: 30 Rhythm: regular Pacemaker: S-A

P wave: normal P-R interval: 0.34 QRS complex: normal

Rhythm 22 Interpretation: 1st Degree H.B.

Rate: 110 Rhythm: irregular Pacemaker: Atria

P wave: Fibrillation P-R interval: none QRS complex: normal

Rhythm 23 Interpretation: Atrial Fibrillation

Rate: 50 Rhythm: irregular Pacemaker: SA

P wave: NORMAL P-R interval: 0.18 QRS complex: NORMAL

Rhythm 24 Interpretation: 2nd Degree H.B (mobitz II)

2I

CARDIOVASCULAR EMERGENCIES

Part III - (pages 683 to 721)

Review of the Objectives for Chapter 2I

After reading this chapter, you should be able to:

23. Name common chief complaints of cardiac patients.

p. 683

Pain

The cardiac patient will most likely present with a dull pain substernally and referred pain radiating into the shoulder, neck, jaw and epigastrium. The pain will generally be dull, constant and range in intensity from just discomfort to severe and debilitating.

Dyspnea

Dyspnea is often associated with the myocardial infarction. It is frequently secondary to pulmonary congestion because of reduced cardiac output.

Syncope

One of the most common causes of syncope is the myocardial infarction. During the heart attack, blood flow to the brain is interrupted. Syncope may be one of the only symptoms presenting in the MI.

Palpitations

Palpitations are sensations of a skipped heart beat or irregular rhythm. They may represent an irritable heart and a dysrhythmia.

24. Describe the appropriate history and physical assessment goals for cardiac patients.

pp. 683 to 688

History

Is the patient taking prescription medications regularly?

Many medications are prescribed for cardiac and related conditions. Their identification can help determine a contributing history or the present problem.

Is the patient currently under treatment for any serious illness?

Current or recent illnesses may contribute to the development of medical problems, including the myocardial infarction and angina.

Does the patient have any history of:

heart attack or angina?
heart failure?
hypertension?
diabetes?
chronic obstructive pulmonary disease?

Does the patient have any allergies?

Any allergy might necessitate careful observation when medications are administered, or the use of alternate drugs.

Physical Assessment

Skin color is a good reflector of peripheral perfusion. It will give a subjective indication of oxygenation.

Capillary refill is a good indicator of tissue perfusion, cardiac output and peripheral resistance.

Jugular vein distention in the semi-seated or seated patient JVD is a good indicator of increased venous pressure; associated with congestive heart failure, right heart failure, etc.

Peripheral or presacral edema found in the dependent areas or behind and above the sacrum reflect heart failure and systemic edema.

Breath sounds may reveal rales, rhonchi or wheezes occurring as fluid backs up in the pulmonary circulation during congestive heart failure.

Heart sounds may reveal anomalies such as valve dysfunction.

Carotid artery bruit will provide evidence of the atherosclerotic process.

Pulse may reveal evidence of an irregular cardiac rhythm or of missed beats when examined with the ECG.

Pulse oximetry may reveal low or erratic values as peripheral vasoconstriction or low flow states occur.

Vital signs may reflect the pathology. The pulse may be bradycardic, tachycardic or irregular. Blood pressure may be hypotensive, normotensive or hypertensive. Respiration may be rapid and shallow.

25. Describe the pathophysiology of atherosclerosis.

pp. 688 to 689

Atherosclerosis is a progressive, degenerative disease of the medium and large arteries. It specifically attacks the aorta and its branches and the coronary and cerebral arteries. It results in fatty deposits collecting under the intimal layer of the artery. The site undergoes inflammation, swelling and, finally, calcium is deposited, forming a plaque. Further injury can occur within the plaque, causing enlargement and partial obstruction of blood flow. As the disease process continues, the entire blood vessel may become occluded.

26. List the major risk factors for atherosclerosis.

p. 689

Modifiable	**Nonmodifiable**
Hypertension	Male gender
Smoking	Advanced age
Elevated blood lipids	Family history
Lack of exercise	Diabetes mellitus

27. Describe the pathophysiology, signs, symptoms, and management of the following patient problems.

pp. 689 to 704

ANGINA PECTORIS

Pathophysiology - angina, or substernal chest pain, occurs transiently when the coronary circulation cannot meet the heart's need for oxygenated circulation. The disease is usually related to stress and abates with rest (stable angina). It may, however, come on with no exertion (unstable angina) and then reflects more arterial restriction. Unstable angina is a precursor to myocardial infarction.

Signs - the angina patient may present with anxiety and diaphoresis. The patient may also display cardiac dysrhythmias.

Symptoms - the patient experiencing angina will often complain of substernal or epigastric pain or discomfort. They may also report that the pain radiates to the shoulder, arm, neck, jaw, or back.

Management - calm and reassure the patient and reduce any stress, either physical or psychological, which he or she may be experiencing. Administer high flow oxygen and nitroglycerin by spray or tablet. Nifedipine may also be indicated. Monitor the ECG, carefully observe the patient and presume this is a myocardial infarction.

ACUTE MYOCARDIAL INFARCTION

Pathophysiology - the myocardial infarction is the death of a portion of the myocardium. It is due to blockage or severe restriction of a coronary artery by a thrombus, emboli or vascular spasm. The myocardium is without oxygen, becomes hypoxic, ischemic and finally necrotic. During the process, the area involved may become irritable and cause dysrhythmias. The myocardial infarction may lead to congestive heart failure, cardiogenic shock and sudden death.

Signs - the signs of the MI include diaphoresis and pallor. The patient may display cardiac dysrhythmias or other ECG changes.

Symptoms - the most common symptom associated with the myocardial infarction is substernal or epigastric pain. The pain may radiate to the shoulder, arm, neck, jaw and back. Some patients, especially the elderly, who experience the MI have no pain at all. Associated symptoms include anxiety, nausea, vomiting, weakness or malaise, and dyspnea.

Management - includes calming and reassuring the patient and limiting any physical exertion. The patient should receive high flow oxygen, an IV line for medications and cardiac monitoring. The following drugs may be considered for administration: nitroglycerin, morphine sulfate or nalbuphine, nitrous oxide, diazepam, lidocaine, procainamide, atropine, isoproterenol, epinephrine, verapamil and bretylium; dependent on the patient's presentation and local protocol.

LEFT VENTRICULAR FAILURE with PULMONARY EDEMA

Pathophysiology - left ventricular failure results in less blood being pumped from the pulmonary circulation by the left ventricle than is pumped into it by the right. Blood backs up in the pulmonary circulation, the pulmonary blood pressure rises and pulmonary edema may develop.

Signs - the patient may experience a productive cough with pink frothy sputum. The patient may have jugular vein distention as well as rales, rhonchi or respiratory wheezes. Vital signs may be normal and there may be dysrhythmias.

Symptoms - the patient may complain of anxiety, dyspnea and may report paroxysmal nocturnal dyspnea. The patient may have a history of a myocardial infarction, may have signs and symptoms of an evolving MI or may have no cardiac signs at all.

Management - calm and reassure the patient, administer high flow oxygen and let the patient sit with his or her feet dangling. Apply rotating venous tourniquets and initiate an IV for venous access. Consider the medications listed for the myocardial infarction and additionally, morphine sulfate (for its hemodynamic properties), nitroglycerin, furosemide, aminophylline, and dobutamine. Treat underlying dysrhythmias and transport rapidly.

RIGHT VENTRICULAR FAILURE

Pathophysiology - right ventricular failure results in blood backing up in the systemic circulation. As the blood backs up in the systemic circulation, the venous pressure rises and edema begins in the peripheral tissues. Right ventricular failure can be caused by left ventricular failure, pulmonary hypertension, myocardial infarction and pulmonary emboli.

Signs - signs include tachycardia, jugular vein distention and liver engorgement. Peripheral edema is a classic sign, especially in the dependent areas. It may be pitting in nature and found systemically including the abdomen (acites), the pericardium and the pleural space.

Symptoms - the patient may complain of the classic signs of the myocardial infarction or those of left heart failure. The history may include the use of digitalis or furosemide or conditions such as an "enlarged" or "weak heart."

Management - right heart failure alone is not usually the dire emergency that the acute MI or left heart failure is. Care should include calming and reassurance, moderate to high flow oxygen, an IV line for medications and monitoring for any associated dysrhythmias.

CARDIOGENIC SHOCK

Pathophysiology - cardiogenic shock is an acute emergency due to the heart's inability to meet the perfusion demands of the body, despite resuscitative measures. It is usually associated with a severe myocardial infarction and carries a poor prognosis.

Signs - cardiogenic shock presents with the signs of the MI which are accompanied by the signs of severe shock. The patient's blood pressure is low and the level of consciousness is often altered. The patient will have cool, clammy and ashen or pale skin, very poor capillary refill and tachycardia. The ECG may show sinus tachycardia or other dysrhythmia.

Symptoms - the patient may display the same symptoms as for the myocardial infarction.

Management - the prognosis for cardiogenic shock is poor and the management is difficult. Rapid transport should be considered with high flow oxygen, an IV line and ECG monitoring. Medications which may be used include: dopamine, norepinephrine, morphine sulfate and furosemide. The PASG may be indicated by protocol in certain cases.

CARDIAC ARREST/SUDDEN DEATH

Pathophysiology - sudden death is a cardiac arrest that occurs within one hour of the onset of cardiac symptoms. In many cases of death, a myocardial infarction is not found, leading authorities to believe a lethal dysrhythmia may be the cause. Sudden death may also be caused by: drowning, electrocution, electrolyte imbalance, acid-base imbalance, drug intoxication, hypoxia, hypothermia, trauma, etc.

Signs - apnea, pulselessness, unresponsiveness are cardinal signs of cardiac arrest.

Symptoms - unresponsiveness

Management - follows the arrest algorithm as set forth by the American Heart Association in their standards for basic and advanced cardiac life support.

PULSELESS ELECTRICAL ACTIVITY (PEA)

Pathophysiology - pulseless electrical activity is a failure of the heart to respond to the electrical impulses of the cardiac electrical pathway. It may be caused by massive myocardial damage, hypovolemia, electrolyte imbalance, cardiac rupture, cardiac tamponade, and acute pulmonary emboli. The prognosis for PEA is grave.

Signs - apnea, pulselessness, and unresponsiveness are cardinal signs of electromechanical dissociation.

Symptoms - unresponsiveness

Management - the management for PEA follows the standards of the American Heart Association for pulseless electrical activity. Should an etiology such as hypovolemia be suspected, treat the underlying problem aggressively.

ABDOMINAL AORTIC ANEURYSM

Pathophysiology - the abdominal aortic aneurysm most commonly involves the abdominal aorta between the renal arteries and the bifurcation of the common iliac arteries. It is much more common in men, especially those between the ages of ages 60 to 70 years.

Signs - hypotension, pulsatile mass, decreased lower extremity pulses and possible GI bleeding are all signs associated with the abdominal aortic aneurysm.

Symptoms The patient may complain of a tearing sensation in the abdomen, back or flank, numbness and tingling in the lower extremities, and possibly the urge to defecate.

Management Treat the patient for shock and expedite transport. Oxygen should be applied at high flow and IVs should be initiated and fluids prepared to run rapidly. PASG may be considered.

DISSECTING AORTIC ANEURYSM

Pathophysiology - a small tear in the aorta, commonly just after the aorta leaves the heart, allows blood to enter. Once the dissection begins, it may extend all the way to the abdominal aorta. The disruption of the vessel can involve the coronary arteries, the aortic valve, subclavian arteries and the carotid arteries. The dissecting aortic aneurysm may cause syncope, stroke, pericardial tamponade or acute myocardial infarction.

Signs - may include hypertension, pulse deficit between the upper extremities and a shocky looking patient.

Symptoms - the patient may complain of a ripping or tearing sensation. It is commonly substernal but may radiate to the back. The patient may experience numbness and tingling in the extremities, most commonly the left.

Management - patient care focuses on rapid transport with special care not to jostle the patient and to keep him or her calm. IVs with crystalloid should be started in anticipation of rapid fluid loss. Trauma tubing should be used and pressure infusers and a PASG should be ready.

ACUTE ARTERIAL OCCLUSION

Pathophysiology - acute arterial occlusion is a sudden occlusion of arterial blood flow to an area due to trauma, thrombosis, tumor or embolus. The occlusion will obstruct the arterial flow to the supplied tissue, causing hypoxia, ischemia and necrosis.

Signs - the area involved, such as an extremity, may become ashen or mottled, cool and clammy, and may be pulseless.

Symptoms - the patient will most commonly complain of severe pain and, if not pain, paresthesia.

Management - should be aggressive only if it involves the mesentery. Oxygen, IVs and the PASG should be prepared while the vital signs are monitored for the signs of developing shock. If the occlusion involves an extremity the patient should be carefully monitored and rapidly transported to definitive care.

ACUTE PULMONARY EMBOLUS

Pathophysiology Acute pulmonary embolism is a clot or other obstructing particle which traveled to the pulmonary circulation from the systemic circulation or from the heart. It blocks the blood flow through the lung and increases pulmonary vascular resistance. It will result in decreased gas exchange.

Signs The patient may display labored breathing, tachypnea, and tachycardia. If the occlusion is significant, the patient may experience the signs and symptoms of right heart failure. The patient may present with rapid deep breathing which may mimic hyperventilation.

Symptoms The patient may complain of sudden dyspnea which may be severe and may be accompanied by pain. They may have a history of prolonged bed rest or immobility, recent surgery or fracture, or phlebitis.

Management Care should concentrate on airway and respiratory care. The patient should receive high flow oxygen via the nonrebreather mask. An IV should be initiated.

DEEP VENOUS THROMBOPHLEBITIS

Pathophysiology - thrombophlebitis is clotting within a vein, usually of the lower extremities. The calf and thigh are most commonly involved. The patient with venous thrombophlebitis may develop pulmonary emboli.

Signs - the patient may present with a limb which is warm, reddened and tender to palpation. The limb may be swollen.

Symptoms - the patient often complains of increasing pain and tenderness.

Management - is directed at rapid transport with supportive care offered enroute.

VARICOSE VEINS

Pathophysiology - varicose veins are dilated superficial veins found in dependent areas, usually the lower extremities. When they rupture they are sometimes accompanied by heavy bleeding.

Signs - the patient will present with moderate blood loss from the rupture of a lower extremity vessel.

Symptoms - the patient will have a history of enlarged superficial veins and swelling and discomfort.

Management - the bleeding can easily be controlled with direct pressure.

PERIPHERAL ARTERIAL ATHEROSCLEROTIC DISEASE

Pathophysiology - chronic peripheral arterial insufficiency is the result of the progression of atherosclerosis. The arterial vessels fail to provide sufficient oxygenated circulation to the distal area, usually an extremity. The end product may be anginal-like pain in the affected area, ulcers or gangrene.

Signs - the patient may display muscle cramping and stiffness in the affected area.

Symptoms - the patient may complain of pain, especially on exertion.

Management - emergency care is limited to transport with care offered to protect the affected area.

HYPERTENSIVE EMERGENCIES

Pathophysiology - a hypertensive emergency is an extreme rise in blood pressure which may threaten life. The pathology in some cases may lead to left ventricular failure.

Signs - the patient may display restlessness, confusion, paralysis, seizures and coma.

Symptoms - the patient will often complain of severe headache, nausea, vomiting, and blurred vision.

Management - patient care includes keeping the patient quiet, administer oxygen, and start an IV. The first line drug is nifedipine. Diazoxide, sodium nitroprusside and labetolol may also be considered to reduce the blood pressure.

28. Describe some common drugs used in cardiovascular emergencies.

pp. 710 to 712

Please review the following drugs from the drug flash cards found at the back of this workbook

atropine sulfate
procainamide
adenosine
epinephrine
isoproterenol
dobutamine
nitrous oxide
morphine sulfate
diazepam
lidocaine
bretylium
verapamil
norepinephrine
dopamine
oxygen
nitroglycerine
furosemide

29. Describe the indications for and the use of the following techniques.

pp. 712 to 721

ECG monitoring should be applied any time the patient may experience any dysrhythmia including: respiratory problems, cardiac problems, severe trauma, stroke, CNS problems and any case where advanced life support skills are applied. The ECG should not be used alone but with all the elements of patient assessment.

Precordial thump is used to stimulate a depolarization within the heart and allow it to resume normal function. It is delivered to a monitored patient who is in ventricular fibrillation. A thump is delivered to the sternum from 10 to 12 inches with the wrist and arm parallel to the long axis of the sternum.

Defibrillation is indicated in the patient who is in pulseless ventricular fibrillation or in nonperfusing ventricular tachycardia. The defibrillator is set to deliver three progressive discharges of 200 joules, 200 to 300 joules and then 360 joules. Modestly jelled paddles are placed on the upper anterior right chest and the left lower lateral chest with firm pressure. When all personnel are safely clear of the patient and adjacent metal, the defibrillator is discharged.

Cardioversion is indicated for perfusing ventricular tachycardia, paroxysmal tachycardia, rapid atrial fibrillation and 2:1 atrial flutter. It is delivered as defibrillation except that is synchronized with the R wave and with energy levels from 50 to 360 joules. The R waves are detected through lead electrodes. Discharge is accomplished by pressing the discharge buttons until the cardioversion energy is delivered.

Carotid sinus massage is indicated for symptomatic paroxysmal supraventricular tachycardia. This procedure is attempted in the patient without carotid bruits by firmly massaging the artery high on the neck for no longer than 15 to 20 seconds while monitoring the ECG.

Transcutaneous cardiac pacing is used in the patient with symptomatic bradycardia such that occur with high degree A-V blocks, atrial fibrillation, etc. The procedure involves monitoring the patient, applying the electrodes, setting the rate (usually 60 to 80), and gradually increasing the voltage until the patient's heart responds.

READING COMPREHENSION SELF-EXAM

21. The first positive deflection of the QRS complex is the ....

    A. R wave.
    B. P wave.
    C. Q wave.
    D. S wave.
    E. T wave.

Answer A

22. The normal P-R interval is ....

    A. 0.04 to 0.12 sec.
    B. 0.10 to 0.20 sec.
    C. 0.12 to 0.20 sec.
    D. 0.20 to 0.24 sec.
    E. none of the above.

Answer C

23. The period in which the myocardium will not respond to stimulation is called the ....

    A. general refractory period.
    B. absolute refractory period.
    C. relative refractory period.
    D. depolarization period.
    E. repolarization period.

Answer B

24. Tachycardia is generally any cardiac rate above ....

    A. 60 beats per minute.
    B. 100 beats per minute.
    C. 120 beats per minutes.
    D. 140 beats per minutes.
    E. none of the above.

Answer B

25. Peripheral edema may be extreme and depress with moderate digital pressure. If the depression remains after the finger is removed it is said to be ....

    A. pitting edema.
    B. cardiogenic edema.
    C. pathologic edema.
    D. dependent edema.
    E. subtle edema.

Answer A

26. Left ventricular failure with pulmonary edema may produce a patient who has which of the following breath sounds on auscultation?

    A. rales
    B. wheezes
    C. rhonchi
    D. all of the above
    E. none of the above

Answer D

27. Dysrhythmias can be caused by which of the following?
    1. hypothermia
    2. hypoxia
    3. acidosis
    4. electrolyte imbalance
    5. myocardial contusion
    6. ischemia

    Select the proper grouping.

    A. 1, 2, 4, 6
    B. 2, 4, 5, 6
    C. 1, 2, 3, 4
    D. 1, 3, 4, 5, 6
    E. 1, 2, 3, 4, 5, 6

    Answer E

28. A carotid bruit is normally the result of decreased cardiac output caused by a dysrhythmia.

    A. True
    B. False

    Answer B

29. Angina is a cardiac-related condition that is milder in presentation than the true myocardial infarction. Hence it is moderately easy to differentiate between the two.

    A. True
    B. False

    Answer B

30. Angina that presents without exertion is referred to as ....

    A. unstable angina.
    B. stable angina.
    C. preinfarction angina.
    D. Prinzmetal's angina.
    E. A and C.

    Answer E

31. The primary drug used to treat angina in the field setting (after oxygen) is ....

    A. nifedipine.
    B. nitroglycerin.
    C. epinephrine.
    D. Procardia.
    E. none of the above.

    Answer B

32. The most common cause of death resulting from myocardial infarction is ....

    A. valvular failure.
    B. muscle loss.
    C. cardiac rupture.
    D. dysrhythmia.
    E. none of the above.

    Answer D

33. Some acute myocardial infarction patients experience no symptoms at all.

A. True
B. False

Answer A

34. During acute myocardial infarction the patient blood pressure is expected to be ....

A. elevated.
B. normal.
C. lowered.
D. any of the above.
E. B or C.

Answer D

35. The only contraindication to high flow oxygen for the heart attack patient is ....

A. suspected hyperventilation.
B. chronic obstructive pulmonary disease.
C. clear lung sounds.
D. numbness and tingling in the fingers and toes.
E. congestive heart failure.

Answer B

36. Which of the following medications are given to the myocardial infarction patient to relieve pain?
   1. procainamide
   2. lidocaine
   3. morphine sulfate
   4. nalbuphine

Select the proper grouping.

A. 1, 2
B. 1, 3
C. 3, 4
D. 1, 2, 4
E. 2, 3, 4

Answer C

37. Which of the following drugs or modalities of care are used for bradycardic dysrhythmias?
   1. atropine sulfate
   2. verapamil
   3. procainamide
   4. epinephrine
   5. transcutaneous pacing

Select the proper grouping.

A. 1, 3
B. 1, 5
C. 2, 3, 4
D. 3, 4, 5
E. 1, 2, 3, 4, 5

Answer E

38. Which of the following represent common signs associated with congestive (left) heart failure?
   1. rales, rhonchi, or wheezes
   2. jugular vein distention
   3. severe dyspnea
   4. elevated blood pressure
   5. pink, frothy sputum

   Select the proper grouping.

   A. 1, 3
   B. 2, 4, 5
   C. 1, 2, 4
   D. 2, 3, 4, 5
   E. 1, 2, 3, 4, 5

Answer E

39. Which of the following statements are true regarding the precordial thump?
   1. it is delivered to the mid sternum
   2. it is delivered with as much force as you can
   3. it is given only to the monitored patient
   4. your hand and forearm are held parallel to, and 12 inches from, the sternum

   Select the proper grouping.

   A. 1, 3
   B. 2, 4
   C. 1, 3, 4
   D. 2, 3, 4
   E. 1, 2, 3, 4

Answer A

40. The best position for the patient experiencing left heart failure with associated pulmonary edema is ....

   A. supine with head slightly elevated.
   B. at 45 degrees.
   C. seated with legs dangling.
   D. seated with legs elevated.
   E. standing.

Answer C

41. Which drugs are indicated for the patient with left heart failure and associated pulmonary edema?
   1. morphine sulfate
   2. nitroglycerin
   3. furosemide
   4. high-flow oxygen
   5. diphenhydramine

   Select the proper grouping.

   A. 1, 3, 4
   B. 2, 3, 5
   C. 1, 2, 4, 5
   D. 1, 2, 3, 4
   E. 1, 2, 3, 4, 5

Answer D

42. Even with aggressive care, the patient who experiences cardiogenic shock still has a very poor prognosis.

A. True
B. False

Answer A

43. The patient who is experiencing a dissecting aortic aneurysm will normally describe the pain as ....

A. dull.
B. sharp.
C. tearing.
D. throbbing.
E. colicky.

Answer C

44. A patient presents with rapid onset dyspnea, a history of recent abdominal surgery and the signs of right heart heart failure including jugular vein distention. You would suspect which of the following pathologies?

A. hyperventilation
B. pulmonary edema
C. left heart failure
D. pulmonary emboli
E. right heart failure

Answer D

45. A patient is found to have extremely elevated blood pressure on assessment. He also complains of a severe headache which was of rapid onset. History identifies that he has chronic hypertension and had an MI two years ago. Which condition is most likely the cause of this patient's current condition?

A. transient ischemic attack
B. stroke
C. right heart failure
D. hypertensive emergency
E. meningitis

Answer D

46. List at least eight of the classic signs and symptoms associated with the myocardial infarction.

Diaphoresis — Syncope | Anxiety — Pallor
nausea — Vomiting | Apprehension — dyspnea
general Weakness | dysrhythmias — malaise
Shoulder, back, jaw, arm pain | Chest Pain (Crushing) — weakness

SPECIAL PROJECTS

The authoring of both the radio message to medical command and the written run report are two of the most important tasks you will perform as a paramedic. Read the following information, reread the case study in your textbook and complete the run report for this call. Ensure that you document the essential information to support the use of protocol and the advanced life support procedures that are performed without direct, on-line medical command.

The call:

Dinner for the crew of Unit 428 is abruptly interrupted at 5:35 p.m. when the auto with the panicked woman and the cardiac arrest victim arrived at the station. Though surprised, your partner, paramedic Albert Darn, picks up the hand-held radio, calls your unit out of service, and requests an engine backup for a possible arrest. He then runs to the unit bay and gathers the primary care and airway bags and the monitor/defibrillator.

After a quick assessment of pulse and breathing, arrest is confirmed and you remove the patient from the car. Once supine on the driveway CPR is begun and Al arrives huffing and puffing with the equipment. The monitor shows ventricular fibrillation via quick look and is confirmed by the absence of a palpable radial or carotid pulse. Al bares the chest, you charge the defibrillator, shout clear and defibrillate (5:39 p.m.). The fibrillation remains through three attempts and the engine company arrives.

The firefighters assume CPR (5:42) while the fire captain calms and reassures and gathers a history from the patient's wife. Your partner starts an IV with D_5W run T.K.O. in the left antecubetal fossa with an 18 gauge angiocath (5:44). After the fire fighters hyperventilate the patient you place a 7.5 mm. endotracheal tube (5:51), and ventilate with 12 L oxygen using the bag-valve with reservoir. Epi. is given at 5:53 p.m., as is the fourth shock. The lidocaine bolus and drip are started 2 minutes later. The patient is quickly loaded into the ambulance via long spineboard and transport is begun at 5:58 p.m.

The fire captain accompanies you to the hospital. He states that the patient, Leonard Thomas, is a 55 year-old male who lives at 1415 Buena Vista and has no history of cardiac problems. He has had diabetes for three years and is on oral medications and a strict diet. He has no other history or any known allergies. He began feeling nauseated with numbness in his left arm at lunch. It progressed to a dull substernal, shoulder and left arm pain about ten minutes before his arrival at the station.

The enroute ECG shows a sinus tachycardia with infrequent PVCs. They are similar, one to another. The vitals are pulse 124, blood pressure 112/78, respirations absent except for the assisted ventilation (6:12). Medical command is contacted and informed of the patient condition (6:13) and of the ten-minute ETA Charity Hospital.

The unit is reported in service at 6:45 p.m.

Using the information contained in the case study and this additional narrative, complete the run report on the following page.

Compare the run report form which you prepared against the example in the answer key section of this workbook. As you make this comparison, realize that there are many "correct" ways to communicate this body of information. Ensure that the information you have recorded contains the major points of your assessment and care, and enough other material to describe the patient and his condition to the receiving physician and anyone else who might review the form. Remember that this document may be the only record of your assessment and care for this patient. When you are done, it should be a complete account of your actions.

Date 4 / 15 / 94 | Emergency Medical Service Run Report | Run # *914*

Patient Information | **Service Information** | **Times**

Name: John DoE | Agency: *PEC Ambulance Serv.* | Rcvd 17 :35

Address: 1415 Dog lane | Location: medic Station | Enrt 17 :35

City: AnAhiem St: CA Zip: 92804 | Call Origin: medic Station | Scne 17 :35

Age: 55 Birth: 04 / 16 / 23 Sex: [X][F] | Type: Emrg[X] Non[ ] Trnsfr[ ] | LvSn 17 :58

Nature of Call: Cardiac Arrest | ArHsp 18 : 23

Chief Complaint: Pulseless nonbreathing Patient brought to Station | InSv 18 : 45

Description of Current Problem:

55 Y/o mAle with no history of heart disease. Experienced nAusea, then Chest PAin (substernAl) And numbness in the left Arm. 10 minutes before Arrival At our station. He became pulseless And apneic Just prior to Arrival, He was in V-Fib And Als Arrest protocol was followed, After fourth Countershock, he converted to An idioventricular Rhythm & Then Sinus Tach w/infrequent unifocal PVCs

Trauma Scr: n/A Glascow: 3

Medical Problems

Past		Present
[X]	Cardiac	[X]
[ ]	Stroke	[ ]
[ ]	Acute Abdomen	[ ]
[X]	Diabetes	[ ]
[ ]	Psychiatric	[ ]
[ ]	Epilepsy	[ ]
[ ]	Drug/Alcohol	[ ]
[ ]	Poisoning	[ ]
[ ]	Allergy/Asthma	[ ]
[ ]	Syncope	[ ]
[ ]	Obstetrical	[ ]
[ ]	GYN	[ ]

Other:

On Scene Care: ALS - Protocol for Arrest
18gA IV left Antecubital - D5W
7.5mm Et tube orally, Defib 2X200 & 2X360
J. Epi 1mg, Lidocaine 100mg / Drip

First Aid: none

By Whom?

O2 @ 12 L 17:51 Via BVM | C-Collar n/A : | S-Immob. n/A | Stretcher 17. :57

Allergies/Meds: Oral hypoglycemic | Past Med Hx: Diabetes for 3 years controlled by oral meds & Diet.

Time	Pulse		Resp.		BP S/D	LOC	EKG
17 : 39	R: 0	[r][i]	R: 0	[s][l]	/	[a][v][p][X]	V-Fib
Care/Comments: Defib - 200, 200 + 360 J, CPR, BVM w/100% O2							
17 : 51	R: 0	[r][i]	R: 0	[s][l]	/	[a][v][p][X]	V Fib
Care/Comments: IV L. Anticubital - D5W, 7.5 Et tube orally Epi 1mg Difib 360 J.							
17 : 55	R: 50	[X][i]	R: 0	[s][l]	110 / p	[a][v][p][X]	Ideoventricular - S - Tach.
Care/Comments: Lidocaine bolus 100mg in drip							
18 : 12	R: 124	[r][X]	R: 0	[s][l]	112 / 78	[a][v][p][X]	S-Tach w/unifocal PVCs
Care/Comments: lidocaine Drip @ 2mg/min							

Destination: Charity Hospital

Reason: [ ]pt [X] Closest [ ] M.D [ ] Other

Contacted: [X] Radio [ ] Tele [ ] Direct

Ar Status: [X] Better [ ] UnC [ ] Worse

Personnel:	Certification
1. C. Robertson.	[X][E][O]
2. John Rookie	[X][E][O]
3. n/A	[X][E][O]

Cardiac Emergencies Crossword Puzzle

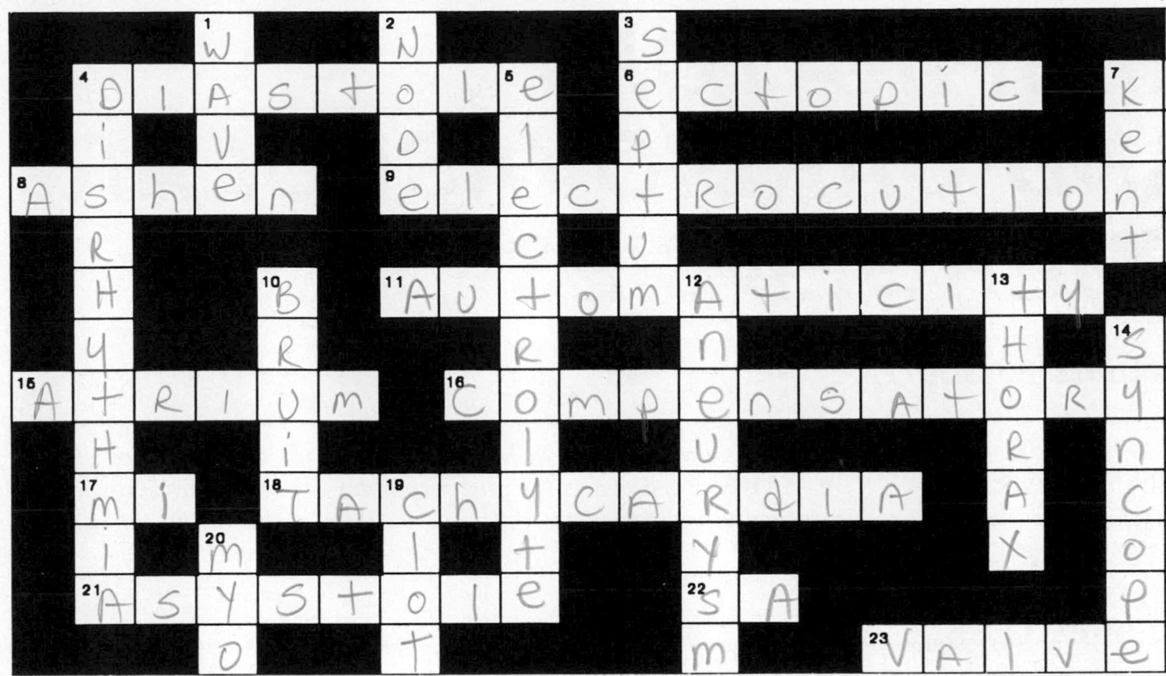

The crossword puzzle above addresses the vocabulary of chapter 21.

ACROSS

4. The phase of the cardiac cycle in which the heart relaxes and fills.
6. Electrical activity occurring outside of its normal origin.
8. A grayish discoloration of the skin secondary to hypoxia.
9. The passage of electricity through the body which induces cardiac arrest.
11. The characteristic of cardiac tissue which permits it to initiate an electrical impulse.
15. An upper chamber of the heart.
16. The longer than usual pause following an ectopic heart beat.
17. The initials for myocardial infarction.
18. A heart rate above 100 beats per mi.
21. The absence of electrical activity.
22. The node which initiates the normal cardiac cycle.
23. The structure between an atrium and a ventricle.

DOWN

1. The form or configuration of the P and T impulses on the ECG.
2. A concentration of specialized tissue that can initiate an electrical impulse in the heart.
3. The structure that divides the left and right heart.
4. A cardiac rhythm that is abnormal.
5. Ionized salts in the blood and body tissues.
7. An accessory AV conduction pathway responsible for some preexcitation dysrhythmias, the bundle of ______.
10. A turbulence heard via stethoscope, usually over the carotid artery.
12. A bulging in a blood vessel wall.
13. The major body cavity in which the heart is found.
14. A fainting or collapse, often caused by cardiac problems.
19. A thrombosis.
20. The prefix meaning muscle.

DIVISION REVIEW

RESPIRATORY AND CARDIOVASCULAR EMERGENCIES

Chapters 20 and 2l

The following scenario based questions are designed to help you review the previous two chapters of **PARAMEDIC EMERGENCY CARE**. *Cardiovascular and respiratory emergencies will account for most of your responses as a paramedic and hence are set aside in this workbook as an independent Division Review.*

Scenario I

On a particularly hot Sunday afternoon the 911 center dispatches your unit to a nearby nursing home to a "difficulty breathing" call. On the third floor of the complex you find an 88-year-old female who is sitting bolt upright in her chair gasping for breath. She is anxious, ashen, sweating profusely, in no apparent pain, and clearly having problems breathing. A quick set of vitals reveals a respiratory rate of 32, shallow breaths, a blood pressure of 132/92, a pulse rate of 98, oxygen saturation of 88, and atrial fibrillation with infrequent PVCs.

1. As a result of these finding which of the following are likely causes of the patient's distress?
   1. pulmonary emboli
   2. asthma
   3. left ventricular failure
   4. pulmonary edema
   5. chronic obstructive pulmonary disease

   Select the proper grouping.

   A. 1, 3, 4
   B. 2, 4
   C. 2, 3, 4
   D. 1, 3, 4, 5
   E. 1, 2, 3, 4, 5

   Answer E

2. An IV line should be established with ....

   A. normal saline run wide open.
   B. normal saline run T.K.O.
   C. D_5W run wide open.
   D. D_5W run T.K.O.
   E. no line should be established.

   Answer D

3. Your early care steps should include which of the following?
   1. high-flow oxygen
   2. supine positioning
   3. lidocaine
   4. aminophylline
   5. atropine

   Select the proper grouping.

   A. 1
   B. 2
   C. 1, 2, 4
   D. 2, 5
   E. 1, 2, 3, 4, 5

Answer A

Patient questioning reveals a complaint of dyspnea for which she has some relief by sitting. Her ankles and lower legs display swelling, which remains indented after finger pressure is released. You question the patient about previous medical history and find that she had a previous MI two months earlier and has been given Lanoxin for her heart. She is also on a water pill (furosemide). She also complains that she is awakened at night with difficult breathing and has been sleeping in a chair for the past three nights. The patient's breath sounds reflect rales in all lung fields and there is a coarse vibration felt in the chest as the patient speaks.

4. The sleep disturbing dyspnea is called ....

   A. chronic obstructive pulmonary disease.
   B. Biot's respirations.
   C. Frank-Starling reflex.
   D. class two rales.
   E. none of the above.

Answer E

5. The distal swelling that indents is called ....

   A. systemic edema.
   B. cardiac related depressions.
   C. pitting edema.
   D. pre-sacral edema.
   E. dependent edema.

Answer C

6. With this additional information, the most probable patient diagnosis is ....

   A. silent myocardial infarction.
   B. left ventricular failure with pulmonary edema
   C. pulmonary edema.
   D. pulmonary embolism.
   E. cor pulmonale.

Answer B

7. The vibration felt in the neck as the patient speaks is called ....

   A. tactile fremitus.
   B. stridor.
   C. rales.
   D. rhonchi.
   E. Bledsoes' hum.

Answer A

8. Which of the following drugs might you consider for this patient?
   1. morphine sulfate
   2. furosemide
   3. nitroglycerin
   4. epinephrine
   5. dobutamine

   Select the proper grouping.

   A. 3, 5
   B. 1, 3, 4
   C. 1, 2, 3, 5
   D. 1, 2, 4, 5
   E. 1, 2, 3, 4, 5

   Answer C

9. Given the severity of the patient's dyspnea and the oxygen saturation it may be appropriate to ventilate the patient using the demand valve or bag-valve mask.

   A. True
   B. False

   Answer A

Shortly after you load the patient onto the stretcher you notice PVCs on the ECG. She begins to cough up pink-tinged fluid, her dyspnea worsens, and her level of consciousness drops. She becomes unresponsive, develops a pulseless ventricular fibrillation, and stops breathing.

10. The best way to assure the airway in this patient is via a(n)....

    A. oral pharyngeal airway.
    B. nasal pharyngeal airway.
    C. oral endotracheal intubation.
    D. nasal endotracheal intubation.
    E. digital intubation.

    Answer C

11. At what level would you first defibrillate this patient?

    A. 50 J.
    B. 100 J.
    C. 200 J.
    D. 300 J.
    E. 360 J.

    Answer C

12. Which of the following drugs should be administered to this patient first?

    A. atropine
    B. epinephrine
    C. lidocaine
    D. bretylium
    E. procainamide

    Answer B

13. After the administration of IV medications, subsequent defibrillation should occur ....

    A. immediately.
    B. within 10 seconds.
    C. within 30 to 60 seconds.
    D. within 1 minute.
    E. within 2 to 3 minutes.

    Answer C

Scenario II

Your rescue squad arrives to attend a patient with "breathing problems." The patient is a 47-year-old overweight and cyanotic male. He complains of shortness of breath and weakness. Patient history reveals a 20 pack/year history of smoking, severe respiratory infections over the past few years, and a chronic productive cough. Rhonchi is noted during auscultation of the chest.

14. The most likely cause of this problem is ....

A. pulmonary embolism.
B. chronic bronchitis.
C. emphysema.
D. asthma.
E. none of the above.

Answer B

15. Oxygen should be administered to this patient at a low-flow rate of about 2 liters per minute while the respiratory rate and volume are watched carefully.

A. True
B. False

Answer A

16. Medications appropriate to the care of this patient include which of the following?
1. metaproterenol
2. isoetharine
3. Solu-Medrol
4. Alupent

Select the proper grouping.

A. 1, 3
B. 1, 4
C. 2, 3, 4
D. 1, 2, 4
E. 1, 2, 3, 4

Answer D

17. Your medical control physician orders a beta antagonist medication to be administered via nebulized inhaler. The pulse rate should be carefully monitored since these drugs are noted for inducing bradycardia.

A. True
B. False

Answer B

After you administer oxygen to this patient, his respiratory rate slows and his level of consciousness drops.

18. You should now begin to assist the patient's respiration with the bag-valve-device.

A. True
B. False

Answer A

22

ENDOCRINE AND METABOLIC EMERGENCIES

Review of the Objectives for Chapter 22

After reading this chapter, you should be able to:

1. Define the term hormone.

p. 726

Hormones are chemical substances released by endocrine glands. They control or affect other glands, organs or body systems.

2. Discuss the location and function of the following endocrine glands.

pp. 726 to 730

The **pituitary** gland is located on a stalk hanging from the base of the brain. It is the master gland and provides control over most of the other endocrine glands as well as many body functions.

The **thyroid** gland is located in the anterior neck on either side of the trachea. It assists in the control of the body's overall metabolic rate.

The **parathyroid** glands are four small pea-shaped glands located near the thyroid. They control the level of calcium in the blood.

The **pancreas** is located in the central and upper abdominal cavity. It produces several digestive juices as well as glucagon and insulin. It is responsible for the control of blood glucose levels.

The **adrenal** glands are located above each of the kidneys. Their products include epinephrine and norepinephrine as well as agents that assist in controlling blood glucose levels and anti-inflammatory responses.

The **ovaries** (the female gonads) are located within the pelvic cavity next to the uterus. They produce the eggs and manufacture the female hormones that cause sexual development.

The **testes** (the male gonads) are contained within the testicular sac or scrotum. They produce sperm and the hormones responsible for the male growth characteristics.

3. List two functions of the islets of Langerhans.

p. 729

The islets of Langerhans are responsible for endocrine production: including insulin, glucagon and somatostatin. Insulin assists glucose in crossing the cell membrane while glucogon controls blood glucose levels. The production of somatostatin inhibits the function of insulin and glucagon.

4. Discuss the function of glucagon.

p. 729

Glucagon is a hormone that stimulates the release of glucose from various locations within the human body. It also stimulates the liver to increase production of glucose. The net effect is a rise in the blood glucose levels.

5. Define diabetes mellitus.

p. 730

Diabetes mellitus is caused by dysfunction of the pancreas and reduced secretion of insulin. The disease causes reduced cellular availability of glucose, a reliable energy source for most body cells.

6. Discuss the function of insulin and its relation to glucose metabolism.

pp. 730 to 731

Insulin causes various cells to take up glucose through facilitated transport. It effectively reduces the blood glucose level and makes glucose available to the body's cells. Insulin must be constantly produced since it is quickly metabolized by the liver.

7. Compare and contrast type I (insulin-dependent) and type II (non-insulin-dependent) diabetes mellitus.

pp. 731 to 732

Type I Diabetes usually occurs early in life. The victim becomes insulin dependent, taking injectable doses of insulin and regulating intake of carbohydrates and sugars. The patient may experience wide variations in the insulin needed, leading to over- and under-dosing.

Type II Diabetes usually occurs later in life and is characterized by reduced insulin production. It develops more gradually and is often associated with obesity. It can be managed by diet, oral medication or both, though insulin may be required. Diabetic ketoacidosis is less likely to develop; however there can be life-threatening emergencies related to hypoglycemia and dehydration.

8. Discuss the osmotic diuresis occurring in diabetes.

pp. 731 to 732

Osmotic diuresis is a general dehydration due to the kidney's eliminating extra glucose, and with it water, in the urine. In diabetes the dehydration can be rapid and severe. The problem may present with warm, dry skin, and dry mucous membranes.

9 . Discuss the presentation, assessment, and management of diabetic ketoacidosis.

pp. 732 to 733

Presentation and Assessment

The patient experiencing diabetic ketoacidosis will display very deep and rapid (Kussmaul) respirations. Thirst, hunger, frequent urination, a general ill feeling, nausea, vomiting, dehydration, and tachycardia and other cardiac dysrhythmias may be present. The patient may have an odor of acetone on his or her breath due to the presence of ketones. Urine or blood glucose levels will be very high as determined by a chem-strip.

Management

Care for the diabetic patient in suspected diabetic ketoacidosis should including drawing blood for later Emergency Department evaluation, evaluation of the current level by a chem-strip, and the administration of dextrose 50% in water, 1 to 2 mg of narcan and 100 mg thiamine. (The dextrose will not harm the diabetic ketoacidosis patient, while failure to administer it to the acute hypoglycemia patient may result in patient death. If the glucose level can be dependably determined in the field, 1 to 2 liters of normal saline should be administered.

10. **Discuss the presentation, assessment, and management of hypoglycemia.**

pp. 733 to 736

Presentation and management

The patient may display abnormal behavior from restlessness, to inappropriate anger, to bizarre actions. Physical signs include diaphoresis and tachycardia. Any patient who displays bizarre or intoxicated behavior should be suspected of hypoglycemia.

Management

If the glucose level can be determined, blood should be drawn, a D_5W drip established and 50 to 100 mL. of dextrose 50% in water administered. If a definitive glucose level cannot be ascertained then 1 to 2 mg Narcan and 100 mg thiamine should also be given. If the patient is conscious, awake and able to protect the airway, then oral glucose sources such as orange juice, sodas or commercial glucose pastes may be administered.

CASE STUDY REVIEW

Reread the case study in **PARAMEDIC EMERGENCY CARE** and then read the discussion below.

This case study presents a rather straightforward diabetic emergency. The paramedics display the normal response to the situation including assessment and pharmacological intervention.

Chapter 22 Case Study

Rescue 21 responds to a typical diabetic emergency. The patient presents with coma, deep respirations, tachycardia, acetone breath and a history of insulin-dependent diabetes. Coma is most likely caused by the ketones and acidosis and their effects on the brain. The deep respirations are the body's attempt to reduce the acidosis by blowing off carbon dioxide. The odor on the patient's breath is probably acetone and is a result of the ketones in the blood which are created as cells metabolize secondary energy sources. This incident is primarily due to the patient's failure to take his prescribed insulin.

The paramedics have access to both pulse oximetry and a glucose determination device. The pulse oximeter reflects that the patient is exchanging respiratory gases but could probably benefit from supplimental oxygen. The glucose reading of "HIGH" establishes that hyperglycemia is the patients problem. IV blood is drawn for more accurate analysis at the emergency department.

As hyperglycemia is confirmed, normal saline administration is initiated to counteract the massive diuresis and dehydration that usually accompanies this pathology. Field administration of insulin is not recommended because it is hard to determine the etiology of diabetic emergencies. Field glucose tests are also relatively inaccurate, and insulin administration can induce acute hypoglycemia if given when not needed.

READING COMPREHENSION SELF-EXAM

1. The primary function of insulin is to ....

A. metabolize glucose at the cellular level.
B. free glucose from the storage sites within the cell.
C. free glucose from the body's storage areas.
D. help transport glucose across the cell wall.
E. assist glucagon in its function.

Answer D

2. Glucagon is a very intense source of glucose. When it breaks down at the cellular level it converts to four glucose molecules.

A. True
B. False

Answer B

3. Which of the endocrine glands produces epinephrine?

A. pituitary
B. thyroid
C. adrenal
D. pancreas
E. gonads

Answer C

4. A common problem associated with the adult-onset (type II) diabetic patient is dehydration secondary to osmotic diuresis.

A. True
B. False

Answer A

5. Diabetic ketoacidosis is caused by low insulin states and results in ....
   1. osmotic diuresis.
   2. dehydration.
   3. the build up of ketones.
   4. metabolic acidosis.

Select the proper grouping.

A. 1, 3
B. 2, 4
C. 1, 4
D. 2, 3, 4
E. 1, 2, 3, 4

Answer E

6. Which of the following signs and symptoms would you expect from a patient found in diabetic ketoacidosis?
   1. warm dry skin
   2. rapid deep breathing patterns
   3. low blood sugar level
   4. tachycardia and weakness

Select the proper grouping.

A. 1, 2
B. 3, 4
C. 1, 2, 3
D. 1, 2, 4
E. 1, 2, 3, 4

Answer D

7. The reason for administering 50% dextrose to the patient suspected of having diabetic ketoacidosis is that it will ....

A. increase the osmolality of the blood.
B. help if the patient is actually hypoglycemic.
C. increase the blood sugar level.
D. increase insulin production.
E. keep the brain alive.

Answer B

8. The early signs of diabetic ketoacidosis include ....
   1. hunger.
   2. thirst.
   3. frequent urination.
   4. malaise.

   Select the proper grouping.

   A. 1
   B. 3
   C. 1, 3
   D. 1, 3, 4
   E. 1, 2, 3, 4

   Answer E

9. Hypoglycemia is often caused because the diabetic ....

   A. consumes too much carbohydrates.
   B. consumes too much sugar.
   C. takes too much insulin.
   D. either A or B.
   E. none of the above.

   Answer C

10. The patient who has a history of diabetes and displays inappropriate behavior is most likely suffering from which of the problems below?

    A. acute hypoglycemia
    B. focal motor seizure
    C. osmotic diuresis
    D. diabetic ketoacidosis
    E. none of the above

    Answer A

SPECIAL PROJECTS

Problem Solving - Diabetic Emergencies

Reread the case study for chapter 3 which dealt with an unruly patient found later to be suffering from hypoglycemia. Based on that case study answer the questions below.

Explain why the patient in this case study was displaying the behavior the paramedics initially noted ("staggering along the road").

a patient with a history of Insulin dependant diabetes overdosed on his Insulin, which Induced Hypoglycemia, that reduced the amount of glucose available to the brain, causing bizzare behavior Staggering and eventually unconsciousness.

Explain why the Glucometer finding was significant.

Normal Blood Sugar Ranges From 75-110mg/dl. A Glucometer Reading of 26mg/dL Is very low + diagnosed Acute Hypoglycemia.

23

NERVOUS SYSTEM EMERGENCIES

Part I - *(pages 741 to 754)*

Review of the Objectives for Chapter 23

After reading this chapter, you should be able to:

1. Identify the parts of the neuron, and give their function.

pp. 741 to 742

The **dendrites** are the short fibers that carry the nervous impulses to the cell body.
The **cell body** is the central mass of the cell.
The **axon** is the long arm of the neuron that carries the nerve impulse away from the cell body.

2. Describe the process of nerve impulse transmission.

pp. 741 to 742

During the resting state the nerve cell is negatively charged inside while positively charged outside. When stimulated, sodium enters and potassium leaves, changing the charge at the point of stimulation. This chemical/electrical impulse then moves rapidly along the nerve fiber. At the axon's end (the synapse) the impulse induces the release of either acetylcholine or norepinephrine which in turn stimulates the next nerve.

3. Identify the protective structures of the brain and the spinal cord.

pp. 742 to 744

The cranial vault of the **skull** forms a fixed volume, rigid container for the brain.
The **vertebral column** provides a skeletal tube, the spinal foramen, that houses the spinal cord.
The **meninges** is a three-layer structure surrounding the brain and spinal column. The dura mater is the outermost layer and lines the inner aspect of the cranial vault and the spinal foramen. The arachnoid is the middle layer. The pia mater is the inner layer and covers the convolutions of the brain and spinal column.
Cerebrospinal fluid (CSF) is a fluid found within the space between the arachnoid and pia mater. It bathes the brain and absorbs shock as the head or spine are jarred.

4. List the major divisions of the brain, and briefly state the function of each.

pp. 744 to 746

The **cerebrum** is the largest portion of the brain. It fills most of the cranial vault and is divided into left and right hemispheres. It is the seat of intelligence and is responsible for learning, analysis, memory, and language.

The **diencephalon** is the most superior portion of the brainstem and contains the thalamus, hypothalamus and the limbic system. It controls many involuntary actions such as temperature regulation, sleep, water balance, stress response and emotions.

The **midbrain**, or mesencephalon, is located between the diencephalon and the pons. It controls a major component of eye movement and certain aspects of motor coordination.

The **pons** lies between the midbrain and the medulla oblongata. It contains the the tracts between the brain and the spinal cord.

The **medulla oblongata** is located between the pons and the spinal cord. It contains the centers for blood pressure, respiration and heart rate.

The **cerebellum** is located in the posterior fossa of the cranium. It is closely related to the brainstem and higher brain centers. It coordinates fine motor movement, posture, equilibrium, and muscle tone.

5. Identify the functions of the spinal cord.

pp. 746 to 747

The spinal cord traverses the spinal foramen from the foramen magnum to the level of the first or second lumbar vertebra. It functions as the major nerve pathway from the brain to the peripheral nerve roots. It permits reflex responses to intense stimuli, such as extreme heat.

6. Identify the location of the brachial plexus.

p. 747

The brachial plexus is a network of nerves located in the posterior neck.

7. Identify the factors to be elicited when evaluating the nervous system, including trauma and non-trauma related problems.

pp. 749 to 754

How long ago did the incident occur?
How did the incident occur?
What was the mechanism of injury?
Was there any loss of consciousness?
What is (was) the patient's chief complaint?
Has there been any change in symptoms?
Are there any complicating factors?
Are there any underlying medical problems?
    Cardiac disease, chronic seizures, diabetes, hypertension
Is there any supporting evidence?
    Medications, Medic-alert, alcohol, drugs

8. Identify the following specific observations and physical findings to be evaluated in a patient with a nervous system disorder:

pp. 749 to 753

Primary assessment

Evaluate and ensure an open and patent airway

Assess the respiratory pattern and identify:

Cheyne-Stokes respiration, central neurologic hyperventilation, ataxic respiration, apneustic respiration, diaphragmatic breathing

Secondary assessment

The **pupils** should be assessed for equality and responsiveness to changes in light intensity.

Extraoccular movements - The eyes should be examined to determine whether the eyes are gazing together or separately (disconjugate gaze). The evaluation should also ensure that the doll's eye reflex is not present. Also check for the patient's ability to follow an object through a full range of motion with their eyes. Do not attempt to move the head in a potential trauma patient.

Spinal evaluation should include examination for any overt sign of injury including contusion, erythema, pain, tenderness or deformity. The evaluation should also examine for motor and sensory function, and position sense in each limb. If loss is noted it is helpful to determine which dermatomes or what anatomic region is involved.

Vital signs - Evaluate the following:

Blood pressure for increase
Pulse for strength increase and rate decrease
Respirations for rate decrease and depth increase
Temperature increase
Level of consciousness decrease

As the intracranial pressure increases, the blood pressure will rise and the pulse rate will decrease.

Neuro evaluation

A - **Alert** - is the patient alert and responding appropriately to questions regarding time, place, person and one's own person?

V - **Verbal** - is the patient able to respond to verbal stimuli, and is the response appropriate?

P - **Painful** - does the patient respond only to painful stimuli? Is the response effective, non-effective, decerebrate or decorticate?

U - **Unresponsive** - does the patient fail to respond to any stimuli?

10. Describe the Glasgow Coma Scale.

pp. 753 to 754

The Glasgow Coma Scale assesses three components of patient responsiveness and awards from one to six points for each response. The responses evaluated are:

Eye opening		Verbal response		Motor response	
Spontaneous	4	Oriented	5	Obeys commands	6
To voice	3	Confused	4	Localizes to pain	5
To pain	2	Inappropriate	3	Withdraws to pain	4
None	1	Incomprehensible	2	Decorticate	3
		None	1	Decerebrate	2
				None	1

CASE STUDY REVIEW

Reread the case study in **PARAMEDIC EMERGENCY CARE** and then read the discussion below.

The patient described in this scenario is typical of many patients a paramedic may be called to treat. He has seizure activity, that could be from many different origins. The paramedics, however, follow the general seizure protocol and safely transport him to the hospital.

Chapter 23 Case Study

The paramedics in this case study are presented with a patient who could be experiencing seizure activity secondary to many etiologies. Among them are head trauma, stroke, acute alcoholism, epilepsy, drug overdose and hypoglycemia, to list just a few. The environment is examined to determine if any drug paraphernalia or medications can be found to suggest the origin of the coma. In the assessment, clear airway and no respiratory odors are noted. Breathing is adequate and the pulse is strong.

Attempts to wake the patient elicit a motor seizure. Note that stimulation, be it your touch, or the sound of the siren, may initiate a seizure. The patient seizes a second time without achieving consciousness, and hence, status epilepticus is encountered. The patient fails to respond to thiamine and dextrose. The paramedics could have attempted naloxone administration but the second seizure called for valium, which successfully terminated it. The patient was transported without lights and sirens because such sensory stimulation can induce seizure activity. During transport the patient was kept on his side to help maintain the airway. Oxygen was administered via a nonrebreather mask to ensure the maximum concentration was received by the patient.

The blood levels of phenobarbitol and Dilantin suggest that this patient has had a history of seizure activity. These medications are commonly prescribed to depress seizures. The sub-therapeutic levels reflect that the patient may have experienced a seizure that resulted in head trauma during the initial collapse or during the clonic phase.

The final diagnosis is one that all emergency medical service personnel should be aware of and concerned about. The chronic alcoholic is very susceptible to head trauma and intracranial hemorrhage. Even though the patient may appear only intoxicated, he or she must be evaluated for reduced level of consciousness. All other causes of reduced level of consciousness must be ruled out (unlikely in the field) before the condition can be solely attributed to alcohol.

READING COMPREHENSION SELF-EXAM

1. The system that is closely associated with the nervous system and assists in the control of the body through hormones is the ....

A. integumentary system.
B. endocrine system.
C. lymphatic system.
D. genitourinary system.
E. lymbic system.

Answer B

2. The sympathetic and parasympathetic nervous systems are best described as opposing divisions of the ....

A. central nervous system.
B. peripheral nervous system.
C. somatic nervous system.
D. autonomic nervous system.
E. none of the above.

Answer D

3. Which of the following are components of the neuron?
   1. synapse
   2. axon
   3. cell body
   4. meninges
   5. dendrites

Select the proper grouping.

A. 1, 3, 4
B. 2, 3, 4
C. 2, 3, 5
D. 1, 3, 4, 5
E. 1, 2, 3, 4, 5

Answer C

4. The cranium is composed of which of the following bones?
   1. frontal bone
   2. occipital bone
   3. parietal bones
   4. temporal bones
   5. sphenoid bones
   6. ethmoid bones

   Select the proper grouping.

   A. 1, 2, 4
   B. 2, 3, 5
   C. 1, 3, 4, 5
   D. 1, 2, 4, 5
   E. 1, 2, 3, 4, 5

   Answer E

5. The middle layer of the meninges is known as the ....

   A. pia mater.
   B. dura mater.
   C. arachnoid.
   D. epidural layer.
   E. subdural layer.

   Answer C

6. The seat of intelligence, learning, analysis, memory and language is the ....

   A. cerebellum.
   B. cerebrum.
   C. pons.
   D. diencephalon.
   E. none of the above.

   Answer B

7. The area responsible for fine motor movement, posture, equilibrium and muscle tone is the ....

   A. diencephalon.
   B. cerebrum.
   C. pons.
   D. medulla oblongata.
   E. none of the above.

   Answer e

8. A dermatome is ....

   A. an area of the body sensed by one peripheral nerve root.
   B. the afferent fiber of a lower spinal nerve root.
   C. the efferent fiber of a lower spinal nerve root.
   D. one of the spaces between vertebrae where the nerve exits.
   E. none of the above.

   Answer A

9. The "fight-or-flight" aspect of the nervous system prepares the body for stressful encounters and is known as the ....

   A. parasympathetic nervous system.
   B. sympathetic nervous system.
   C. visceral sensory motor afferent.
   D. somatic sensory motor afferent.
   E. vertebrobasilar nervous system.

   Answer B

10. The breathing pattern characterized by prolonged inspiration without effective exhalation attempts is termed ....

A. apneustic respirations.
B. central neurologic ventilation.
C. Cheyne-Stokes respiration.
D. ataxic respiration.
E. none of the above.

Answer A

11. If you are caring for a patient who shows signs and symptoms of increasing intracranial pressure, you should ....

A. hypoventilate the patient to retain CO_2.
B. ventilate normally.
C. ventilate normally with supplemental oxygen.
D. hyperventilate the patient to blow off CO_2.
E. none of the above.

Answer D

12. The classic signs of increasing intracranial pressure include ....

A. increasing blood pressure.
B. decreasing pulse rate.
C. decreased respiratory rate.
D. increasing temperature.
E. all of the above.

Answer E

13. Which of the common vital signs move in the same direction in both shock and increasing intracranial pressure?

A. blood pressure
B. pulse strength
C. pulse rate
D. level of consciousness
E. respiration rate and depth

Answer D

14. The P of the AVPU neurologic evaluation stands for ....

A. proprioception.
B. posturing.
C. proper response to questioning.
D. painful stimuli.
E. pupillary responsiveness.

Answer D

15. Decorticate posturing occurs when the patient's arms and legs are extended.

A. True
B. False

Answer B

16. A patient is found to open her eyes only to pain, mumble incomprehensibly, and withdraws to pain. You would assign which Glasgow Coma Scale value?

A. 9
B. 8
C. 6
D. 5
E. 4

Answer B

17. A patient which you are caring for is conscious and alert with no identifiable central nervous system deficit. What Glasgow Coma Score would you assign?

A. 10
B. 15
C. 25
D. 30
E. 50

Answer B

18. You are caring for a patient who was hit on the head by a baseball bat. He was unconscious but is now completely alert. During assessment you notice that one pupil is greatly dilated but still responds to light. You should suspect ....

A. possible increasing intracranial pressure.
B. a normal condition found in 10% of the population.
C. doll's eye reflex, a drug-induced problem.
D. serious brain anoxia.
E. none of the above.

Answer A

CNS PHARMACOLOGY

Emergency management for nervious system emergencies utilizes some of the pharmacologic agents which are available to the paramedic. Please begin to review and memorize the various names, indications, therapeutic effects, contraindications, side effects, routes of administration, and recommended dosages for the following. (See the drug cards at the back of this workbook.)

dextrose 50 %

oxygen

methylprednisolone (Solu-Medrol)

diazepam (Valium)

thiamine

naloxone (Narcan)

23

NERVOUS SYSTEM EMERGENCIES

Part II - (pages 754 to 767)

Review of the Objectives for Chapter 23

After reading this chapter, you should be able to:

10. Describe the use of the following drugs in relation to CNS problems. **pp. 757 to 764**

Dextrose 50% in water is administered when hypoglycemia is suspected or a possible contributor to unconsciousness. For the adult, 25 gm (50 mL) are usually given IV.

Naloxone (Narcan) is a narcotic antagonist which is given if narcotic overdose might be a cause of unconsciousness. It is administered in a dose of 1 to 2 mg IV, ET, IM or SQ. If no response is obtained the dose may be repeated several times.

Thiamine (Thiamine or vitamin B1) assists the brain in obtaining energy from glucose. Its administration is recommended for the patient who is suspected of alcoholism. It is usually administered in a dose of 100 mg IV.

Dexamethasone (Decadron) is a steroid designed to reduce cerebral inflammation and swelling. It is given IV in dosages ranging from 4 to 24 mg.

Diazepam (Valium) is indicated in the seizure patient because of its sedative and anticonvulsant effects. The adult usually receives 5 to 10 mg of diazepam IV slowly, no more than 1 mL per minute.

11. Describe the pathophysiology, assessment, and management of the following: **pp. 754 to 767**

Altered mental status

Pathophysiology - the most serious altered mental status, coma is a deep unarousable state of unconsciousness. It originates from two major categories of insult: structural lesion and toxic-metabolic states.

Assessment of the patient in coma must attempt to identify the cause and severity of the coma. Past medical history should be obtained, as should the history of the present problem and any pre-existing medical problems that could account for or contribute to the development of the coma.

Management of the coma patient should begin with spinal immobilization if there is a potential for injury and need for airway care. Breathing should be supported with high-flow oxygen and assisted ventilations as needed. Intubation may be necessary to secure the airway; however, it may transiently increase intracranial pressure so it should be accomplished quickly and atraumatically. An IV should be initiated and blood drawn for both on scene and emergency department analysis. Dextrose 50%, Narcan, and possibly thiamine.

Seizure

Pathophysiology - the seizure is a temporary alteration in behavior due to massive electrical discharges in the brain. They are either generalized or involve a portion of the body. The major types of seizures include grand mal, psychomotor, petit mal and hysterical.

Assessment attempts to isolate the cause or precipitating factors of the seizure. Previous history of seizure activity and non-compliance to prescribed medications is important.

Management - seizures are managed by calming relatives and friends, administering oxygen, and maintaining the airway. The patient should be protected from striking objects during the seizure. Body temperature should be maintained. Following the event, calm and quiet transport to the hospital should be provided.

Status epilepticus

Pathophysiology - status epilepticus is a series of two or more grand mal seizures occurring without an interim period of patient consciousness. It is a life threatening event due to the hypoxia experienced.

Assessment of status epilepticus is the same as for the grand mal seizure though the seizures are repetitive.

Management - the repeating seizure should be treated with aggressive airway care, including airway maintenance, 100% oxygen and assisted ventilation. An IV should be established and 50% dextrose and 5 to 10 mg diazepam administered.

Cerebrovascular accident (CVA)

Pathophysiology - the stroke is an injury to brain tissue due to interruption of blood flow. CVA is usually due to atherosclerosis or hypertension, or both. Two methods of insult are common: occlusion and hemorrhage. If the blood supply is halted by embolus or thrombosis, the portion of the brain supplied by the artery receives an inadequate supply of blood and nervous tissue dies. In hemorrhage, blood seeps into the nervous tissue or the cerebral spinal fluid and may paralyze vital centers.

Assessment may reveal labored breathing with the cheeks puffing with expiration and possibly snoring due to relaxed muscle tone in the respiratory tract. The level of consciousness will likely be reduced and the patient may have difficulty with speech due to motor, speech and sensory area impairment. Paralysis is common and often involves one side of the body. Pupil dilatation may be noted unilaterally.

Management - the stroke patient should be kept supine with the head slightly elevated. Oxygen should be administered liberally and special attention should be directed to ensuring the airway remains clear and unobstructed. Blood should be drawn, the cardiac rhythm monitored and 50% dextrose may be considered. The patient's paralyzed extremities need protection and a special effort should be made to calm, comfort and reassure the patient.

Transient ischemic attack (TIA)

Pathophysiology - the transient ischemic attack is the result of small emboli which present with stroke-like symptoms. The problem is generally transient, but warns that a more significant event may follow.

Assessment - as with stroke, the TIA presents with acute symptoms though they tend to be more limited than with the stroke. Obtain a complete history similar to that gained in the assessment of a CVA patient.

Management of the patient with the suspected transient ischemic attack is identical to the stroke.

12. List the possible causes of altered mental status.

p. 755

Pharmacological
- barbiturates
- narcotics
- hallucinogens
- depressants

Structural
- trauma
- brain tumor
- epilepsy
- intracranial hemorrhage
- space-occupying lesions

Cardiovascular
- hypertensive encephalopathy
- shock
- anaphylaxis
- dysrhythmias
- cardiac arrest
- cerebrovascular accident

Metabolic
- thiamine deficiency
- anoxia
- hypoglycemia
- diabetic ketoacidosis
- hepatic failure
- renal failure

Respiratory
- chronic obstructive pulmonary disease
- toxic inhalation

Infectious
- menigitis
- encephalitis

13. Describe and differentiate the major types of seizures.

pp. 760 to 761

Grand mal is the general tonic-clonic seizure. The victim experiences the classic aura, tonic phase, clonic phase and a post-ictal period of disorientation and confusion.

The **petit mal** seizure is a brief loss of conscious awareness. Some eye fluttering and occasional loss of muscle tone may be experienced. Often the episode is not recognized as a seizure.

Focal motor seizures are characterized by dysfunction of one particular body region. They often spread or progress into a generalized clonic seizure.

Psychomotor seizures are characterized by sensory disturbances including unusual sounds, smells or sights. They may also account for sudden personality changes. They last about 1 to 2 minutes.

Hysterical seizures are psychologically, rather than physiologically, induced. They can mimic any other seizure activity, and the victim may be very difficult to differentiate from the true seizure patient.

14. Describe the different phases of a grand mal seizure.

pp. 760

Aura - the patient experiences a heralding sensation or taste that warns of the oncoming seizure.

Loss of consciousness - the patient becomes unconscious immediately before the active seizure begins.

Tonic phase The patient becomes rigid as the muscles tense.

Hypertonic phase The patient displays extreme hyperextension, including arching of the back.

Clonic phase The patient alternately flexes and extends the limbs and neck with violent force.

Post-ictal The post-ictal period is a time when the patient returns from the seizure state. It is a time of progression from confusion and disorientation to a complete alert state.

15. Differentiate between syncope and seizures.

p. 762

Syncope is a collapse due to reduced blood supply to the brain. It generally results in a transient weakness or collapse. The patient will recover quickly and display a slow, weak pulse and cool and clammy skin.

Seizure is a central nervous system disturbance which leaves the patient confused and disoriented. It often involves tonic, clonic or other motor or sensory dysfunction.

READING COMPREHENSION SELF-EXAM

19. Which of the following are possible causes of altered mental status?
    1. diabetic ketoacidosis
    2. stroke
    3. trauma
    4. renal failure
    5. hypoglycemia
    6. epilepsy

    Select the proper grouping.

    A. 1, 3, 5, 6
    B. 1, 2, 4, 5
    C. 1, 2, 3, 5, 6
    D. 1, 3, 4, 5, 6
    E. 1, 2, 3, 4, 5, 6

    Answer E

20. In the care for the coma patient, three drugs are commonly given IV. They are ....
    1. insulin.
    2. epinephrine.
    3. dextrose 50%.
    4. naloxone.
    5. thiamine.

    Select the proper grouping.

    A. 1, 2, 4
    B. 1, 3, 4
    C. 2, 4, 5
    D. 2, 3, 4
    E. 3, 4, 5

    Answer E

21. The common dosage for dextrose 50% is 25 gm. What volume of the drug would you administer?

A. 12 mL
B. 25 mL
C. 50 mL
D. 75 mL
E. 100 mL

Answer C

22. The drug naloxone can be administered by which of the following routes, safely?

A. IV
B. IM
C. SQ
D. ET
E. all of the above

Answer E

23. Thiamine is indicated for an unconscious patient who is suspected of coma due to ....

A. epilepsy
B. chronic alcoholism
C. acute hypoglycemia
D. cerebral edema
E. B and C

Answer E

24. For suspected increasing intracranial pressure the medical control physician may order which of the following drugs for diuresis?

A. mannitol
B. decadron
C. thiamine
D. naloxone
E. none of the above

Answer A

25. Place the events of a grand mal seizure chronologically as they are expected to occur.

5 1. post-ictal
3 2. tonic phase
1 3. aura
4 4. clonic phase
2 5. loss of consciousness

Select the proper grouping.

A. 3, 5, 4, 2, 1
B. 4, 5, 2, 3, 1
C. 1, 3, 2, 4, 5
D. 3, 5, 2, 4, 1
E. 2, 1, 3, 5, 4

Answer D

26. Which seizure disorder begins at one location and may progress to a generalized seizure?

A. psychomotor
B. focal motor
C. petit mal
D. grand mal
E. hysterical

Answer B

27. Which of the following elements of history would be important in evaluating a patient who experienced a seizure?

A. recent history of head trauma
B. alcohol or drug abuse
C. diabetes, heart disease
D. fever, stiff neck or headache
E. all of the above

Answer e

28. Status epilepticus is repeated seizures ....

A. lasting over 10 minutes
B. without an interim consciousness
C. with more than three in a row
D. not broken by valium
E. all of the above

Answer B

29. Valium is administered to the status epilepticus patient ....

A. IV 5 to 10 mg rapidly.
B. IV 20 to 40 mg rapidly.
C. IV 50 mg slowly.
D. IM in two 12 mg doses.
E. none of the above.

Answer E

30. The major mechanisms of stroke include ....

1. emboli or blood vessel occlusion
2. electrical disruption of the cerebral cortex
3. primary breakdown of the CSF circulation system
4. hemorrhage

Select the proper grouping.

A. 1, 2
B. 3, 4
C. 1, 4
D. 2, 4
E. 2, 3, 4

Answer C

PHARMACOLOGY MATH WORKSHEET III

Formulas

Rate = Volume/Time	mL/min = gtts per min/gtts per mL
Volume = Rate x Time	gtts / min = mL per min x gtts per mL
Time = Volume/Rate	mL = gtts/gtts per mL

Concentration = Weight/Volume	1 Kg = 2.2 lb.
Weight = Volume x Concentration	1 gm = 1,000 mg
Volume = Weight/Concentration	1 mg = 1,000 mcg

Please complete the following drug and drip math problems:

[1] You are asked to run a drip at 25 gtts/min. through a 45 mcgtts/mL set. What amount of fluid would you infuse during a ....

A) twenty minute run?

B) 36 minute call?

C) 47 minute call?

What would be the volume with a 60 mcgtts/mL set for the above?

A)

B)

C)

[2] Medical control asks that you infuse 250 mL of fluid during the transport to the hospital. What rate would you set your 10 gtts/mL administration set for if your ETA was ....

A) 12 minutes?

B) 37 minutes?

C) 1 hour and 23 minutes?

With a 60 mcgtts/mL set what would your rate be for the above?

A)

B)

C)

[3] You are asked to mix a dopamine drip with a concentration of 1.6 mg/mL. The only bag of D_5W you have is a 250 mL one. How much of the drug would you add?

What drip rate would you administer for a 2mcg/kg/min drip ....

A) for a 100 lb. patient @ 60 mcgtts/mL?

B) for a 220 lb. patient @ 45 mcgtts/mL?

C) for a 165 lb. patient @ 60 mcgtts/mL?

24

GASTROINTESTINAL, GENITOURINARY, AND REPRODUCTIVE SYSTEM EMERGENCIES

Review of the Objectives for Chapter 24

After reading this chapter, you should be able to:

1. Describe the structures of the abdominal cavity.

p. 771

The abdomen is bordered superiorly by the diaphragm, a domed sheath of muscle tissue that moves dynamically with respiration. The lower border of the abdominal cavity is an imaginary plane over the pelvis that separates the abdominal and pelvic cavities. The organs of the abdomen include ....

Stomach	Small Bowel
Large Bowel	Liver
Pancreas	Spleen
Kidneys	

2. Discuss the topographical anatomy of the abdomen and describe which organs lie within each quadrant.

pp. 771

The abdomen can be divided into four quadrants by drawing one line across the abdomen through the umbilicus and one superior to inferior, again, through the umbilicus. The areas defined are the right upper quadrant, the left upper quadrant, the right lower quadrant and the left lower quadrant.

Right upper quadrant	**Left upper quadrant**
liver and gall bladder	spleen
head of the pancreas	tail of the pancreas
part of the duodenum	stomach
right kidney	left kidney
hepatic flexure of the colon	splenic flexure of the colon

Right lower quadrant	**Left lower quadrant**
appendix	small intestine
ascending colon	descending colon
small intestine	left ovary
right ovary	left fallopian tube
right fallopian tube	

3. Describe the organs of the gastrointestinal system.

pp. 772 to 773

The **mouth** or oral cavity contains the teeth, tongue, gums, lips and cheeks. It begins the digestive process by physically breaking down the food and mixing it with the first digestive secretion, amylase.

The **esophagus** is a hollow, muscular tube designed to transport food from the mouth to the stomach.

The **stomach** is a hollow, muscular organ that physically mixes the digesting food. It also subjects the food to its secretions, including hydrochloric acid.

The **small intestine** is intended to continue the digestive process and to absorb nutrients. The small intestine is divided into three subdivisions. They are the duodenum, the jejunum, and the ileum.

The **large intestine** is where digesting food enters the final stage of digestion. Here water is released and absorbed from the digesting matter. As with the small intestine, the large intestine is also divided into three sections: the cecum, the colon and the rectum.

The **liver** is the largest of the solid abdominal organs. It secretes bile to assist in fat digestion, produces proteins, detoxifies many substances, and stores glycogen (a form of glucose).

The **pancreas** is responsible for the production of some digestive enzymes as well as insulin, glucagon and somastatin.

The **appendix** is a blind narrow pocket of the cecum. It has no known function.

4. Name the two major blood vessels found within the abdominal cavity.

p. 773

Abdominal aorta — Inferior vena cava

5. Describe the organs of the genitourinary system.

p. 774

The **kidneys** are paired organs located within the retroperitoneal space. They filter blood and concentrate waste products as urine. They are also responsible for assisting in blood pressure regulation and maintaining fluid and electrolyte balance.

The **ureters**, which are also retroperitoneal, extend from each kidney to the bladder.

The **urinary bladder** is located within the pelvic cavity and is responsible for the collection of urine.

The **urethra** is a tube extending from the bladder to the outside. It is considerably shorter in the female than the male.

6. Describe the organs of the male and female reproductive system.

pp. 775 to 776

Male

The male gonads are the **testes**. They are responsible for producing sperm and the male hormones.

The **epididymis** is a small appendage located on each teste. They collect and store sperm.

The **prostate** is a small gland located where the male ureter exits the bladder. It provides the fluid medium for the sperm.

The **vas deferens** are small muscular tubes which transport sperm from the testes to the ureter.

The **penis** is the male organ of copulation.

Female

The **ovaries** are the female gonads and are small, walnut-sized structures, located in the abdominal and abdominopelvic cavity. They are responsible for ovum production and some of the female hormones.

The **fallopian tubes** are hollow tubes connecting the abdominal cavity with the uterus. The fallopian tubes' distal opening is in the proximity of the ovary.

The **uterus** is a hollow muscular organ located in the lower pelvis. During pregnancy it will enlarge to accommodate the developing fetus and expel it at term.

The **vagina** is the female organ of copulation, extends from the outside to the uterus and serves as the birth canal.

7. Discuss the causes of acute abdominal pain originating in the gastrointestinal system.

pp. 776 to 779

Peptic ulcer disease is caused by erosions (ulcers) on the lining of the esophagus, stomach or duodenum. It may be caused by excess secretion of stomach acid or the breakdown of the digestive system lining by drugs, alcohol or other agents. The pain is usually epigastric or in the left upper quadrant and will frequently diminish with eating or antacids.

Appendicitis is inflammation of the appendix due to obstruction or other cause. The onset of pain is abrupt, usually begins around the umbilicus, and migrates to the right lower quadrant. It is often associated with nausea, vomiting, fever and anorexia.

Diverticulitis is the formation of pouches in the large intestine which develop with age. They become inflamed in much the same manner as the appendix, though symptoms are usually left-sided.

Pancreatitis is an inflammation of the pancreas. It is frequently associated with alcohol abuse, elevated blood cholesterol or triglycerides, or unknown causes. The pain begins abruptly in the central abdomen, then radiates to the back and shoulders. It is often accompanied by nausea and vomiting, and is cared for with fluid, pain medication and nasogastric tube placement.

Cholecystitis is an inflammation of the gall bladder which is frequently associated with a stone lodging in the bile duct. If the obstruction is severe, it may cause liver congestion and possibly pancreatitis. The pain is located in the right upper quadrant and will increase with ingestion of fatty foods. Treatment is commonly removal of the gall bladder.

Hepatitis is an inflammation of the liver, which may be the result of infection, or alcohol or other substance abuse. It normally presents with dull right quadrant pain and upper abdominal tenderness. It may be accompanied by anorexia, malaise, clay colored stool, and jaundice.

8. Discuss the causes of abdominal pain originating in the genitourinary system.

pp. 779 to 781

The genitourinary disorders are usually related to inflammation, infection, obstruction or hemorrhage. Disorders may also be related to reduced kidney efficiency or failure.

Kidney stone are crystallized salts which obstruct the ureter as they pass. Their passage is quite painful and colicky in nature. Pain will start in the upper back and move lower as the stone moves. Kidney stones can cause excruciating pain and their passage is facilitated with IV fluids and pain medication.

Pyelonephritis is an infection of the kidney caused by an infection that originated in the bladder. The patient will present with fever and low back pain. The patient may also display with pain at the costrovertebral angle. Care normally involves the administration of intravenous antibiotics.

9. Discuss the causes of acute abdominal pain originating in the reproductive system.

pp. 781 to 782

Epididymitis is an inflammation of the epididymis which may occur secondary to gonorrhea, syphilis, tuberculosis, mumps, urethritis or use of an indwelling catheter. The patient will generally present with chills, inguinal pain and have a swollen epididymis.

Testicular torsion occurs when part of a blood vessel becomes twisted and circulation to the testes is interrupted. The patient will experience severe pain.

Pelvic inflammatory disease normally results from a sexually transmitted disease and usually will affect the vagina, cervix, uterus, fallopian tubes, and the broad ligaments. The patient may experience fever, chills, lower abdominal pain, and possibly vaginal discharge or hemorrhage.

Ectopic pregnancy is a pregnancy which is outside the uterus and induces bleeding when the location of implantation ruptures. The patient may have a history of missed or irregular periods, lower abdominal pain, vaginal hemorrhage and the signs and symptoms of shock.

An **ovarian cyst** is a fluid filled sac located on the ovary that may, on occasion, cause pain.

10. Describe the signs and symptoms of upper and lower gastrointestinal hemorrhage.

p. 778

Upper Gastrointestinal Hemorrhage - results from hemorrhage in the esophagus, stomach, or duodenum. Signs and symptoms include hematemesis (vomiting blood), melena (dark stools resembling coffee grounds), and possibly epigastric pain.

Lower Gastrointestinal Hemorrhage - results from hemorrhage in the distal duodenum, colon, or rectum. Signs and symptoms include rectal bleeding, increased stool frequency, and in some cases, crampy, diffuse abdominal pain.

11. Describe the method of assessment for patients complaining of abdominal pain.

pp. 783 to 786

Primary Assessment is as with any emergency patient. Assure the airway, breathing, circulation, disability, and expose for head, neck, chest, and abdominal injury

Secondary Assessment in the stable patient follows the head to toe order with a focus on signs and symptoms of abdominal pathology. Inspect the abdomen for distension, asymetry, signs of trauma, or pulsing. Palpate the abdomen for guarding, tenderness, and rebound tenderness. Determine the vital signs and look for signs of shock that might be attributed to abdominal hemorhage. Evaluate the patient history for, or for suggestion of, abdominal problem.

12. Discuss the field management of acute abdominal pain.

pp. 786 to 787

In general, the patient with abdominal pain should be kept supine, given supplemental oxygen, monitored for oxygen saturation and ECG abnormalities, and given crystalloid fluid at a to-keep-open rate. If the patient is actively bleeding or displays the signs of shock, the fluid infusion rate should be wide open, high flow oxygen given and the PASG considered. Rapid transport should be provided.

13. Discuss hemodialysis and peritoneal dialysis.

pp. 787 to 788

Hemodialysis is a medical procedure which is employed to rid the body of wastes which the kidney is unable remove. Blood is processed through a machine which permits the diffusion and then elimination of waste products. In some cases the dialysis occurs within the peritoneal cavity. The peritoneal dialysis process may cause or be associated with hemorrhage at the vascular access site, peritonitis, infection, dehydration, air emboli, or dysrhythmias.

14. Discuss assessment, management, and complications of the dialysis patient.

pp. 788 to 790

The patient who is on renal dialysis should be carefully monitored to identify any problems with the vital signs or any dysrhythmias. Fluid access should be accomplished through a site other than the dialysis shunt, and any medical problem treated as for any other patient. Special concern should be provided to ensure no hemorrhage occurs at the vascular access site.

CASE STUDY REVIEW

Reread the case study in **PARAMEDIC EMERGENCY CARE** and then read the discussion below.

The case study for chapter 24 is a classical presentation of the acute abdomen. It affords us the opportunity to review assessment and management for the patient with abdominal complaints.

Chapter 24 Case Study

Steve Fletcher has the signs, symptoms and history commonly associated with acute appendicitis. He has the central abdominal pain that moves toward the right lower quadrant. He has the malaise, loss of appetite, nausea and vomiting. While this is a classical presentation of appendicitis and the paramedics in this case were right, it is much safer to assume nothing and resist the temptation to find a cause for the patient's presentation. Abdominal pain is very difficult to relate to one specific cause. The appendix, for example, is reasonably mobile within the abdomen and may present pain in almost any quadrant when inflamed. Fifteen percent of abdominal pain is caused by a problem outside the abdominal cavity including heart attack, pulmonary emboli, spinal column problems, etc. Glen, and any paramedic, should keep from forming an opinion as to the cause of a patient's symptoms and instead continue to assess and gather information to support or rule out several causes. If care is not taken, the paramedic may suffer from tunnel vision and miss other significant signs, symptoms and the true underlying problem.

Glen did approach a fellow worker in an appropriate way. It is very hard to objectively treat someone you know. It would be ideal to step aside and let someone else provide care but we don't often have that option in emergency medical service. If confronted by a relative, an acquaintance, or a co-worker, the paramedic must divorce him or herself from the relationship, take charge as Glen did, and provide the care that would be offered someone who was unknown.

The care offered to Steve Fletcher is that given any other patient with the same presentation. He is given oxygen at a modest rate. He is placed in the position of comfort while a complete history was taken. Rapid but safe transport is provided while Glen watches for the signs and symptoms of developing shock.

READING COMPREHENSION SELF-EXAM

1. The pain felt by a patient when palpation of the abdomen is released is called ....

   A. tenderness.
   B. rebound tenderness.
   C. guarding.
   D. peritonitis.
   E. Collig's sign.

   Answer ______

2. Epigastric pain is often associated with ....
   1. cholecystitis.
   2. peptic ulcer.
   3. esophagitis.
   4. appendicitis.

   Select the proper grouping.

   A. 1, 2
   B. 1, 3
   C. 2, 3
   D. 1, 3, 4
   E. 2, 3, 4

   Answer ______

3. Place the components of the digestive tract in order as digesting food would travel through them.
   1. duodenum
   2. cecum
   3. esophagus
   4. descending colon
   5. rectum

   Select the proper grouping.

   A. 3, 1, 2, 4, 5
   B. 2, 4, 3, 1, 5
   C. 3, 5, 4, 1, 2
   D. 1, 3, 2, 4, 5
   E. 3, 2, 1, 4, 5

   Answer ______

4. The blood vessels which drain blood from the intestine and transport it to the liver are the ....

   A. esophageal varices.
   B. vena cavae.
   C. renal veins.
   D. portal veins.
   E. hepatic veins.

   Answer ______

5. Pouches that are found in the large intestine and may become inflamed, similar to appendicitis, are called ....

   A. cholecystitis.
   B. ovarian cysts.
   C. diverticuli.
   D. pyelonephritis.
   E. varices.

   Answer ______

6. Which of the following conditions would be most likely to cause clay colored stool?

A. peptic ulcer disease
B. esophageal varices
C. hepatitis
D. rectal bleeding
E. pancreatitis

Answer C

7. If a pulsatile mass is found in the abdomen, the area should be thoroughly palpated to approximate the exact location and size of the mass.

A. True
B. False

Answer B

8. The tilt test to determine if a patient is hypovolemic is considered to be positive if the pressure when supine is how much greater than the reading for the patient in the seated or standing position?

A. 15 mm Hg
B. 25 mm Hg
C. 35 mm Hg
D. 50 mm Hg
E. 75 mm Hg

Answer A

9. Which of the following would you employ if a patient displayed a positive tilt test or other signs of intra-abdominal hemorrhage?
   1. high-flow oxygen
   2. crystalloid IVs run wide open
   3. PASG
   4. monitor ECG

Select the proper grouping.

A. 1, 3
B. 2, 4
C. 1, 2, 4
D. 2, 3, 4
E. 1, 2, 3, 4

Answer E

10. Acute renal failure can be caused by which of the following?
   1. reduction in blood flow to the kidneys
   2. shock
   3. kidney infection
   4. diverticulitis
   5. enlarged prostate

Select the proper grouping.

A. 1, 3, 5
B. 2, 4, 5
C. 1, 2, 3, 5
D. 1, 3, 4, 5
E. 1, 2, 3, 4

Answer C

11. Chronic renal failure may be expected to cause all of the following except ....

A. ascites.
B. jugular vein distention.
C. pericardial tamponade.
D. rales.
–E. severe dehydration.

Answer E

12. A patient you have been called to treat and transport is a 35-year-old male, has a history of gout, and is complaining of severe flank pain. The most likely cause of the problem is ....

A. renal failure.
B. pancreatitis.
C. pelvic inflammatory disease.
–D. kidney stone.
E. testicular torsion.

Answer D

13. A patient undergoing dialysis experiences headache, lethargy, and then coma. What problem should you suspect?

–A. disequilibrium syndrome
B. air emboli
C. cardiac dysrhythmias
D. uremic intoxication
E. profound hypotension

Answer A

14. Even though venous access is difficult, the dialysis shunt should not be used for infusion in the renal failure patient.

A. True
B. False

Answer A

15. The condition in which the blood vessel supplying the testicle becomes twisted is called ....

A. epididymitis.
B. vasectomy.
C. gonadal extremus.
D. testicular torsion.
E. none of the above.

Answer D

16. Identify the general elements of care for a patient who is experiencing abdominal pain.

Keep patient Supine / Administer Cryptalloid Solution IV – TKO
monitor Vital Signs / Supply O'2 Via N.C. / Provide Imediate transport.

17. Identify five elements of the PQRST mnemonic for abdominal physical assessment and give an example of a question you might ask regarding each.

PAin – what Provocted this.
Quality – Describe How it feels.
Radiation – Does the Pain travel to Any place else.
Severity – Scale of 1–10 of Pain
Time – when did this Start – how frequant is it.

25

ANAPHYLAXIS

Review of the Objectives for Chapter 25

After reading this chapter, you should be able to:

1. Define anaphylaxis.

p. 794

Anaphylaxis is an extreme allergic reaction to an antigen by the body's immune system. The reaction threatens life.

2. Define antigen.

p. 795

An antigen is any substance that is capable of inducing an immune response. Examples include drug molecules, serum, animal secretions and blood.

3. List ways an antigen can be introduced into the body.

p. 795

Antigens can be injected, ingested, inhaled or absorbed through the skin.

4. Define antibody.

p. 795

An antibody is a protein manufactured by the immune system which combines with the invading antigen and renders it harmless.

5. Describe the pathophysiology of allergic reactions and anaphylaxis.

pp. 796 to 798

An antigen enters the body and triggers a severe response. Histamine is released in high quantities causing severe bronchoconstriction, vasodilatation and very likely, shock. The bronchoconstriction may lead to severe dyspnea and hypoxia.

Vasodilatation may induce peripheral pooling of blood and hypotension. It may also cause tachycardia. The end result is a rapid onset, life threatening emergency that calls for immediate intervention.

6. Discuss the effects of allergic reactions and anaphylaxis on the following body systems:

p. 798

Skin

The skin, especially of the face and mucous membranes, may display edema.

Respiratory

The respiratory system is affected by severe bronchoconstriction. Edema affecting the larynx may cause partial or complete obstruction of the airway.

Cardiovascular

The cardiovascular system undergoes vasodilatation and vascular pooling. The net result is hypotension, tachycardia and reduced cardiac output.

Gastrointestinal

The gastrointestinal manifestations of anaphylaxis include nausea, abdominal cramping, vomiting, and diarrhea.

Nervous

The patient may experience CNS manifestations including headache, unconsciousness and possibly convulsions.

7. Describe the clinical presentation of the patient suffering an allergic reaction and anaphylaxis.

pp. 798 to 799

The classical signs of the patient who is experiencing anaphylaxis include dyspnea, stridor, and possibly hypoxia. He or she may also display local or systemic edema, hypotension and tachycardia. Gastrointestinal problems may be apparent as may unconsciousness and seizures. The patient who is experiencing an anaphylactic reaction will generally display anxiety and fear.

8. Discuss the assessment of the patient suffering an allergic reaction and anaphylaxis.

p. 799

The assessment of the anaphylaxis patient moves quickly to identify the life-threatening manifestations of the emergency and ensure they are rapidly corrected. Assess the airway for the development, or potential development, of laryngeal edema. Assess the lungs by evaluating breath sounds. Assess the pulse strength and rate to determine the effect anaphylaxis is having on the cardiovascular system. Observe the skin for the presence of hives (urticaria). Constantly monitor the level of consciousness.

9. Describe the management of a patient with a severe allergic reaction.

pp. 800 to 802

The airway should be secured. If necessary, an endotracheal tube or transtracheal ventilation should be used. Monitor the pulse, blood pressure, oxygen saturation and cardiac rhythm. Initiate an IV with normal saline or lactated Ringer's solution and consider epinephrine, diphenhydramine, and methylprednisolone.

10. Describe the actions of the following medications and relate their usage in the management of allergic reaction and anaphylaxis.

pp. 800 to 802

Oxygen is primarily used to ease hypoxia and improve the efficiency of respiratory effort. It should be used early and freely in anaphylaxis.

Epinephrine is the first line drug in combating anaphylaxis. It counteracts the effects of histamine. It should be administered subcutaneously (0.3 to 0.5 mg of 1:1000) in the mild reaction and intravenously (3 to 5 ml of 1:10,000) for the severe reaction.

Diphenhydramine (Benadryl) is used after the administration of epinephrine. It blocks histamine's effects on lungs and vascular system.

Methylprednisolone (Solu-Medrol) is a corticosteroid and the third line drug for anaphylaxis. It is an anti-inflammitory. It slows histamine release and the leakage of fluid from the capillaries.

CASE STUDY REVIEW

Reread the case study in **PARAMEDIC EMERGENCY CARE** and then read the discussion below.

This case study describes a severe and life threatening anaphylactic reaction. It is aggressively treated through protocol and illustrates effective care in a dire emergency.

Chapter 25 Case Study

The crew in this scenario was fortunate because they arrive early in the development of anaphylaxis and the history of the incident is preserved by the bystanders. The dispatch information about bee stings and "can't breathe" allows them to prepare the airway kit and ready the drugs they may need for the problem. They also review the local protocol for anaphylaxis and identify the care steps they will take upon arrival.

The A-B-C-D-E of the primary assessment reveals some of the classic signs of the severe allergic reaction. The airway is compromised by the swelling of angioneurotic edema as noted by the stridorous respirations. Breathing is compromised by bronchoconstriction. The cardiovascular system also displays signs of compromise including the absent pulse and weak rapid carotid pulses. The rapid pulse may indicate excitement, or more likely, shock; one of the body's first compensatory mechanisms. The absent radial pulse (which is checked bilaterally) gives further cause to suspect hypovolemia secondary to vasodilatation. At the end of the primary assessment the paramedic is certain he has a critical patient. Transport will occur quickly with most care enroute. The administration of oxygen is increased and equipment for endotracheal intubation is prepared, just in case it is needed.

The secondary survey is quickly applied in an abbreviated fashion. It reveals a patient who is rapidly deteriorating. The pulse rate has risen by 10 in just a few minutes. The stridor is growing worse and threatening complete obstruction. The paramedic employs protocol and administers epinephrine and Benadryl. The epinephrine is given IV because of the urgency of the patient's condition. Intramuscular Benadryl injection is not used because peripheral circulation, as noted by the pale and diaphoretic skin, may be slow and absorb the medication unpredictably. The heart is monitored, not only because of the administration of epinephrine in the presence of tachycardia but because dyspnea and hypoxia may also cause heart disturbances. The crew also administers Solu-Medrol to reduce edema, both systemic and laryngeal.

The effect of drug therapy is dramatic and positive. The stridor decreases, breath sounds increase and, no doubt, the patient's sensorium and ability to communicate improve. Endotracheal intubation is no longer considered and the paramedic contacts medical control to provide a patient report, let them know that protocol was used, and request further orders.

READING COMPREHENSION SELF-EXAM

1. Anaphylaxis is a rapid and extreme allergic reaction due to an ingested, injected, absorbed or inhaled antigen.

   A. True
   B. False

   Answer 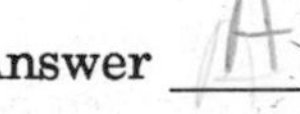

2. Antigen responsible for the induction of an allergic reaction may be which of the following?
   1. drug molecules
   2. animal secretions
   3. whole blood
   4. mast cells

   Select the proper grouping.

   A. 1, 3
   B. 2, 3
   C. 1, 2, 3
   D. 1, 2, 4
   E. 1, 2, 3, 4

   Answer C

3. The substance released from mast cells during an anaphylactic reaction, which causes bronchoconstriction and vasodilatation is ....

A. neutriphil.
B. attenuated bacteria.
C. macrophage.
D. histamine.
E. hydrocortisone.

Answer D

4. Which of the following responses may occur during an anaphylactic reaction?
1. vasodilatation
2. bronchodilatation
3. peripheral edema
4. increased gastric secretion
5. diarrhea
Select the proper grouping.

A. 1, 2, 4
B. 2, 3, 5
C. 1, 2, 3, 4
D. 1, 3, 4, 5
E. 1, 2, 3, 4, 5

Answer D

5. The stridor associated with anaphylaxis is caused by ....

A. mucosal edema.
B. bronchodilatation.
C. respiratory center depression.
D. spasm of the vocal cords.
E. all of the above.

Answer A

6. In the patient suffering from a possible anaphylactic reaction, the primary concern is for the ....

A. airway.
B. bronchoconstriction.
C. vasodilatation.
D. histamine release.
E. peripheral edema.

Answer A

7. If the site of antigen injection is known, as it may be in a bee sting, what special step may the rescuer provide?

A. pack the site in ice
B. wash and scrub the wound with soap and water
C. inject the site with epinephrine (1:10,000)
D. place a venous constricting band between the site and the heart
E. place an arterial constricting band between the site and the heart

Answer D

8. The epinephrine dosage for subcutaneous injection in anaphylaxis is ....

A. 0.3 to 0.5 ml (1:1,000).
B. 0.3 to 0.5 mg (1:1,000).
C. 3 to 5 ml (1:10,000).
D. 3 to 5 mg (1:10,000).
E. either A or B.

Answer E

9. In severe and life-threatening anaphylaxis which of the following would you administer and in which order?
   1. epinephrine (1:1,000)
   2. methylprednisolone
   3. Benadryl
   4. atropine
   5. epinephrine (1:10,000)

   Select the proper grouping.

   A. 1, 5, 2, 3
   B. 5, 3, 2
   C. 2, 3, 1
   D. 5, 2, 3, 4
   E. 5, 1, 2, 3, 4

   Answer B

10. Which of the following are corticosteroids that may be given to the anaphylaxis patient to slow histamine release and capillary leakage?
   1. neutrophil
   2. Solu-Cortef
   3. Decadron
   4. methylprednisone
   5. aminophylline

   Select the proper grouping.

   A. 1, 3, 5
   B. 2, 3, 5
   C. 2, 3, 4
   D. 1, 3, 4, 5
   E. 2, 3, 4, 5

   Answer C

11. List the signs and symptoms expected from a patient experiencing anaphylaxis.

Signs	Symptoms
dyspnea - hypotension	dyspnea - History of 1. ingestion
Coughing - vasodilation	Abdominal cramping 2. injection
Sneezing - vomiting	nausea 3. Allergies
Stridor - diarrhea	headache, 4. Anaphylaxis
tachycardia - uticaria (Hives)	lump in throat

DRUGS USED IN THE CARE OF ANAPHYLAXIS:

Emergency management for anaphylaxis utilizes many of the pharmacologic agents which are available to the paramedic. Please review and memorize the various names, indications, therapeutic effects, contraindications, side effects, routes of administration and recommended dosages for the following.

aminophylline	diphenhydramine (Bendryl)
epinephrine (1:10,000) (adrenalin)	epinephrine (1:1,000) (adrenalin)
oxygen	

26

TOXICOLOGY AND SUBSTANCE ABUSE

Review of the Objectives for Chapter 26

After reading this chapter, you should be able to:

1. Discuss the importance of toxicologic emergencies in prehospital care.

p. 806

Over 1 million persons are poisoned annually
10% of all emergency responses
70% of accidental poisonings are in children under six
Accidental ingestion in children has a repeat rate of 25%
80% of attempted suicides involve a drug overdose

2. Describe the various entry routes of toxic substances into the body.

pp. 807 to 809

Ingestion is the most common route for entry of toxic substances. The effects can be both immediate and delayed. They may damage the mouth, throat and esophagus immediately through the corrosive effects of the agent. Absorption will occur from the small intestine and, to a lesser degree, the stomach.

Inhalation results in the rapid absorption of toxins through the alveoli-capillary membrane. Inhalation of toxins can also result in airway burns as the toxin combines with tissue fluids to form corrosive chemicals.

Injection introduces an agent into the dermal, subcutaneous, intramuscular or intravenous tissue. The rate of entry into the vascular system is dependent on the site of injection and the level of circulation.

Absorption through the body's surface is slow and unpredictable. Agents such as poison ivy and oak are well known. Chemical agents, such as the organophosphates, may also be absorbed through the skin.

3. Discuss the role of poison control centers within the EMS system.

pp. 809

Poison control centers are staffed with specially trained personnel who have reference materials on all types of poisoning. They can provide information on the expected effects and recommended care for specific poisonings.

4. Describe general principles of toxicologic management.

p. 809

The general principles of management for toxicologic emergencies include surveying the scene for evidence of the toxic material and any evidence of attempted suicide. Ensure the scene is clear of hazards, then perform the primary assessment, assuring that the airway is clear and breathing is adequate. As appropriate for the poison, limit absorption, enhance elimination, and administer the antidote.

5. Relate general principles for assessing and managing patients who have ingested poison.

pp. 812 to 817

Patient assessment

What was ingested? (container, contents or sample emesis)
How long since ingestion?
How much was taken?
Have attempts been made to induce vomiting?
Has charcoal or an antidote been administered?
Does the patient have a psychiatric or suicide history?

Management

Induce vomiting with ipecac (30 mL) and two to three glasses of water
Activated charcoal may be administered (50 to 100 g in water)
Consider $D_{50}W$, naloxone and thiamine

6. Discuss the factors affecting the decision to induce vomiting in a patient who has ingested poison.

pp. 812 to 813

Induce vomiting unless:

more than 3 to 6 hours since ingestion
the patient is stuporous or unconscious
the patient is pregnant
the patient has a history of heart disease or might be having an MI
a corrosive substance has been ingested
hydrocarbon substances have been ingested

(In cases of pesticides, heavy metals, halogenated hydrocarbons, chamfer-based hydrocarbons or aromatic hydrocarbons, vomiting should be induced.)

7. Describe the signs, symptoms, and management of patients who have ingested the following toxins.

pp. 814 to 817

Antiemetics

Induce vomiting if the patient is conscious, and it has been less than 30 minutes since ingestion. Also consider an NG tube and activated charcoal if transport is prolonged.

Contaminated food

The patient may display various abdominal complaints including nausea, vomiting, diarrhea, and diffuse pain. Establish and maintain the airway, administer high-flow oxygen, intubate and assist respirations as needed, establish venous access, and consider ipecac.

Poisonous plants

The patient may display many gastro-intestinal signs. Treat as for contaminated food.

Niacin

The patient will have a history of vitamin B ingestion and profuse flushing, itching, burning, and tingling sensations. This experience is self-limiting and usually requires only supportive care.

Ethylene glycol/methanol

Signs and symptoms include abdominal pain, nausea, vomiting, intoxication, and tachypnea/hyperpnea. Care should include establishing an airway, high-flow oxygen, intubation and assisted ventilation as needed. Establish venous access and consider sodium bicarbonate and possibly oral ethanol.

8. Describe the presentation and treatment of the following toxic conditions.

pp. 817 to 834

Inhaled poisons

Signs - the patient may display tachypnea, rales, rhonchi, wheezes, hoarseness or stridor. The patient may also present with dizziness, confusion, seizures, coma or cardiac dysrhythmias.

Symptoms - the patient may complain of dyspnea, headache, hallucinations or chest tightness or pain.

Treatment - safely remove the patient from the environment and maintain the airway. High-flow oxygen should be given and an IV route obtained. The airway must be continuously monitored since the inhalation injury may progressively obstruct it.

Injected poisons

Signs - evidence of the sting or injection site may be visible as may erythema and edema. In severe or anaphylactic reactions the patient may experience dyspnea and systemic signs.

Symptoms - the patient will relate a history of the incident and may complain of localized pain, and possible systemic complications.

Treatment - remove the stinger with a scraping motion and wash the area. Cool the site and watch for the possible development of anaphylaxis.

Surfaced absorbed poisons

Signs - the patient may have residue on the skin or erythema.

Symptoms - the patient may reveal a history of exposure or identify CNS or other symptoms.

Treatment - safely decontaminate and remove the patient from the source. The patient should receive oxygen and airway control as needed. An IV should be established.

9. Discuss the presentation and management of the following bites or stings

pp. 821 to 828

Bees, hornets, wasps, or yellow jackets - the bee or other insect sting will generally present with local irritation only. Observe the patient for the development of respiratory embarrassment or other signs of anaphylaxis.

Brown recluse spiders - the bite of the brown recluse spider presents with a small bleb surrounded by a white ring. It may cause some pain and swelling. The patient may experience chills, fever, nausea, vomiting, joint pain or bleeding disorders. Only supportive care is recommended in the prehospital setting.

Black widow spiders - the black widow spider bite will present with immediate pain, redness and swelling. There may be accompanying large muscle group pain and spasm with nausea, vomiting, seizures, paralysis, hypertension and diminished LOC. The patient should be calmed and valium, or calcium gluconate, considered.

Scorpions - the scorpion sting is accompanied by mild to sharp pain, numbness, restlessness, slurred speech, salivation, muscle twitching, abdominal pain and cramping, nausea, vomiting, and seizures. Care should include reassurance and a constricting band, proximal to the bite. Analgesics should be avoided.

Rattlesnake, copperhead or cotton-mouth water moccasins - the bite of any of these pit vipers will be reddened, painful and display fang marks at the site of injection. The patient may complain of weakness, dizziness, sweating, chills, thirst, nausea, vomiting, diarrhea, and numbness and tingling around the face and head. There may also be tachycardia, hypotension and bloody urine. The patient may have shallow breathing which may progress to respiratory failure. Management includes supine positioning, immobilization of the site and a constricting band between the bite and heart. Initiate oxygen, an IV line, and respiratory support.

Coral snakes - the coral snake bite may not exhibit any local or systemic signs immediately. The patient may experience numbness, weakness, drowsiness, ataxia, slurred speech, difficult swallowing, double vision, dilated pupils, abdominal pain, nausea, vomiting, seizures, unconsciousness, respiratory failure and hypotension. Care includes aggressive and immediate washing of the wound, a venous tourniquet, oxygen, an IV and rapid transport.

Marine animals - the site of a marine animal sting will be intensely painful and will swell. The victim may experience weakness, nausea, vomiting, dyspnea, tachycardia, and in severe cases hypotension and shock. Care should include maintaining the airway, oxygen, warming the sting site, and a venous tourniquet. Remove any stinger still in place.

10. Discuss the general principles regarding the recognition and management of substance abuse.

pp. 830 to 836

The drugs of abuse include alcohol, cocaine, opiates, marijuana, amphetamines, halluciogens and sedatives. The presentation will depend on the substance used while management, in general, is as for any other ingested poison.

11. Identify some of the physiological signs and effects of chronic drug abuse

pp. 830 to 836

Alcohol is a central nervous system depressant and a potent vasodilator. Its chronic use can result in enlarged liver, dehydration, otherwise unexplained gastroinestinal bleeding, flushed face and palms, dry mouth, vomiting, tremors, etc. Effects of chronic abuse may include ....

hepatitis
esophageal varices
loss of cerebral function
upper GI hemorrhage
liver cirrhosis
loss of sensation in hands and feet
pancreatitis
subdural hematoma

CASE STUDY REVIEW

Reread the case study in **PARAMEDIC EMERGENCY CARE** and then read the discussion below.

The case study in this chapter presents a frequent problem related to drug overdose. It provides a chance to look at the problems associated with caring for an overdose patient who does not want care and some of the concerns the paramedic should have while attending the patient.

Chapter 26 Case Study

This scenario is relatively common to emergency medical service. The patient is found unconscious with the environment suggesting the potential for drug overdose. Street drugs are notorious for causing overdose because of the varying concentration of the active ingredient. If a particularly pure batch hits the streets, there will be a rash of overdoses.

The paramedics are asked to employ Narcan (naloxone) in response to the environment conditions, which were communicated to the medical control physician. Narcan is a narcotic antagonist and will bind to the narcotic receptors thereby preventing any natural or synthetic narcotic from acting. The glucose level is found to be within normal tolerances. If it were not or a glucometer was not available, glucose would be given to correct any hypoglycemia and yet not appreciably affect either the normo-glycemic or hyperglycemic patient. The paramedics may also consider thiamine if the history suggested chronic alcoholism. Thiamine is essential to the metabolism of glucose and may be depleted in the chronic alcoholic.

Narcan is administered and is dramatically effective. It can then be assumed that the unconsciousness was caused by a narcotic overdose. The paramedics must be carefully observe the patient for two reasons. The administration of Narcan can cause an immediate and extreme withdrawal from chronic narcotic use. The patient may become very violent and assault the crew. Narcan also is shorter acting than most narcotics. Hence, the patient may return to unconsciousness after the Narcan is no longer effective. The patient may then experience respiratory depression or arrest. The paramedics must be careful to ensure the patient does not endanger them and he receives continued observation and care until well after the effects of the illicit drug wear off.

READING COMPREHENSION SELF-EXAM

1. What percentage of attempted suicide is attributable to drug overdose?

   A. 80 %
   B. 70 %
   C. 60 %
   D. 50 %
   E. 25 %

   Answer A

2. The most common route of poisoning is ....

   A. injection.
   B. ingestion.
   C. inhalation.
   D. absorption.
   E. none of the above.

   Answer B

3. Most absorption of ingested toxins occurs within the ....

   A. mouth.
   B. esophagus.
   C. stomach.
   D. small intestine.
   E. large intestine.

   Answer D

4. The absorption of toxins inhaled through the respiratory system is usually very slow because it takes a prolonged period of time for the toxin to cross the alveolar-capillary membrane.

   A. True
   B. False

   Answer B

5. Frequently, poisoning histories are inaccurate because of drug induced confusion, misinformation, or deliberate attempts at deception.

   A. True
   B. False

   Answer A

6. Which of the following are true regarding poison control centers?
   1. they are available by phone 24 hours a day
   2. they have computers to rapidly access information
   3. they can suggest field care for about 10% of cases
   4. they can determine the potential toxicity of the ingestion

   Select the proper grouping.

   A. 1, 3
   B. 2, 4
   C. 1, 2, 4
   D. 1, 3, 4
   E. 1, 2, 3, 4

   Answer C

7. Which of the following are contraindications to the use of ipecac?
   1. stuporous or comatose patient
   2. a late pregnancy patient
   3. pesticide ingestion
   4. heavy metal ingestion
   5. halogenated hydrocarbon ingestion

   Select the proper grouping.

   A. 1, 2
   B. 1, 2, 5
   C. 1, 3, 4
   D. 1, 3, 4, 5
   E. 1, 2, 3, 4, 5

   Answer A

8. The adult dose of ipecac is ....

   A. 10 mL.
   B. 15 mL.
   C. 30 mL.
   D. 50 to 100 g.
   E. 20 to 50 g.

   Answer C

9. The recommended dose of ipecac for the child under one year is ....

   A. 5 mL.
   B. 10 mL.
   C. 15 mL.
   D. 30 mL.
   E. 50 mL.

   Answer B

10. The adult patient who is to receive charcoal should receive what amount mixed with water?

    A. 10 mL
    B. 30 mL
    C. 20 to 50 g
    D. 50 to 100 g
    E. none of the above

    Answer D

11. What volume of water should follow the administration of ipecac in the adult patient?

A. 1 glass
B. 2 to 3 glasses
C. 4 to 5 glasses
D. 1 liter
E. 2 liters

Answer B

12. If a suspected poisoning patient is unconscious, what medication may be considered?

A. oxygen
B. naloxone
C. dextrose 50%
D. thiamine
E. all of the above

Answer e

13. The patient who has inhaled a toxic substance may be expected to display with or complain of ....

A. hoarseness.
B. wheezing.
C. chest tightness.
D. tachypnea.
E. any of the above.

Answer e

14. Calcium gluconate may be considered for which of the following injected poisonings?
   1. yellow jacket sting
   2. rattlesnake bite
   3. coral snake bite
   4. scorpion sting
   5. black widow spider bite

Select the proper grouping.

A. 1
B. 3
C. 5
D. 1, 3
E. 1, 4, 5

Answer C

15. You have been called to attend a snake-bitten patient. The patient states that the snake had a triangular head and elliptical pupils. The site displays swelling and severe pain. To which of the poisonous snakes would you attribute this bite?

A. pit viper
B. coral snake
C. elapidae
D. cannot differentiate from this information
E. either A or B

Answer A

16. Which of the following are care steps for the poisonous snake-bite patient?
   1. cooling of the wound site
   2. immobilization of limb
   3. IV started with crystalloid
   4. transport to hospital for possible antivenin administration
   5. a constricting band proximal to bite
   Select the proper grouping.

   A. 1, 3
   B. 2, 4, 5
   C. 3, 4, 5
   D. 2, 3, 4, 5
   E. 1, 2, 3, 4, 5

   Answer ____

17. The venom of most marine animals is deactivated by the application of heat.

   A. True
   B. False

   Answer ____

18. In treating a patient who was stung by a marine animal you notice a stinger is still impaled in the patient. You should ....

   A. leave it where it lies.
   B. remove it.
   C. apply cool compresses.
   D. cut off the protruding portion.
   E. none of the above.

   Answer ____

19. Which of the following are consequences of chronic alcohol ingestion?
   1. hepatitis
   2. liver cirrhosis
   3. hypoglycemia
   4. pancreatitis
   5. upper GI hemorrhage
   Select the proper grouping.

   A. 1, 2
   B. 1, 3, 5
   C. 2, 3, 4
   D. 1, 2, 4, 5
   E. 1, 2, 3, 4, 5

   Answer ____

20. Delirium tremens is a minor complication of alcohol withdrawal that occurs about 24 to 30 hours after sudden abstinence of alcohol intake.

   A. True
   B. False

   Answer ____

PHARMACOLOGY MATH WORKSHEET IV

Formulas

Rate = Volume/Time
Volume = Rate x Time
Time = Volume/Rate

mL/min = gtts per min/gtts per mL
gtts / min = mL per min x gtts per mL
mL = gtts/gtts per mL

Concentration = Weight/Volume
Weight = Volume x Concentration
Volume = Weight/Concentration

1 Kg = 2.2 lb.
1 gm = 1,000 mg
1 mg = 1,000 mcg

Please complete the following drug and drip math problems:

[1] What are the concentrations of the following drugs?
A) 500 mg in 10 mL?

B) 1 G in 100 mL?

C) 25 mg in 2 mL?

D) 150 mg in 500 mL?

[2] What weight (dose) of the drug would you be administering to a patient if you gave ....
A) 5 mL of a 10 mg/mL solution?

B) 1 mL of a 200 mg/5mL solution?

C) 10 mL of a 2% solution?

D) 5 mL of a 1:10,000 solution?

E) 3 mL of a 1:1,000 solution?

[3] What volume of a drug would you draw into a syringe to obtain ....
A) 2 mg of a 1:1,000 solution?

B) 15 mg of a 1:10,000 solution?

C) 7 mg of a 5% solution?

D) 5 mg of a 15 mg/30mL solution?

27

INFECTIOUS DISEASES

Review of the Objectives for Chapter 27

After reading this chapter, you should be able to:

1. Define the following terms:

pp. 841 to 842

Bacteria are small unicellular organisms that are capable of living without other organisms. They are responsible for many common infections.

Antibiotics are drugs which inhibit the growth of or kill bacteria. They have no effect on viruses.

Viruses are smaller than bacteria and cannot grow without the assistance of another organism. They invade a cell and take over its function. They are very difficult to treat.

Fungi are more like plants than animals; they rarely cause human disease other than skin and some vaginal infections.

Antigens are proteins on the surface of a virus or bacteria which identifies it as foreign to the body.

2. Define toxin and give examples of endotoxins and exotoxins.

p. 841

Toxins are poisonous chemicals released by bacteria. The endotoxin is released as the cell dies, as in septic shock. Exotoxins are released by the bacteria while it is alive and may cause serious consequences, such as the muscle spasm in tetanus.

3. Describe the difference between bacterial and viral infections.

p. 841

Bacterial infections are caused by cells that can support themselves alone. They are common but relatively easy to combat.

Viral infections are caused by very small organisms that must have another organism to assist their growth. They invade the cells of the organism they infect. Viruses are difficult to treat because the host cell must be killed to kill the virus.

4. Briefly discuss the body's immune system.

pp. 842 to 843

The human immune system recognizes foreign antigens and initiates a response to the invading agent. Antibodies are formed and transported to the site of infection, and attach to the antigens, deactivating the agent. White blood cells are also transported to the site and engulf the pathogen.

5. Define the following terms.

p. 842

Leukocytes are the white blood cells and assist in disease fighting by engulfing the foreign cell and then dying.

Cell-mediated immunity involves the leukocytes that engulf the invading cell and render it ineffective.

Humoral immunity involves the production of five specialized proteins called antibodies. These agents attach to the surface of the foreign cell, inactivating it and allowing scavenger cells to remove it.

Macrophages are scavenger cells which remove the cells inactivated by the humoral immunity process.

6. Identify factors that increase the risk of disease.

pp. 843 to 844

The **type of organism**, such as bacteria and viruses, are more easily transmitted than others such as parasites and fungi.

Virulence is the strength of an organism to infect. Hepatitis B is very virulent while HIV dies when exposed to light or air.

Dosage is the amount of infectious material, specifically the number of organisms. In most cases, there is a minimum number before infection will take hold.

Host resistance is the ability of the host to fight off the infection.

7. Describe meningitis, its presentation, prehospital care, and appropriate safety precautions.

pp. 850 to 851

Meningitis is the most common infection of the central nervous system encountered in prehospital care. It is an inflammation of the meninges. Meningitis normally begins as a cold that spreads to the brain and spinal cord. In the infant, meningitis presents with fever, irritability and poor feeding. In the older child or adult the problem may cause malaise, headache, and a stiff or sore neck. It is usually accompanied by nausea and vomiting. In acute cases, the patient may present with confusion, seizures or coma. Management is supportive with gloves and masks employed to reduce the risk of disease transmission. The ambulance should be decontaminated, the laundry properly bagged and medical follow-up should be performed.

8. Describe tuberculosis, its presentation, prehospital care, and appropriate safety precautions.

pp. 851 to 853

Tuberculosis is a serious respiratory infection spread through droplet contamination. It initially presents as a cough, then chills, fever, fatigue, weight loss, profuse sweating at night and hemoptysis. The patient should be cared for with support for the signs and symptoms of the disease. Care should be taken to minimize the possibility of disease transmission. The patient and paramedic should be masked and the patient area should be well ventilated. Avoid contact with body fluids, especially sputum.

9. Describe scabies and lice.

pp. 853 to 854

Scabies are a species of mite which are very infectious. They burrow into the skin and cause a severe itch.

Lice are parasites slightly larger than mites. They attach to hair folicles and lay their eggs there. Lice also cause severe itching.

10. Describe common childhood diseases and their implications for prehospital care.

pp. 854 to 855

Measles are a common childhood disease with an incubation period of 8 to 13 days. It manifests as a red rash that typically appears on the face and spreads from there. It is transmitted through the respiratory tract.

Mumps is an infectious disease affecting the salivary glands and inducing fever. Its incubation period is 12 to 26 days. Transmission is usually through saliva.

Varicelli, or chicken pox, is a form of herpes infection. It is transmitted through the respiratory tract. It has an incubation period of 10 to 21 days. It begins with fever, followed by crops of skin erruptions

11. Describe gastroenteritis, its presentation, prehospital care, and appropriate safety precautions.

pp. 855

Gastroenteritis is a common infection of the stomach and intestine. More commonly called food poisoning, it occurs minutes to hours after ingesting contaminated food. The patient will present with vomiting, diarrhea, abdominal pain and possible dehydration. Care should be primarily supportive with fluids given via IV line if dehydration is moderate to severe. The paramedic should wear gloves and wash the ambulance and equipment thoroughly after transport.

12. Describe hepatitis, its presentation, prehospital care, and appropriate safety precautions.

pp. 855 to 857

Hepatitis is a very dangerous and contagious disease of the liver. There are three forms: hepatitis A, hepatitis B, and hepatitis non A, non B. Hepatitis A is a self-limiting disease which ends in lifetime immunity to the disease and does not provide a carrier state. Hepatitis B is more serious and will result in a carrier state for life. Non A, non B hepatitis is similar to hepatitis B though the actual agent causing it is unknown. The patient with hepatitis will present with weakness, loss of appetite, and jaundice. Hepatitis may lead to cirrhosis of the liver and eventual death. Care for the hepatitis patient should be supportive with the paramedic utilizing some precautions against disease transmission. Wear gloves at all times and wash hands after all contact. Bag and clean all laundry properly and wash the ambulance and all equipment. All emergency personnel should be vaccinated against hepatitis B.

13. Explain the reasons that hepatitis B poses a serious health threat to medical personnel.

pp. 855 to 856

Hepatitis B, commonly called serum hepatitis, is a highly infectious blood borne agent. It is transmitted by contact with blood or body secretions. It is a virulent disease.

14. Identify common sexually transmitted disease, and describe prehospital management.

pp. 857 to 861

Sexually transmitted diseases are infectious diseases transmitted from one person to another through sexual intercourse. They include syphilis, gonorrhea and chlamydia, herpes and AIDS. When you care for a patient with a suspected sexually transmitted disease, wear gloves at all times, clean the ambulance thoroughly, notify emergency personnel, sterilize all instruments used, and bag and wash all linen properly.

15. Explain Acquired Immune Deficiency Syndrome (AIDS).

pp. 858 to 859

Acquired Immune Deficiency Syndrome is a syndrome caused by the human immunodeficiency virus (HIV). AIDS is a breakdown in the body's disease defense system which leave it unable to combat even the simplest of infections.

16. Describe methods of HIV transmission.

pp. 858 to 859

HIV transmission occurs through blood, vaginal secretions and semen. Though not common, transmission may also be possible through tears, cerebrospinal fluid, saliva, breast milk, amniotic fluid or urine. The virus can enter the body through breaks in the skin, mucous membranes or the eyes.

17. List precautions that should be employed to protect prehospital personnel from HBV and HIV.

pp. 860 to 861

The paramedic should employ the "universal precautions" whenever transporting a patient with an infectious disease. The precautions include:

Barrier protection

Gloves, changed for each patient contacted.

Masks and protective eye wear for any contact where blood or body fluids may be splashed.

Gowns should be worn where splashing body fluids are expected.

Hand washing

Hands and other body surfaces in contact with the patient should be thoroughly washed immediately after the contact.

Needle stick prevention

Care should be exercised to prevent needle sticks. Needles should not be recapped and care should be observed in the use and disposal of sharp objects such as scalpels.

Resuscitation

Where possible, resuscitation should be accomplished via mouthpiece, bag valve mask or oxygen powered ventilator.

Weeping wounds

Any health care worker with a weeping wound or other exudate should refrain from patient contact.

18. Define "Universal Precautions."

pp. 860 to 861

The universal precautions, as described above, are precautions that health care professionals can employ to significantly reduce their exposure to and chance of contracting a communicable disease. They are simple procedures that should be used whenever caring for a patient with suspected communicable disease.

CASE STUDY REVIEW

Reread the case study in **PARAMEDIC EMERGENCY CARE** and then read the discussion below.

This case presents a relatively typical scenario involving a contagious disease. It allows for discussion of the dangers of failing to use the universal precautions and other actions that could protect the paramedic from serious debilitating disease.

Chapter 27 Case Study

The paramedics respond to a call, which could be anything from a routine "taxi ride" to a critical emergency. The home is run-down and should suggest that universal precautions might be considered even before entering. Gloves could protect against lice, scabies or contagious diseases that might exist in the unsanitary environment. Their application before arrival at the patient's side allows immediate care and prevents delay if the patient is in need of immediate resuscitation.

The sunlight reveals the jaundiced patient's skin and suggests hepatitis. This conclusion is supported by the patient's loss of appetite and taste for cigarettes. The history of dark brown urine and tenderness under the border of the right rib margin also support hepatitis as the cause of the patient's problem. The needle tracks place the patient in a very high risk group for hepatitis and HIV diseases.

In caring for this patient the paramedics must be very careful not to needlessly or carelessly expose themselves to the patient's disease. Hepatitis is a very serious disease process, which can be debilitating and in some cases life-threatening. Immunization, which these paramedics have already received, is a modest cost for important protection.

The hospital should be alerted to the patient's condition early. This will allow them to take the proper precautions for staff and allow isolation so other emergency department visitors are not exposed to the disease unnecessarily. The staff should be alerted about the patient's girl friend who is also infected and employed in a role that would allow her to expose others to the disease.

As the patient responsibilities are completed, the paramedics wash and clean the ambulance with a strong disinfectant. They bag all linen and set it aside for proper cleaning or disposal. All equipment is sterilized or cleaned appropriately. These efforts protect both the paramedics who will be staffing the unit and the patient's they will be caring for.

Lastly, the paramedics will record the call and, specifically, their exposure to hepatitis. This will document that the exposure existed in case one of the team members becomes symptomatic in the next few months.

READING COMPREHENSION SELF-EXAM

1. The proteins found on the surface of bacteria and viruses that are recognized by the immune system are called ....

   A. T bodies.
   B. antibodies.
   C. antigens.
   D. pathogens.
   E. phagocytes.

   Answer ____

2. A patient is assessed to find a general ill feeling, headache, stiff neck, and nausea with some vomiting. Which of the following contagious diseases would you suspect?

   A. mumps
   B. hepatitis
   C. meningitis
   D. chlamydia
   E. herpes zoster

   Answer ____

3. The respiratory disease that occurs most frequently in crowded and unsanitary conditions and presents with cough, chills, fever, fatigue weight loss, and profuse night sweats is most likely ....

   A. meningitis.
   B. chlamydia.
   C. herpes zoster.
   D. tuberculosis.
   E. varicella.

   Answer ____

4. Your patient is complaining of general malaise and loss of appetite. You notice that she has a yellowish hue to her skin and a moderately tender right upper quadrant. Her problem is most likely related to which disease process?

A. hepatitis
B. herpes
C. tuberculosis
D. human immunodeficiency virus
E. scabies

Answer A

5. Which of the following is not a sexually transmitted disease?

A. chlamydia
B. herpes simplex
C. human immunodeficiency virus
D. scabies
E. gonorrhea

Answer D

6. During your assessment of a pregnant mother near term, she states that she has herpes simplex and active lesions. What effect might this have on delivery?

A. elective delivery ought to be by cesarean section
B. the vagina canal should be carefully draped
C. this condition should not affect the delivery process
D. the vaginal canal should be sprayed with a topical antibiotic
E. B and D

Answer A

7. HIV virus has been commonly linked to transmission through which of the following body fluids?
   1. urine
   2. blood
   3. semen
   4. vaginal secretions

   Select the proper grouping.

A. 1, 3
B. 2, 4
C. 1, 2, 3
D. 1, 2, 4
E. 2, 3, 4

Answer E

8. The universal precautions against the transmission of contagious diseases include which of the following care steps?
   1. gloves when encountering any body fluids
   2. eye shields when airborne fluid droplets are expected
   3. gowns worn when fluid splashing is likely
   4. hands washed thoroughly after each patient contact
   5. all needles recapped before being placed in a sharps container

   Select the proper grouping.

A. 1, 4, 5
B. 2, 3, 4
C. 1, 2, 4, 5
D. 1, 2, 3, 4
E. 1, 2, 3, 4, 5

Answer D

9. The universal precautions should be observed by EMS personnel ....

A. when HIV infection is suspected.
B. when sexually transmitted disease is encountered.
C. during any IV initiation procedure.
D. when a patient is bleeding.
E. when caring for any patient. Answer E

10. After caring for a patient with a suspected infectious disease, you should do which of the following?
1. cleanse the ambulance thoroughly
2. bag and mark all the linen
3. clean and sterilize all equipment used
4. alert ED personnel to the disease
5. wash hands thoroughly

Select the proper grouping.

A. 1, 2
B. 2, 5
C. 1, 3, 4
D. 2, 3, 4, 5
E. 1, 2, 3, 4, 5 Answer E

SPECIAL PROJECTS

11. You are dispatched to an auto accident and find a patient with numerous wounds and in need of an IV line. During the patient history the patient identifies that she is HIV positive. What care precautions, under the categories listed below, would you take to protect yourself against disease transmittion?

Barrier protection:

Gloves wren for Protection Changed After each Patient
Protective eye wear - prevent splash exposure
Gowns - may also be considered

Needlestick protection:

Needles should not be recapped, bent, dicarded or removed
From a syringe they should be placed in a Puncture Resistant
Container for disposal

Hand washing:

Hands should be washed - immediatly if contacted body fluids.
Also washed immediately after gloves are removed.

28

ENVIRONMENTAL EMERGENCIES

Review of the Objectives for Chapter 28

After reading this chapter, you should be able to:

1. Describe the four ways in which the body loses heat.

p. 865

Radiation accounts for about 60% of normal heat loss and occurs as the body gives off infrared rays.
Conduction occurs as heat is transferred from one object to another as when the body contacts cold metal.
Convection occurs when the heat is transferred to a medium such as air or water next to it. Currents then carry the warmed medium away and replace it with cooler air or water.
Evaporation is the conversion of a liquid to a vapor. It takes a large amount of heat energy and cools the body efficiently.

2. Describe mechanisms used by the body to maintain a core temperature in both warm and cold environments.

pp. 865 to 867

Warm environment
The body dissipates heat energy by shunting it to the surface via peripheral vasodilation temperature and increasing the rate of heat loss. As the heat gradient between the air and the skin become close, sweat is released on the skin's surface to evaporate and take heat energy with it.

Cold environment
The body uses three mechanisms to maintain body temperature in a cold environment. Vasoconstriction reduces the flow of blood through the skin, allowing it to cool and reducing the heat loss through it. Piloerection causes the hairs to stand on end and provide a better insulation factor where the hair still exists. Lastly, the body increases muscular activity (shivering) to increase heat production.

3. Distinguish between hyperthermia and hypothermia.

pp. 867 to 876

Hyperthermia is a general raising of the core temperature caused by transfer of heat from the environment. Hypothermia is a general lowering of the core temperature due to transfer of heat energy from the body to the environment.

4. Identify the signs, symptoms and recommended management techniques for heat cramps, heat exhaustion, water intoxication, and heat stroke.

pp. 869 to 871

Heat cramps - in heat cramps the patient will experience muscle cramping while he or she remains normotensive, diaphoretic, and alert. The patient should be removed from the hot environment and activity is to be limited. Severe heat cramps may require IV fluid replacement with normal saline and electrolyte supplements.

Heat exhaustion - the patient with heat exhaustion will present with weakness, tachycardia, diaphoresis and pallor. The patient may complain of nausea, vertigo, thirst and anxiety. The patient will have a history of prolonged exposure to heat and probably humidity. Management is accomplished by removing the patient from the hot environment, modest cooling, and replacing lost fluids and electrolytes. Normal saline or lactated Ringer's solution are preferred.

Water intoxication - the patient with water intoxication will have a history of fluid intake and yet does not intake sufficient electrolytes. Signs and symptoms include nausea, vomiting, headache, and alterations in mental status. Care involves encouraging the patient to eat food high in sodium and restrict fluid intake. Unconscious patients should receive an IV of normal saline, run T.K.O.

Heat stroke - the patient will have an elevated core temperature and may no longer be sweating as the cooling mechanisms cease to function. The patient may be hypotensive and will display a lowered level of consciousness. Care should include removing the patient from the environment and rapid cooling until the body temperature is below 102 degrees. Administer oxygen and start one to two IV lines with normal saline or lactated Ringer's solution. Monitor the ECG for dysrhythmia.

5. Discuss the pathology of hypothermia, and cold-related injuries.

pp. 871 to 877

Mild hypothermia is a general cooling of the core temperature below 95 degrees. The patient with mild hypothermia has a good prognosis.

Severe hypothermia occurs when a patient has a core temperature below 90 degrees. It is a serious condition because the body metabolism slows, as does heat production.

Frostbite is the frank freezing of a distal body part. It may be superficial or deep. It damages the tissue as ice crystals form and destroy the cell membranes.

6. Identify the stages of systemic hypothermia, and describe the physical signs and symptoms associated with them.

pp. 873 to 874

As a patient is exposed to a cold environment the body reduces heat loss by vasoconstriction and cooling of the skin. Muscular activity increases (shivering) to raise heat production. If heat loss exceeds production the core temperature begins to drop.

Mild hypothermia is considered a core body temperature of 97° to 94° while a core temperature of 93° to 86° is considered moderate hypothermia. In both cases, the patient will shiver, experience muscle stiffness and walk with a staggering gait. The patient may also exhibit a lowered level of consciousness.

Severe hypothermia is a core temperature below 86°. The patient may be disoriented and confused progressing into stupor and unconsciousness. The ECG may display J waves, atrial fibrillation, bradycardia, and ventricular fibrillation.

7. Identify non-environmental causes of hypothermia.

pp. 874

Hypothermia may be caused by hypothyroidism, brain tumors, or head injury. Other conditions that may cause hypothermia are myocardial infarction, diabetes, hypoglycemia, drugs, poor nutrition, sepsis, or old age.

8. Discuss the concerns and precautions involved in rewarming a hypothermia patient in the field.

pp. 874 to 876

Attempts to rewarm the patient externally will cause the peripheral vessels to dilate, allowing the cold peripheral blood to enter the core, further reducing the body's temperature. If transport will be prolonged, all attempts must be made to warm the core through warm humidified oxygen, warm IV fluids and possibly warmed gastric lavage. Localized warming, for frostbite, should be accomplished via warm water immersion, provided there is no chance of re-freezing. The water should be at 102 degrees and constantly monitored.

9. Describe the events that occur during the near-drowning emergency.

pp. 877 to 879

As the patient slips below the surface of the water the patient experiences a period of apnea while blood is shunted to the heart, lungs and brain. Hypoxia develops and eventually induces panic and violent inspiration. If laryngospasm occurs, the vocal folds will close off (dry drowning). If it doesn't, water will enter the lungs (wet drowning). Continued submersion leads to anoxia, deep coma, swallowing and gastric distention, hypotension, bradycardia and death.

10. Identify the sources of ionizing radiation, and relate their relative penetrating potential.

pp. 880 to 881

Alpha radiation is low energy radiation that will not penetrate cloth or paper. Its greatest danger is in ingestion or inhalation.

Beta radiation is medium energy radiation that can be stopped by metals or thick clothing. It generally causes less damage than alpha particles though it can still be harmful if inhaled or ingested.

Gamma radiation is a high energy radiation that will penetrate clothing and the entire body. It is very harmful and can induce extensive cell damage.

Neutron radiation is the most powerful, penetrating and dangerous radiation. Fortunately it exists only in the close proximity of a nuclear reactor.

11. Name some of the factors that can help reduce the exposure to a radiation source.

pp. 881 to 882

Time - the greater the time of exposure to ionizing radiation, the greater the damage. The rescuer should limit the exposure time to the minimum required to effect the rescue.

Distance - the greater the distance from the source of radiation the less strength it has. The rescuers should stay as far away as practical from the radiation source.

Shielding - the greater the matter between the source and the rescuer, the less exposure to the ionizing radiation. Place as much steel, lead, concrete and earth between the rescuers and the source as is possible.

12. Identify prehospital management of the patient who has been exposed to ionizing radiation.

pp. 883 to 884

The primary concern is to remove the patient from the source of radiation since exposure is cumulative. It is also important to decontaminate the patient if any dust or other radioactive material is on their person. Otherwise, the care is directed at any signs or symptoms of underlying disease or injury.

13. Identify common diving/hyperbaric emergencies.

pp. 886 to 890

Decompression sickness, or the bends, is a disease process that occurs as nitrogen comes out of the blood and tissues as small bubbles. These bubbles travel through the vascular system and collect in joint areas, causing pain (type I decompression sickness). Should the patient display paresthesia, paralysis, headache, dizziness or vertigo, loss of consciousness, nausea, hemoptysis, or chest pain, the patient should be considered as having the more serious type II decompression sickness.

Air embolism is the introduction of air bubbles into the blood stream during or immediately after ascent. As the diver rises in the water, the pressure dramatically decreases. If the air in the lungs is not allowed to escape, it may be forced into the circulation and travel to the heart and brain, causing vascular obstruction.

Pneumomediastinum is gas, usually air, released into the mediastinum. The problem is caused when air is forced into the mediastinum during diving because of the increased pressures.

14. Describe the signs and symptoms of diving related emergencies.

pp. 886 to 890

Decompression sickness - the patient suffering from decompression sickness will have a history of a recent dive. He or she will present with symptoms ranging from minor joint pain and fatigue to vertigo, paralysis, priapism, frothy reddish sputum and dyspnea.

Air embolism - the patient will have a history of a dive with onset of signs and symptoms upon surfacing. He or she may present with sudden sharp tearing pain, paralysis (often hemiplegic) and possible cardiopulmonary collapse.

Pneumomediastinum - the pneumomediastinum patient will have a history of a recent dive and will display hoarseness, chest pain, irregular pulse, abnormal or distant heart sounds, reduced blood pressure, jugular vein distention and a narrowed pulse pressure.

15. Describe the management of the patient with a diving-related emergency.

pp. 889 to 890

Decompression sickness - the patient with decompression sickness should be given high-flow oxygen, and intubated if unconscious. The patient should be placed on the left side with the head low. Normal body temperature should be maintained. An IV should be started with lactated Ringer's solution or normal saline, not D_5W. The patient should be transported to the nearest recompression chamber quickly.

Air embolism - the patient suspected of air embolism should be placed in the left lateral, head low position and transported with high flow oxygen to the nearest recompression facility. An IV should be started enroute and Solu-Medrol considered.

Pneumomediastinum - the patient is observed for the signs and symptoms of decompression sickness, air embolism and pericardial tamponade. He or she must receive high-flow oxygen, an IV, and transport to the nearest medical facility.

CASE STUDY REVIEW

Reread the case study in **PARAMEDIC EMERGENCY CARE** and then read the discussion below.

This case presentation relates a near-drowning that goes on to death secondary to multiple organ failure. It addresses several of the concerns regarding the resuscitation of the near-drowning patient and also presents an arrest resuscitation.

Chapter 28 Case Study

One of the problems associated with the resuscitation of a near-drowning patient is vomiting and the threat of aspiration. As the patient struggles during the drowning process, he swallows large volumes of water. It is not uncommon for the patient to vomit copious amounts of water and gastric contents as mouth-to-mask ventilation and chest compressions begin. The paramedic is well advised to have suction ready and to accomplish early intubation to protect the airway.

The defibrillator paddles are applied for a quick look. The rhythm is ventricular fibrillation, which is common for a hypoxia induced arrest. The paramedics rapidly defibrillate with 200 joules of power. They need to be very careful in their defibrillation attempts because of all the water and fluids around the patient. If care is not taken, the defibrillation attempt may affect not only the patient but the rescuers.

The paramedics are unsuccessful in their initial attempts to defibrillate so they initiate an IV and intubate. Should attempts to start an IV fail, the drug epinephrine could be given via the endotracheal tube. You will note that the dosage of epinephrine is 1 mg, more than the current standards indicate but still a reasonable order.

This patient is probably not the victim of a cold water drowning so rewarming is not instituted. Cold water drowning does carry a better prognosis for resuscitation, even after prolonged emersion. Expect that the patient may not respond to therapy until the body is rewarmed in the hypothermic drowning.

READING COMPREHENSION SELF-EXAM

1. Temperature regulation is generally centered within the ....

A. medulla oblongata.
B. hypothalamus.
C. pituitary gland.
D. cerebellum.
E. ascending reticular activating system.

Answer B

2. Which of the following is a way the body maintains temperature in a hot environment?
   1. induces peripheral vasoconstriction
   2. increases perspiration
   3. decreases heat production
   4. increases cardiac output
   5. increases the respiratory rate

   Select the proper grouping.

A. 1, 3, 5
B. 1, 2, 4
C. 1, 3, 4, 5
D. 2, 3, 4, 5
E. 1, 2, 3, 5

Answer D

3. Heat cramps are usually due to ....

A. loss of electrolytes.
B. decreased circulation.
C. water losses.
D. all of the above.
E. A and C.

Answer ____

4. Heat exhaustion may present with which of the following?
1. bradycardia
2. hypertension
3. syncope or dizziness
4. nausea
5. weakness
Select the proper grouping.

A. 1, 2, 5
B. 2, 3, 4
C. 1, 2, 3, 4
D. 3, 4, 5
E. 1, 2, 3, 4, 5

Answer ____

5. A patient presents with tachycardia, dry hot skin, hypotension, and is noticeably confused after prolonged heat exposure. Which temperature disorder would you suspect?

A. heat cramps
B. heat exhaustion
C. heat stroke
D. pyrexia
E. none of the above

Answer ____

6. A patient collapsed while exercising in the hot summer sun. The patient is fully conscious but weak, nauseated, tachycardic and profusely sweating. What heat related problem would you suspect?

A. heat cramps
B. heat exhaustion
C. heat stroke
D. pyrexia
E. none of the above

Answer ____

7. The patient who is experiencing heat stroke should have his or her temperature rapidly lowered to a target temperature of ....

A. 110 degrees.
B. 102 degrees.
C. 98.6 degrees.
D. 98 degrees.
E. 95 degrees.

Answer ____

8. The heat stroke patient is likely to have hypotension. Vasopressors like dopamine may be helpful in raising the blood pressure, and improving the patient's condition.

A. True
B. False

Answer ____

9. Which of the following are signs of moderate to severe hypothermia?
   1. uncontrolled shivering
   2. cardiac dysrhythmias
   3. lowered level of consciousness
   4. muscle stiffness
   5. staggering gait
   Select the proper grouping.

   A. 1, 2, 4
   B. 2, 3, 4
   C. 1, 2, 4, 5
   D. 2, 3, 4, 5
   E. 1, 2, 3, 4, 5

   Answer E

10. Hypothermia should only be suspected when the environmental temperature is below freezing.

   A. True
   B. False

   Answer B

11. In general, care for the mild hypothermic patient should include which of the following?
   1. giving the patient coffee
   2. handling the patient gently
   3. insulation from heat loss
   4. rewarming of the extremities
   5. warm humidified oxygen
   Select the proper grouping.

   A. 1, 2, 4
   B. 2, 3, 5
   C. 1, 3, 4, 5
   D. 2, 3, 4, 5
   E. 1, 2, 3, 4, 5

   Answer B

12. Which of the following are true regarding frostbite?
   1. it normally involves the extremities, head and face
   2. it requires subfreezing temperatures
   3. the affected area progresses from cold to painful to numb
   4. the site is always rigid and unyielding
   Select the proper grouping.

   A. 1, 2
   B. 2, 4
   C. 3, 4
   D. 1, 2, 3
   E. 2, 3, 4

   Answer D

13. Drowning refers to the patient who is submerged and does not survive the experience for more than 24 hours.

   A. True
   B. False

   Answer A

14. The patient who has salt water in the alveoli is expected to have ....

A. a bacterial infection.
B. a viral infection.
C. relatively dry lungs.
—D. significant pulmonary edema.
E. none of the above.

Answer D

15. Which of the following types of nuclear radiation has the greatest ability to penetrate and hence is the most dangerous?

A. alpha
B. beta
C. gamma
D. neutron
E. none of the above

Answer D

16. Which of the following should be used to reduce exposure to a radiation source?

A. increased distance from source
B. decreased time of exposure
C. increased shielding from source
D. all of the above
E. none of the above

Answer D

17. A properly decontaminated patient will not expose the rescuers to a radiation hazard.

A. True
B. False

Answer A

18. Decompression sickness, or the bends, is caused by ....

A. air bubbles in the blood stream.
B. joint pain and stiffness.
C. nitrogen bubbles in the blood stream.
D. nitrogen intoxication.
E. none of the above.

Answer C

19. A patient with a recent history of diving is assessed by paramedics and found to have joint pain, headache, vertigo and nausea. Care should include ....

A. recompression.
B. oxygen.
C. positioning in the left lateral head low position.
D. maintenance of body temperature.
E. all of the above.

Answer E

20. A diver arrives at the surface and immediately exhibits stroke-like signs and symptoms. What pathology would you suspect?

A. the bends
B. air embolism
C. the chokes
D. pneumomediastinum
E. nitrogen narcosis

Answer B

SPECIAL PROJECTS

Problem Solving - Environmental Emergencies

You are called to the airport to care for a patient who became ill during flight. The patient has joint pain, some numbness and tingling in the extremities, nausea, vertigo and dyspnea. He states that he just returned from the Caribbean where he had been scuba diving for the past two days.

Identify what you consider to be this patient's problem and why.

Problem: The bends II Nitrogen Emboli

The patients Scuba Diving has allowed Nitrogen gas to disolve in the blood and body tissue. The reduced pressure of flight has caused the gas to come out of solution to rapidly and form Bubbles. The result is mutiple emboli which occlude the small arterioles, causing the signs and symptoms.

Identify the care you would provide for this patient.

ABC'S 100% oxygen via NRM
Positioned on his left side with head down 10-15% Give patient liquids and infuse NS or LR. If air evacuation is considered ensure the altitude is kept to a minimum

29

EMERGENCIES IN THE ELDERLY PATIENT

Review of the Objectives for Chapter 29

After reading this chapter, you should be able to:

1. Discuss statistics on aging and the elderly population in the United States.

pp. 894

It is the fastest growing segment of our population because the birth rate is declining, mean survival of older persons is increasing, and because of an absence of wars, and improvement in health care. Nearly 36% of all EMS calls are related to the elderly patient.

2. Discuss age-related systemic decline as it relates to the following body systems.

p. 896

Respiratory system - vital capacity is reduced by up to 50%; maximum oxygen intake may be reduced by up to 70% and there is a more frequent incidence of respiratory infection and pulmonary disease.

Cardiovascular system - stroke volume and heart rate decrease; the conduction system degenerates (resulting in blocks and dysrhythmias); the left wall may thicken by as much as 25%; and fibrosis and ASHD may result in hypertension and decreased cardiac function.

Renal system - there may be a reduction of up to 40% of renal nephrons, renal blood flow may be reduced by 45% and there may be a resultant increase in waste products remaining in the blood.

Nervous system - the nervous system may lose up to 45% of its cells in certain areas. There may be an overall loss of 6 to 7% of its weight, reduced cerebral oxygen use may occur and there may be up to a 15% reduction in nerve conduction velocity.

Musculoskeletal system - there may be a 2 to 3 inch reduction in height, an increased curvature of the thoracic spine, loss of mineral content and softening of the bone, increased incidence of fractures and decreased skeletal muscle weight.

Gastrointestinal system - saliva volume may decrease by up to 33%, gastric secretions may be reduced by 80% and esophageal motility may decrease.

3. Explain the need to distinguish the chief complaint from the primary problem among the elderly.

p. 897

The **chief complaint** is the major discomfort or problem about which the patient is concerned.

The **primary problem** is the underlying medical problem affecting the patient.

4. List four factors that complicate the clinical evaluation of an aged patient.

p. 897

Effects of aging are difficult to separate from the consequences of disease.

Geriatric patients are more likely to suffer from more than one disease at a time.

The geriatric response to illness is different than that of the younger patient.
The patient's emotional evironment may greatly effect his or her health.

5. List some factors that complicate gathering a history from an aged patient.

pp. 898 to 899

multiple diseases
medication errors
noncompliance
confusion
multiple medications
drug interactions
reduced senses

6. Describe reasons the elderly are more susceptable to trauma

p. 899

Trauma is more prevalent in the elderly for many reasons including slower reflexes, diminishing eyesight and hearing, arthritis, loss of elasticity in blood vessels, and fragile tissues and bones.

7. Discuss common respiratory problems among the aged.

pp. 900 to 901

Pneumonia is an infection of the lung that effects the elderly more frequently due to reduced effectiveness of the cough reflex and immobility.

Pulmonary embolism usually originates in the deep veins of the legs following periods of immobilization or due to atrial fibrillation.

Pulmonary edema can develop rapidly in the elderly. It is frequently associated with the MI.

Chronic obstructive pulmonary disease is a frequent complaint of the elderly.

Cancer occurs more frequently in the elderly with progressive dyspnea as the presenting symptom.

8. List two causes of cardiac dysrhythmias in the elderly.

pp. 902

Degeneration of the electrical pathways - as the aging process continues, the electrical conduction system of the heart begins to function less efficiently. Many dysrhythmias occur, including atrial fibrillation, bradycardias, and heart blocks.

Reduced tolerance of rate variations - rate extremes are not as well tolerated in the older patient. Tachycardias and bradycardias, as may be caused by bowel movement (valsalva), may cause a drop in cardiac output and an interruption of blood flow to the coronary and cerebral arteries.

9. Define syncope.

p. 902

Syncope is a transient unconsciousness or decreased level of consciousness caused by a decrease or complete interruption in the blood flow to the brain. It may be caused by many etiologies including vasodepressive, orthostatic, vasovagal, cardiac, seizures, and transient ischemic attacks.

10. Discuss the following kinds of syncope.

pp. 902 to 903

Vasodepressor syncope is more commonly called fainting and occurs secondary to emotional stress, mild hypovolemia, anemia, etc.

Orthostatic syncope is caused by a reduction in the vascular volume that is manifest when the patient attempts to rise from the supine to seated or seated to standing positions. It may also be caused by the body's inability to rapidly adjust to position change because of prolonged bed rest, autonomic dysfunction, or medications.

Cardiac syncope is caused by cardiac output irregularities. Etiologies may include the silent myocardial infarction or cardiac dysrhythmias such as bradycardias, tachycardias, heart blocks and sick sinus syndrome.

11. Define vertigo, and discuss the progression of events associated with it.

pp. 904

Vertigo is a disruption of the positional sense centers located in the auditory centers of the brain. The patient feels as though the room, or his/her head, is spinning. It is often accompanied by nausea, vomiting, sweating and pallor.

12. Define dementia as it applies to the elderly.

pp. 905

Dementia is the loss of memory, thought processing, and behavior control mechanisms which may be either acute or gradual in onset. It can be caused by many etiologies and should be considered a serious symptom if the onset is acute and the deficit noticeable.

13. Define Alzheimer's disease.

pp. 905

Alzheimer's disease is the gradual progression of dementia associated with aging. While there is some expected mental loss associated with the aging process, that loss is very dependent on the individual. It is important to remember that acute loss of mental faculties may be due to a specific pathology.

14. Identify causes of gastrointestinal bleeding in the elderly.

pp. 906 to 907

Gastrointestinal hemorrhage is a common and serious medical emergency in the elderly population. Causes include peptic ulcer, gastritis, esophageal varices, Mallor-Weiss tear, diverticulosis, tumors, ischemic collitis, and artrio-venous malformation.

15. Discuss the general management of gastrointestinal bleeding in elderly patients.

pp. 906 to 907

Gastrointestinal hemorrhage should be managed aggressively. This is especially true in the geriatric patient who may not tolerate hypovolemia well. Care should include high-flow oxygen, airway management, fluid replacement, PASG and transport.

16. Discuss the impact of environment changes on the elderly.

pp. 907 to 908

The elderly are especially susceptible to the effects of both the physical and emotional environment.

Physical environment - the elderly patient is less tolerant of environmental extremes. They are more likely to succumb to heat exhaustion and stroke or hypothermia. They have lower body reserves and may suffer from dehydration more quickly than younger patients.

Emotional environment - because of the reduced ability of the elderly patient to cope with disease and environmental extremes, emotional stress such as the loss of a spouse or retirement may result in the worsening of disease or death.

17. Discuss elderly abuse and neglect of the elderly, and determine resources available in your community to address this problem.

p. 909

The elderly, as well as children, are occasionally abused or neglected by those responsible for caring for them. Abuse often occurs when care for the geriatric patient places a strain on the already stressful life of the care giver. There are often local resources that can assist in these circumstances. Consult your instructor.

18. Recognize the need to be familiar with state and local laws regarding abuse or neglect of the elderly.

p. 909

The elderly are protected from abuse by state laws. It is important that you be aware of those laws and the appropriate authorities and process through which you report cases of suspected abuse. Each state, and in some cases local, laws protect the elderly from abuse and neglect. Consult your instructor for the specific applicable laws in your location.

CASE STUDY REVIEW

Reread the case study in **PARAMEDIC EMERGENCY CARE** and then read the discussion below.

This case study presents a typical geriatric patient and the circumstances in which the paramedic might expect to find her. It focuses upon a common presentation and describes the care that might be expected.

Chapter 29 Case Study

As do many elderly, Mrs. Robertson lives by herself, and is checked in upon by her family occasionally. EMS is called when she displays a syncopal episode in front of her daughter.

The initial patient presentation provides a patient who looks pale but has a respectable blood pressure. The pulse is rapid due either to excitement or a medical problem. The ECG reflects atrial fibrillation, a common dysrhythmia in the elderly, which may account for the patient's inability to tolerate rapid position change. The blood pressure, taken in the seated position, suggests a probable hypovolemia, which is confirmed by a directed history. The history of diarrhea and melena support both fluid and blood loss as a cause of the problem. The history of increased aspirin consumption (which reduces coagulation) supports the suspicion of a gastrointestinal bleed. These elements of assessment and a good patient history are essential for the care of the elderly. Due to reduced pain perception and the increased physical complaints of growing old, the geriatric patient may not recognize important signs and symptoms of their disease. The paramedic must be especially conscientious in the assessment of the geriatric patient.

The care of the geriatric patient must be just as conscientious. The geriatric patient is unable to respond to the stress of disease or trauma as is the younger patient. Over-care may be just as endangering for the patient as is the initial medical problem. Medications may cause a more significant effect or a much longer effect than for the younger patient.

This patient is provided with rapid fluid resuscitation. Her blood pressure and pulse are observed and her lung fields carefully auscultated to ensure over-hydration does not occur. Oxygen is administered to maintain a high oxygen saturation though the readings remain low because of the relative anemia. The PASG is applied, though not inflated. Inflation might be considered to assist in controlling the hemorrhage and increasing the blood pressure if initial fluid therapy is ineffective.

During the entire care process, the paramedic speaks to the patient and explains what is going on and why. The language is clear and simple and the communication is empathetic. Older patients need to know that they still are considered in the care decisions and that they still maintain some control over their lives.

READING COMPREHENSION SELF-EXAM

1. It is often difficult for the paramedic to differentiate between the effects of aging and the consequences of disease.

   A. True
   B. False

Answer A

2. Which of the following is true of the aging process?
   1. total body water decreases
   2. body fat decreases
   3. the metabolic rate decreases
   4. vital lung capacity decreases
   5. the left ventricular wall thickens

   Select the proper grouping.

   A. 1, 4, 5
   B. 2, 3, 4
   C. 1, 2, 4, 5
   D. 1, 2, 3, 4
   E. 1, 2, 3, 4, 5

   Answer C

3. Factors which contribute to increased risk of trauma for the elderly include all **except** which of the following?

   A. high incidence of risk taking
   B. slower reflexes
   C. failing eyesight
   D. more fragile tissues and bones
   E. frequently targeted for crime

   Answer A

4. Elements of aging that may confound assessment include ....
   1. diminished pain perception.
   2. depressed temperature regulation mechanisms.
   3. diminished sight and hearing.
   4. dementia.

   Select the proper grouping.

   A. 1, 3
   B. 1, 4
   C. 2, 4
   D. 1, 2, 3
   E. 1, 2, 3, 4

   Answer E

5. The reduced size and weight of the the brain in the elderly accounts for which of the following in head trauma?
   1. increased incidence of brain injury
   2. decreased incidence of brain injury
   3. increased signs and symptoms of brain injury
   4. decreased signs and symptoms of brain injury

   Select the proper grouping.

   A. 1, 3
   B. 1, 4
   C. 2, 3
   D. 2, 4
   E. none of the above

   Answer B

6. Which of the following types of syncope is caused by the body's inability to compensate for movement from the supine to seated or from the seated to standing position?

A. orthostatic syncope
B. vasovagal syncope
C. simple syncope
D. vasodepressor syncope
E. cardiac syncope

Answer A

7. The older patient is at a higher risk for stroke because of an increased incidence of ....

A. atherosclerosis.
B. hypertension.
C. atrial fibrillation.
D. congestive heart failure.
E. all of the above.

Answer E

8. Medication problems are common in the elderly population because of ....
   1. decreased excretion.
   2. increased medication use.
   3. multiple disease processes occuring simultaneously.
   4. patient forgetfulness.

   Select the proper grouping.

A. 1, 3
B. 2, 4
C. 1, 2, 4
D. 1, 3, 4
E. 1, 2, 3, 4

Answer E

9. In the case of suspected geriatric abuse, the paramedic should carefully confront the family to determine if abuse did occur and to determine who was the offender.

A. True
B. False

Answer B

10. Which of the drugs or classes of drugs listed below commonly cause toxicity in the elderly?

A. digitalis
B. anticoagulants
C. Inderal
D. theophyline
E. all of the above

Answer E

DYSRHYTHMIA RECOGNITION

It may be helpful to review the steps of dysrhythmia analysis described on page 232 of this workbook. The five step analysis process found there may assist you in analyzing the next 15 rhythms.

DYSRHYTHMIA RECOGNITION EXERCISE - B

Rate: 120 Rhythm: Regular Pacemaker: S-A.

P wave: Normal P-R interval: 0.14 QRS complex: Normal

Rhythm 1 Interpretation: Sinus Tachycardia

Rate: 30 Rhythm: Regular Pacemaker: Ventricles

P wave: Normal P-R interval: unrelated QRS complex: wide 0.14

Rhythm 2 Interpretation: 3rd Degree H.B.

Rate: none Rhythm: none Pacemaker: Ventricles

P wave: none P-R interval: none QRS complex: Fibrillation

Rhythm 3 Interpretation: V-Fib

DYSRHYTHMIA RECOGNITION EXERCISE - B (cont.)

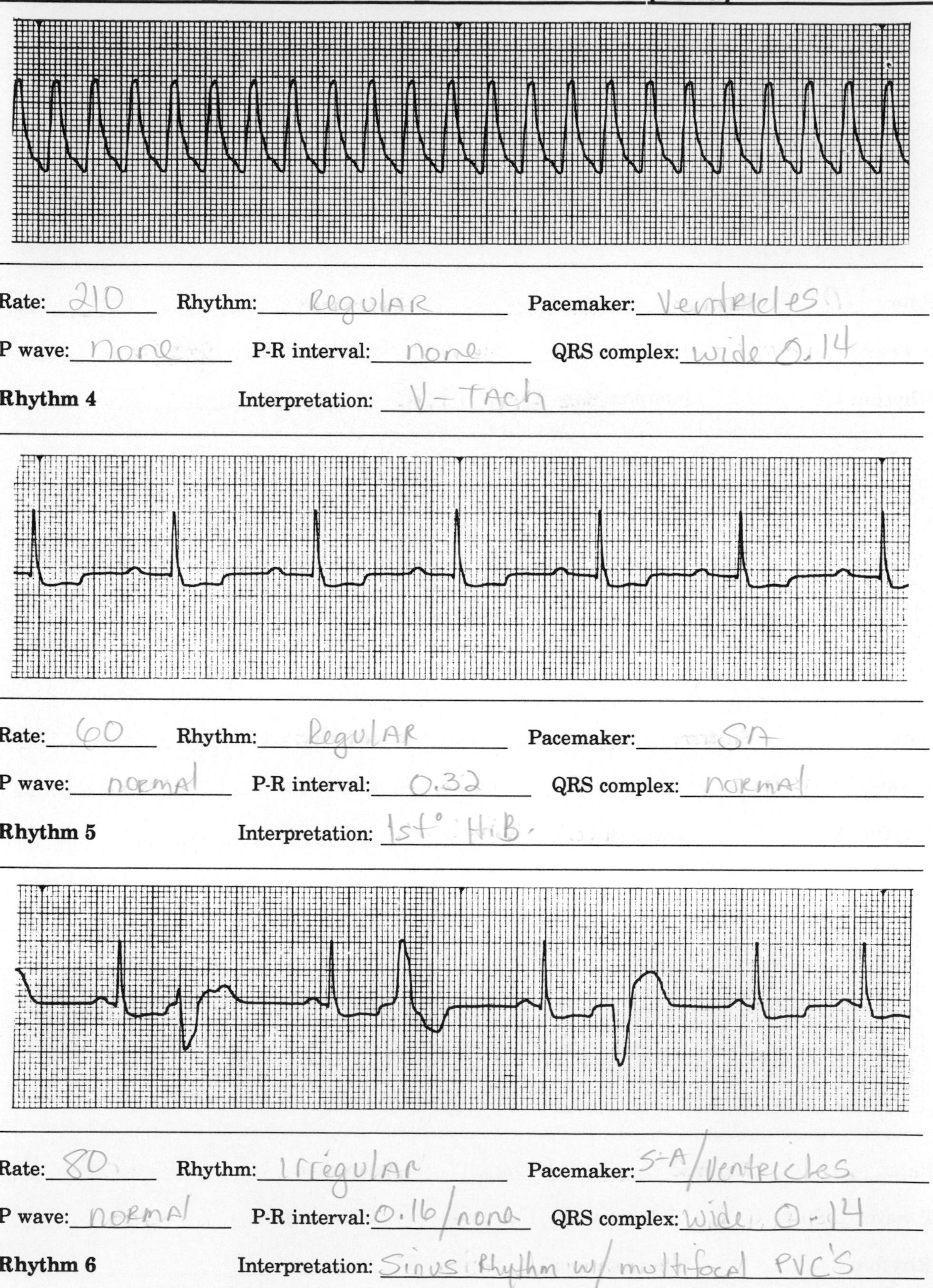

Rate: 210 Rhythm: Regular Pacemaker: Ventricles

P wave: none P-R interval: none QRS complex: wide 0.14

Rhythm 4 Interpretation: V-Tach

Rate: 60 Rhythm: Regular Pacemaker: SA

P wave: normal P-R interval: 0.32 QRS complex: normal

Rhythm 5 Interpretation: 1st° HB.

Rate: 80 Rhythm: Irregular Pacemaker: S-A/ventricles

P wave: normal P-R interval: 0.16/none QRS complex: wide 0.14

Rhythm 6 Interpretation: Sinus Rhythm w/ multifocal PVC'S

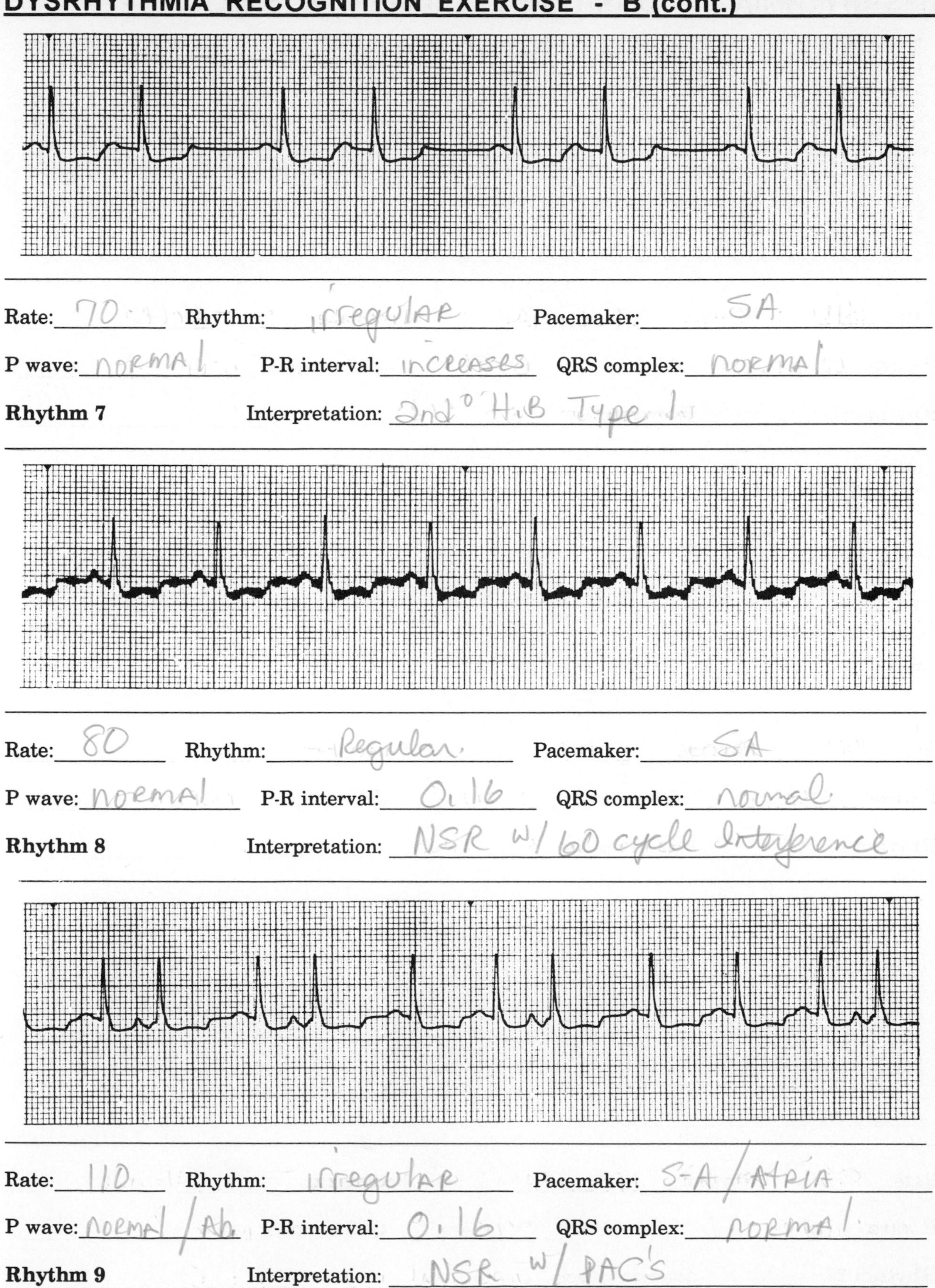

Rate: 70 Rhythm: irregular Pacemaker: SA

P wave: normal P-R interval: increases QRS complex: normal

Rhythm 7 Interpretation: 2nd° H.B Type I

Rate: 80 Rhythm: Regular Pacemaker: SA

P wave: normal P-R interval: 0.16 QRS complex: normal

Rhythm 8 Interpretation: NSR w/ 60 cycle Interference

Rate: 110 Rhythm: irregular Pacemaker: S-A / Atria

P wave: normal / Ab. P-R interval: 0.16 QRS complex: normal

Rhythm 9 Interpretation: NSR w/ PAC's

DYSRHYTHMIA RECOGNITION EXERCISE - B (cont.)

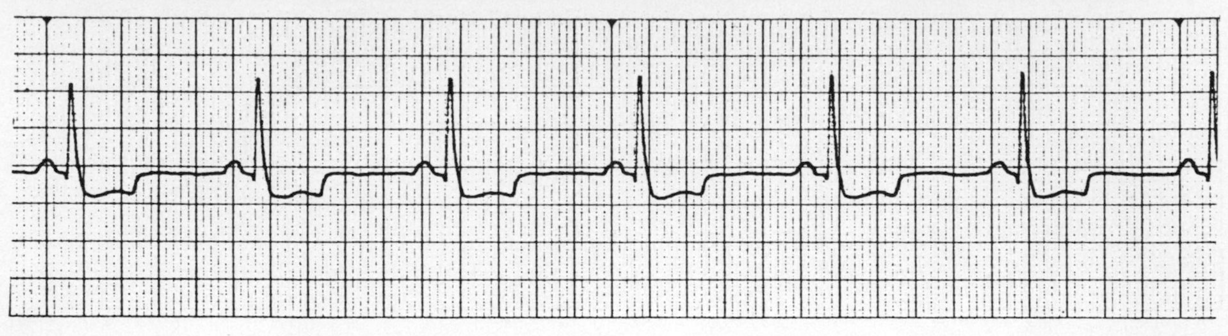

Rate: 60 Rhythm: Irregular Pacemaker: S-A / Atria

P wave: normal / Ab P-R interval: 0.16 QRS complex: normal

Rhythm 10 Interpretation: NSR w/ PAC's

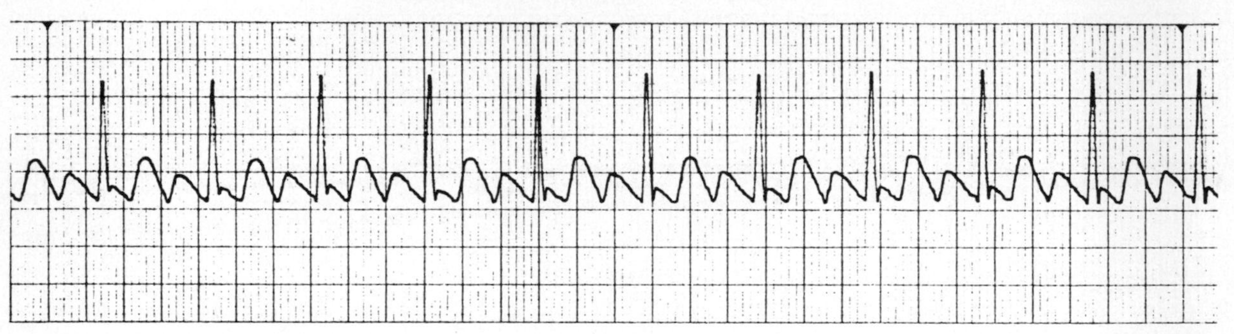

Rate: 100 Rhythm: Regular Pacemaker: Atria

P wave: Sawtooth P-R interval: 0.20 QRS complex: Normal

Rhythm 11 Interpretation: A-Flutter 3:1

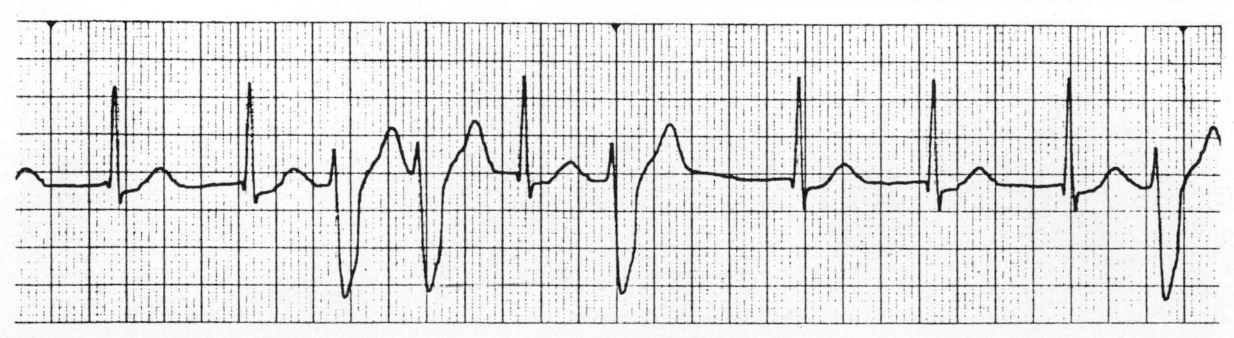

Rate: 95 Rhythm: irregular Pacemaker: Junction / Ventricles

P wave: none P-R interval: none QRS complex: normal / wide

Rhythm 12 Interpretation: Junctional Rhythm w/ PVC's

DYSRHYTHMIA RECOGNITION EXERCISE - B (cont.)

Rate: 50 Rhythm: Irregular Pacemaker: SA / Ventricles

P wave: normal / none P-R interval: 0.16 / none QRS complex: normal / wide

Rhythm 13 Interpretation: Sinus Brady w/ PVC's

Rate: 80 Rhythm: irregular Pacemaker: SA / Junction

P wave: normal / none P-R interval: 0.16 / none QRS complex: normal

Rhythm 14 Interpretation: NSR w/ PJC's

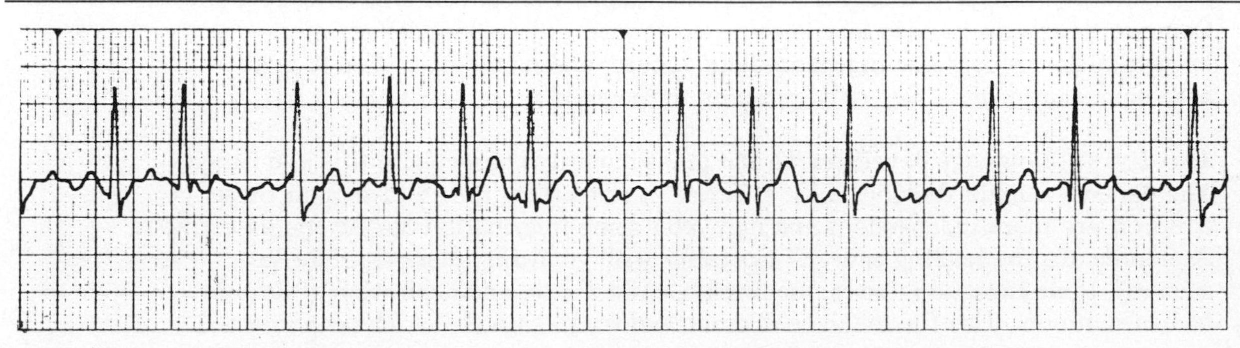

Rate: 110 Rhythm: grossly Irregular Pacemaker: Atria

P wave: Fibrillation P-R interval: none QRS complex: normal

Rhythm 15 Interpretation: A-Fib

30

PEDIATRIC EMERGENCIES

Review of the Objectives for Chapter 30

After reading this chapter, you should be able to:

1. Describe a typical child's emotional response to an emergency.

pp. 912 to 913

The child's primary emotional response to the emergency, and the care you offer, is fear. Children commonly experience fear of separation from their parents, fear of the unknown, and fear of mutilation or disfigurement.

2. List appropriate developmental milestones for each age group of children and relate the appropriate approach to patient assessment.

pp. 913 to 917

Birth to 1 mo. (Neonate) - this stage is often accompanied by a weight loss of up to 10% as well as the development of reflexes and personality. History should be gained from the parents. Premature infants may not be as well developed as the full-term baby. During assessment watch for fever, skin color and tone, and respiratory activity.

1 to 5 mo. - children in this stage develop muscle control and usually double their birth weight. History is still best determined from the parents. Common problems are vomiting, diarrhea, dehydration, SIDS, meningitis, child abuse, and household accidents.

6 to 12 mo. - the 6 to 12 month old child is able to ambulate and continues to develop a personality. He or she begins to exhibit stranger anxiety and will cling to a parent. Common problems include febrile seizures, vomiting, diarrhea, dehydration, bronchiolitis, croup, toxic ingestion, falls, abuse, and meningitis. Toe-to-head assessment order may be less frightening to the child than head-to-toe.

1 to 2 yrs. - language development and great mobility characterize this age range. The parents remain the ones most effective at comforting the child though these children are more independent and may offer some information during the assessment. Accidents are the leading cause of mortality with vomiting, diarrhea, febrile seizures, toxic ingestion, croup, meningitis, child abuse, and aspiration of foreign bodies common. Use the toe-to-head order and try to gain the child's confidence.

3 to 5 yrs. - fine motor control and language development occur during this stage. The child may possess a temper, and a vivid imagination may scare the child and cause him or her to fear mutilation. More information may be gained from the questioning of the child though imagination may distort the facts. Allow the child to participate in the assessment. The use of a doll may serve to distract the child. Common medical problems include croup, asthma, epiglottitis, febrile seizures, burns, drowning, meningitis, and child abuse.

6 to 12 yrs. - children in this age group are becoming independent and very active. They may be much more helpful in the assessment but may be reluctant to disclose information if their activity was forbidden. Respect their privacy and modesty during the exam. Common medical problems include drowning, accidents, burns, and child abuse.

12 to 15 yrs. - the personality and physical stature of persons in this group is well developed. They are independent and concerned with their body image. These patients are good historians and will respond well to exam if their modesty is respected. Common problems are mononucleosis, asthma, accidents, drug and alcohol problems, suicide gestures, sexual abuse, and pregnancy.

3. Discuss the typical parent's response to a pediatric emergency.

p. 917

The parents of the pediatric patient will usually respond with grief, guilt, fear, shock, denial, anger, or complete loss of control. Your objective should be to care for the child and assure the parents. If appropriate, transport a parent with the child.

4. Describe pediatric patient assessment.

pp. 917 to 920

With the pediatric patient, it may be worthwhile to question the patient regarding history before the physical assessment. This will gain the confidence of the patient and distract him or her from some of the fear. Use simple sentences honesty, and a calming voice. Initiate the physical exam without instruments and actively involve the child. The exam should progress as would the adult assessment. Assure blood pressure is taken with the appropriate sized cuff, assure the patient is as close to a resting state as possible during vital sign assessment, and monitor the pulse and respirations for at least 30 seconds each.

5. Describe the normal and abnormal appearance of the anterior fontanelle in the infant.

pp. 918 to 919

The anterior fontanelle is a diamond shaped opening in the top of the newborn's skull, along the midline and slightly anterior. It is normally level with or slightly below the level of the skull and may pulsate. With head trauma or meningitis it may bulge outward while dehydration may cause it to sink inward.

6. Identify normal age-related vital signs in the pediatric patient.

pp. 919 to 920

Age	Pulse rate	Blood pressure	Resp. rate
Newborn	100 - 160	50 - 70	30 - 60
1 - 6 Wks	100 - 160	70 - 95	30 - 60
6 Months	90 - 120	80 - 100	25 - 40
1 Year	90 - 120	80 - 100	20 - 30
3 Years	80 - 120	80 - 110	20 - 30
6 Years	70 - 110	80 - 110	18 - 25
10 Years	60 - 90	90 - 120	15 - 20

7. Describe the role of non-invasive monitoring in prehospital pediatric emergency care.

p. 920

Pulse oximetry is a valuable tool in the assessment of the effectiveness of respiration and circulation in the pediatric patient. Assure that you use a proper sized sensor probe.

ECG monitoring is appropriate for any seriously ill child. It will quickly identify the pulse rate and the effectiveness of medications.

8. Discuss pediatric trauma emergencies, and compare them to trauma seen in adult patients.
pp. 921 to 923

Trauma is the leading cause of death in the child over one year of age. Most deaths are caused by auto accidents, burns and drowning and are blunt in nature.

Head, Face and Neck Injuries are common, partly due to the proportionately larger and heavier head. Injuries are caused by falls, bicycle accidents, auto accidents, and auto-pedestrian accidents. Facial injuries are more common than for the adult population while neck injuries are less common.

Chest and Abdominal Injuries are the second cause of child mortality. Pneumothorax and hemothorax can occur and present much as in the adult. Abdominal trauma frequently results in spleen injury, the most commonly injured pediatric organ. The liver is also frequently injured. Any blunt trauma to the child should result in transport to a pediatric trauma center.

Extremity Injuries are typically limited to fractures and lacerations, and rarely involve amputations or serious injury. Young children often suffer incomplete fractures such as the greenstick fracture.

Burns are the second leading cause of pediatric death. Scalds often occur when the child pulls hot liquids off a stove. Burn surface area approximation is different for the child than the adult. In the small child the head is about twice the surface area of the adult.

9. Describe the characteristics of the abused child and of the child abuser.
pp. 923 to 924

The abused child may be seen as "special" or different and is often handicapped or has special needs. Premature infants and twins are at higher risk.

The child abuser may come from any ethnic or socio-economic background. The individual was usually abused as a child and is in the role of parent or guardian.

10. Describe signs and symptoms suggestive of child abuse or neglect.
pp. 924 to 926

The **abused child** may present with numerous injuries in various states of healing. They may also have unexplained injuries, vague explanations, or injuries that do not fit the explanation. Any child under 2 years with a fracture should be suspected of child abuse.

The **neglected child** will usually exhibit malnutrition, multiple insect bites, or extreme lack of cleanliness.

11. List the management techniques to use when treating an abused child.
pp. 926 to 927

Manage the abused child as any other patient. However obtain a complete history in a non-judgemental way and provide a report of the incident to the emergency department staff. Assure that the child is transported to the hospital by someone other than the suspected abuser.

12. Discuss the pathology, assessment, and management of the following pediatric neurological emergencies.
pp. 927 to 929

Seizures

Pathology - pediatric seizures may be caused by hypoxia, infection, trauma, hypoglycemia, toxic ingestion, tumors, and electrolyte disturbances. Often the etiology may be unknown.

Assessment - a complete history should be taken and the patient should be transported to the hospital to rule out other causes.

Management - the seizure should be managed as prescribed in earlier chapters of this text.

Febrile Seizures

Pathology - febrile seizures are most common in children and occur as the body temperature rises very rapidly.

Assessment - the patient will generally be between 6 months and 6 years with a high fever. The fever will have just risen very rapidly.

Management - remove excess clothing and consider administering acetaminophen.

Meningitis

Pathology - meningitis is a bacterial or viral infection of the meninges.

Assessment - it generally presents with a child who has been sick for one to a few days, history of a recent ear or respiratory infection, fever, lethargy or irritability, and possibly a stiff neck (in the older child).

Management should include rapid transport with oxygen and IV fluids as needed. As with all infectious diseases, universal precautions should be used.

Reye's Syndrome

Pathology - Reye's syndrome is a disease of unknown origin which attacks children from newborn to 15 years. Its occurrence has been related to outbreaks of flu, the use of aspirin, a recent history of gastroenteritis, and other circumstances.

Assessment - Physical examination may reveal rapid deep and irregular respirations, dilated and sluggish pupils, and cardiac dysrhythmias.

Management should include rapid transport and respiratory support.

13. Discuss the pathology, assessment, and prehospital management of the following pediatric respiratory emergencies.

pp. 930 to 935

Aspirated foreign bodies

Pathology - children, especially those from 1 to 3 years of age, are prone to aspirate foreign objects. These emergencies are often associated with running or falling while eating.

Assessment - the child may present with a history of respiratory distress or apnea. The child may display stridor, or other distress, or may be aphonic. Tracheal deviation may occur if the object occludes or acts as a valve in one of the mainstem bronchi. Cyanosis, costal retraction, and abnormal chest expansion may be present.

Management should include airway and respiratory support and may employ the "Heimlich Maneuver." If these are unsuccessful, visualization of the vocal cords or offending object may be attempted. The needle or surgical cricothrodomy may be indicated.

Croup

Pathology - croup is a viral infection which causes edema of the upper airway and narrowing of its lumen.

Assessment - the child will have a history of a respiratory infection and present with a barking cough during the evening hours. The patient will have an inspiratory stridor, will insist on sitting rather than lying down. He or she may exhibit nasal flaring, tracheal tugging, and costal retraction. Severe cases may develop tachycardia, cyanosis, and complete airway obstruction.

Management should focus on patient comfort, the administration of humidified oxygen, the possible administration of racemic epinephrine, and rapid transport.

Epiglottitis

Pathology - epiglottitis is an acute infection and inflammation of the epiglottis.

Assessment - you will find a child, usually over 4 years of age, who has been awakened with a brassy cough and high fever. The child will have pain on swallowing and may drool with the mandible jutted forward.

Management should include maintaining the child's position of comfort, humidified oxygen, and rapid transport. If the obstruction becomes complete, intubation must be attempted immediately. If intubation is not successful, high pressure bag-valve-masking or needle cricothyrotomy must be attempted.

Bronchiolitis

Pathology - bronchiolitis is differentiated from asthma in that it is normally associated with children under 1 year of age. It is a respiratory infection affecting the medium-sized bronchioles.

Assessment - the patient will present with rales and wheezes, and may also have a history of a recent infection.

Management should include placement in a semi- or full-seated position, support of ventilations as necessary, cardiac monitoring, the administration of a bronchodilator such as albuterol.

Asthma

Pathology - asthma is a common respiratory disease that causes bronchospasm and airway obstruction.

Assessment - the patient experiences difficulty in exhaling air, the lungs become hyperinflated, and respiratory distress and hypoxia become pronounced. On examination, the child will be seated, tachypneic, and have an unproductive cough. Wheezing may be audible or absent in severe cases.

Management should include airway maintenance, humidified oxygen therapy, and respiratory support. The patient may also benefit from the administration of epinephrine or aminophylline by infusion or albuterol, terbutaline or isoetharine by nebulizer.

Status Asthmaticus

Pathology - status asthmaticus is a severe and prolonged asthma attack that cannot be broken by epinephrine. It is life-threatening.

Assessment - the child will often have a hyperinflated and distended chest. Wheezing and breath sounds may be absent and the child will be severely dyspneac.

Management is the same as for asthma with anticipation of the need for endotracheal intubation. Transport should be immediate with aggressive care enroute.

14. Discuss the pathology, assessment, and management of the following pediatric gastrointestinal emergencies.

p. 935

Nausea and vomiting

Pathology - nausea and vomiting are symptoms of other disease processes. The concern is for the dehydration, which may result in severe dehydration since the fluid reserves for the child is minimal.

Assessment - the child will display with vomiting and dehydration. The child will have difficulty keeping fluids down.

Management - care is primarily supportive. If the patient is unable to keep fluids down, consider intravenous fluid therapy. If capillary refill time is prolonged, a 20 mL/kg fluid bolus of normal saline may be ordered.

Diarrhea

Pathology - diarrhea is a common occurance in infants and children. It is often due to viral or bacterial infections.

Assessment - significant diarrhea is 10 or more loose stools per day and is often associated with nausea and vomiting.

Management - care is primarily supportive. If dehydration is severe, administer fluids with 20 mL/kg bolus of normal saline.

15. Discuss the pathophysiology, assessment, and management of the following pediatric cardiovascular emergencies.

pp. 936 to 939

Dehydration

Pathology - dehydration is a common childhood problem which is complicated by the child's inability to independently obtain fluids, a high body surface to weight ratio, and low body reserves.

Assessment - diarrhea, vomiting, poor fluid intake, fever or burns may precipitate the problem. Decreased urination (fewer diapers), poor skin turgor, weight loss, absent tears and sunken, dull looking eyes may be revealed during the assessment.

Management - ensure the ABCs, monitor the vital signs, and infuse fluids as needed.

Sepsis

Pathology - septicemia is the presence of an infectious agent in the blood stream that causes a generalized infection.

Assessment - the patient commonly displays diffuse symptoms including fever, lethargy, irritability, and possibly shock.

Management should include oxygen, respiratory support as needed, IV fluids, and rapid transport.

16. Define Sudden Infant Death Syndrome (SIDS), including the theories of etiology and management in the prehospital setting.

p. 940

SIDS is the death of an infant (up to one year) from an unknown etiology. There are several current theories including an immature respiratory center, upper airway obstruction, pharyngeal relaxation during sleep, and an enlarged tongue. Care should be offered to the baby and the family. Resuscitation should begin while the parents are comforted and ensured that everything possible is being done.

17. Discuss the concept of Pediatric Advanced Life Support (PALS).

pp. 941 to 945

The emphasis of ACLS for the pediatric patient (PALS) is placed on preventing cardiopulmonary arrest. The origin of life-threatening problems in the infant and young child are usually vascular volume related or respiratory in nature. With the exception of congenital conditions, rarely is the problem of cardiac origin. PALS, as with ACLS for the adult, is focused upon the major sources of patient death and the best approach to care for the age group.

18. Describe the modifications required for pediatric advanced life support, including drug dosage, endotracheal intubation, defibrillation, and IV therapy.

pp. 945 to 951

Drug dosages are generally reduced and administered by patient weight. Please see Table 30-7.

Endotracheal intubation is accomplished with an uncuffed tube beginning at 2.5 mm for the newborn and up to 6.0 mm for the 8 year old. The straight blade should be used for the infants while either the straight or curved may be used after one year.

Defibrillation is delivered at 2 joules/Kg initially and up to 4 joules/Kg with paddles sized appropriately.

IV therapy is basically the same as for adults though the volume of fluid required is less. There are additional IV sites available including the interosseos site.
Fluid boluses may be administered up to 20 mL/Kg for hypovolemia and repeated as needed.

CASE STUDY REVIEW

Reread the case study in **PARAMEDIC EMERGENCY CARE** and then read the discussion below.

This case study addresses the pediatric patient and the variations in assessment and care approach that are necessary with the younger patient. This study also points out the need and value of caring for the parents as well as the child.

Chapter 30 Case Study

The crew of Medic one is responding to a typical pediatric respiratory emergency. The time of year is most likely the fall or winter as noted by the "cold but clear morning." This is the time of the year most frequently associated with pediatric respiratory problems.

The patient the paramedics are attending is in serious condition. She is ill in appearance and turns cyanotic with bouts of coughing. The barking cough focuses the attention toward an upper respiratory restriction such as croup or epiglottitis. Because of the age of the child, under 4, it is most likely croup. The epiglottitis patient would also displace his or her jaw forward and experience painful swallowing (which results in drooling).

The child is left in the mother's arms to calm both the mother and the child and maintain a comfortable position for the little girl. The paramedics, correctly, choose not to examine the throat. Doing so might aggravate the swelling and lead to increased or complete obstruction. A stridor is noted, most likely on expiration.

Axillary rather than oral temperature is taken because of the throat irritation. The blood pressure is taken using a small cuff (approximately 2/3 the width of the child's arm). The chest is auscultated to assess air movement and to rule out any other pathology. Care for the child is limited to humidified oxygen, guided by pulse oximetry.

The mother is calmed and reassured. The child is very aware of the mother's concern and normally will respond well to her mother's relaxing anxieties. Transport is effected quickly with intubation equipment readied in case the airway restriction becomes a complete obstruction.

READING COMPREHENSION SELF-EXAM

1. Which of the following heart rate ranges would you expect for a 10-year-old pediatric patient?

   A. 50 to 100
   B. 60 to 90
   C. 85 to 205
   D. 100 to 190
   E. less than 60

Answer B

2. The proper sized cuff for determining the blood pressure of a pediatric patient should be ....

A. 2 inches up to age 8.
B. equal in width to the child's upper arm.
C. 2/3 the width of the child's upper arm.
D. it does not matter.
E. the cuff should cover 1/2 the length of the upper arm.

Answer C

3. For which of the following age groups would the paramedic not begin the physical assessment with the head and face?
1. 1 to 5 months
2. 6 to 12 months
3. 1 to 3 years
4. 3 to 5 years
Select the proper grouping.

A. 1, 2
B. 2, 3
C. 1, 2, 3
D. 2, 3, 4
E. 1, 2, 3, 4

Answer D

4. Current theories suggest that Sudden Infant Death Syndrome (SIDS) may be due or related to ....

A. a mild respiratory infection.
B. an immature respiratory center.
C. a posterior pharyngeal airway obstruction.
D. winter months.
E. all of the above.

Answer E

5. Which of the circumstances listed below would suggest child abuse?
1. fractures in children under two years of age
2. injuries in various stages of healing
3. injuries to various parts of the body
4. an injury that does not fit the explanation
Select the proper grouping.

A. 1, 2
B. 3, 4
C. 1, 3, 4
D. 2, 3, 4
E. 1, 2, 3, 4

Answer E

6. A pediatric patient is seen by paramedics for a seizure. Assessment and history identify that the child has a fever of 101 degrees, was lethargic and irritable before the seizure, and has had no previous seizure activity. The child complained of a stiff neck and headache earlier in the day. Which of the etiologies listed below is the most likely cause of this episode?

A. fever or febrile convulsions
B. meningitis
C. hypoglycemia
D. hypoxia
E. none of the above

Answer B

7. If valium cannot be administered IV because a line is not available in the pediatric patient, it can be administered rectally.

A. True
B. False

Answer A

8. You are caring for an ill child with a history that includes a recent case of the flu and aspirin ingestion followed by severe nausea and vomiting. You would be most suspicious of ....

A. meningitis.
B. Reye's syndrome.
C. croup.
D. bronchiolitis.
E. septicemia.

Answer B

9. A 5-year-old patient is experiencing a severe respiratory problem which awakened her from sleep. She is displaying a brassy cough with fever, finds it very painful to swallow, and is drooling. The most likely cause of this problem is ....

A. croup.
B. bronchiolitis.
C. asthma.
D. epiglottitis.
E. status asthmaticus.

Answer D

10. A pediatric patient has severe upper respiratory swelling, either due to epiglottitis or croup. The paramedic should electively intubate if nasal flaring or costal retraction is present.

A. True
B. False

Answer B

11. Cardiopulmonary arrest in the pediatric patient is not usually of cardiac origin.

A. True
B. False

Answer A

12. Which of the following signs would be indicative of acute distress in the pediatric patient?
1. respiratory rate greater than 60
2. heart rate below 80 (child under 5)
3. heart rate above 180
4. heart rate above 160 (child over 5)
Select the proper grouping.

A. 1, 4
B. 1, 3
C. 1, 2, 3
D. 1, 2, 4
E. 1, 2, 3, 4

Answer C

13. Which of the following is false regarding airway protection devices for pediatric patients under 8 years?

A. EOAs are not recommended
B. nasal pharyngeal airways are not recommended
C. the straight laryngoscope blade is recommended for infants
D. endotracheal tubes should be cuffed
E. all of the above are true

Answer D

14. A venous access location not available in the adult but used for the pediatric patient is the ....

A. jugular vein.
B. anticubital vein.
C. femoral vein.
D. intraosseos site.
E. intrasplenic site.

Answer D

15. The appropriate initial defibrillation charge for a 13 kilogram pediatric patient is ....

A. 7.5 joules.
B. 13 joules.
C. 26 joules.
D. 39 joules.
E. none of the above.

Answer C

PEDIATRIC PHARMACOLOGY

Emergency management of the pediatric patient may involve the use of medications. To effectively administer the correct dose for the patient the paramedic must approximate the patient's weight and then infuse a bolus based upon the recommended doses below.

Epinephrine	1:10,000 0.01 mg/kg	Sodium bicarbonate	1 mEq/kg
Epinephrine	0.1 to 1.0 mcg/kg/min	Atropine sulfate	0.02 mg/kg
Dopamine	2 to 20 mcg/kg/min	Calcium chloride	20 mg/kg
Dobutamine	2 to 20 mcg/kg/min	Glucose	0.5 to 1 g/kg
Isoproterenol	0.1 to 1.0 mcg/kg/min	Lidocaine (bolus)	1 mg/kg
Lidocaine	20 to 50 mcg/kg/min	Bretylium toslate	5 mg/kg
Adenosine	0.1 to 0.2 mg/kg	Diazepam	0.2 to 1 mg

Remember that there is an additional route for drug administration in the pediatric patient. That route is intraosseous.

PHAMACOLOGY MATH WORKSHEET V

Formulas

Rate = Volume/Time	mL/min = gtts per min/gtts per mL
Volume = Rate x Time	gtts / min = mL per min x gtts per mL
Time = Volume/Rate	mL = gtts/gtts per mL

Concentration = Weight/Volume	1 Kg = 2.2 lb.
Weight = Volume x Concentration	1 Gm = 1,000 mg
Volume = Weight/Concentration	1 mg = 1,000 mcg

Please complete the following drug and drip math problems:

[1] A three-year-old 14 kilogram child exhibits a profound bradycardia. Please identify the amount of the following drugs you would administer

A) Atropine

B) Isoproterenol
(initially)

(maximum dose)

[2] You respond to a pediatric cardiac arrest to find a six-year-old 20 kg patient. In attempts to resuscitate the patient you would administer how much of each of the following drugs?

A) Epinephrine

B) Sodium bicarbonate

C) Calcium chloride

D) Lidocaine (bolus)

[3] What drip rate range would you use for a 25 kg pediatric patient for the following?

A) lidocaine mixed by adding 400 mg in 100 mL and running through a 60 mcgtts/mL administration set.

B) dopamine mixed by adding 60 mg in 100 mL and run through a 60 mcgtts/mL administration set.

C) Isuprel mixed by adding 15 mg in 100 mL and run through a 60 mcgtts/mL administration set.

DIVISION REVIEW

MEDICAL EMERGENCIES

Chapters 22 through 30

The following scenario based questions are designed to help you review the previous nine chapters of **PARAMEDIC EMERGENCY CARE**. *They combine the knowledge gained thus far through your reading and course work.*

Scenario I

You are caring for a 15-year-old patient who has been drinking, was acting "rather wild," and now is responsive only to painful stimuli. He has a vial of insulin in his refrigerator and a few syringes in the bathroom.

1. Based on the history above this patient's disease is best described as ....

   A. pancreatitis.
   B. type I diabetes.
   C. type II diabetes
   D. diabetic ketoacidosis
   E. nonketotic hyperosmolar coma

   Answer B

2. The above described condition is best controlled by diet.

   A. True
   B. False

   Answer B

3. The patient above would most likely respond dramatically to which of the following?

   A. naloxone
   B. thiamine
   C. insulin
   D. $D_{50}W$
   E. magnesium sulfate

   Answer C

Scenario II

A patient is found in a back alley of a poorer section of town. His clothing is tattered and soiled with fecal material and he smells of alcohol. The patient is unresponsive even to painful stimuli. Respirations are 12 and shallow, the pulse is 100 and weak, and the blood pressure is 110/68. A glucometer is unavailable.

4. You should anticipate this patient to experience seizures during your care.

   A. True
   B. False

   Answer A

5. Which of the following should you suspect as the problem of the patient in this scenario?

A. hypoglycemia
B. drug overdose
C. head injury
D. alcohol overdose
E. all of the above

Answer E

6. Which of the following drugs would be indicated in the care of this patient?
1. naloxone
2. Valium
3. glucose
4. thiamine
5. dexamethasone
Select the proper grouping.

A. 1, 4
B. 2, 3
C. 3, 5
D. 2, 3, 5
E. 2, 3, 4

Answer E

7. Assuming that this patient is a chronic alcoholic, what are the consequences of that disease?

A. hepatitis
B. liver cirrhosis
C. esophageal varices
D. pancreatitis
E. all of the above

Answer e

8. Which of the following precautions against infectious disease should be observed in caring for this patient?
1. gloves
2. goggles
3. gown
4. hand washing after care
5. bagging all linen
Select the proper grouping.

A. 2, 5
B. 1, 4
C. 1, 4, 5
D. 2, 3, 5
E. 1, 2, 3, 4, 5

Answer C

Scenario III

Temperatures have been in the lower 30s for the past few days and you are called to a small home on the outskirts of town. There you find a 79-year-old female patient in a chilly apartment. She has a noticeably altered level of consciousness, speaks with slurred speech, and displays slow reflexes. She is embarrassed that you were called and identifies no history of any recent medical problems. Physical assessment reveals no signs of disease or injury and a blood pressure of 112/88, pulse of 58 and weak, and respirations of 20 and shallow. The patients temperature is 93°F. The ECG shows atrial fibrillation.

9. Given this patient's body temperature, her hypothermia would be considered ....

   A. very mild.
   B. mild.
   C. moderate.
   D. severe.
   E. critical.

   Answer C

10. Geriatric patients are prone to hypothermia because of ....

    A. increased muscular mass.
    B. slowed reflexes.
    C. endocrine disorders.
    D. inadequate fluid intake.
    E. all of the above.

    Answer C

11. The dysrhythmia in this scenario is one that might be expected in the hypothermia patient.

    A. True
    B. False

    Answer A

Scenario IV

A local restaurant calls for a man who collapsed while eating. You arrive to find a 56-year-old male who is trying to speak but cannot be understood. He is moving his left extremities but not the right. His wife states that he left the table earlier complaining of a severe and sudden headache.

12. What is the suspected cause of this patient's problem?

    A. epilepsy
    B. cerebrovascular accident
    C. diabetic coma
    D. acute airway obstruction
    E. hypertensive encephalopathy

    Answer B

13. The best position to place this patient in is ....

    A. supine.
    B. supine with head elevated 15 degrees.
    C. left lateral recumbent.
    D. prone.
    E. semi-seated.

    Answer B

31

GYNECOLOGICAL EMERGENCIES

Review of the Objectives for Chapter 31

After reading this chapter, you should be able to:

1. Identify the location and function of the following organs.

pp. 954 to 956

Ovaries are located at the lateral ends of the fallopian tubes. They produce the female hormones, estrogen and progesterone, and produce and release the eggs for reproduction.

Fallopian tubes are hollow structures that extend from the upper uterus laterally to the ovaries. They are the most common location of egg fertilization.

The **uterus** is a pear-shaped muscular organ located in the lower abdominal cavity and pelvis. It connects with the vagina and fallopian tubes. It is the organ that accepts the fertilized egg and supports its development. Its contractions cause labor and the eventual delivery of the infant.

The **endometrium** is the lining of the uterus that is sloughed each month if the uterus does not receive a fertilized egg. Its passage is the menstrual period which occurs about once every 28 days.

The **cervix** is the neck of the uterus. It is a muscular valve that dilates to permit the passage of the infant during delivery.

The **vagina** is a hollow tube extending from the uterus to the outside. It is the female organ of copulation.

The **perineum** is the tissue area between the vaginal opening and the anus.

The **labia** are fleshy folds that serve to cover and protect the opening of the vaginal canal.

2. Describe the stages of the menstrual cycle.

p. 957

The normal menstrual cycle is 28 days in length. The first 14 are dominated by the hormone estrogen and the thickening of the endometrium. About midpoint in the cycle an ovary releases an egg (ovulation) which travels through the fallopian tube to the uterus. If the egg is fertilized during its trip (approximately 24 hours) it will implant on the uterine wall and the development of a fetus will begin. If it is not fertilized, the endometrium will slough at the end of the cycle.

3. Discuss assessment of the gynecological patient.

pp. 957 to 958

The assessment of the gynecological patient should include the standard primary and secondary assessment. The patient will normally present with either lower abdominal pain or discomfort or vaginal bleeding or discharge. The assessment should investigate any history of kidney stones, previous pregnancies, the last menstrual period, and any use of birth control devices or medications. If pregnancy is suspected the patient should be asked about any bloating, breast tenderness, nausea, vomiting or increase in urinary frequency. Any vaginal discharge should be described, including volume and frequency. Do not perform any internal vaginal exam.

4. Discuss the recognition and management of pelvic inflammatory disease (PID).

pp. 959

The patient with pelvic inflammatory disease will most commonly complain of lower abdominal pain. It is an infection and inflammation of the female reproductive system, often related to sexually transmitted disease. The pain is often made worse by sexual intercourse and may vary with the monthly period. Severe PID may be accompanied by fever, chills, nausea, vomiting and yellow vaginal discharge. Management involves making the patient as comfortable as possible and transporting.

5. Discuss nontraumatic causes of abdominal pain in the female.

pp. 959 to 960

Ectopic pregnancy is a potentially life-threatening emergency caused by the fertilized egg implanting at a location other than the uterus. The egg grows until the location can no longer support its development and then hemorrhage, often severe, occurs. The patient may present with lower one-sided abdominal pain, late or missed period, vaginal bleeding and possibly the signs and symptoms of shock. Care should address support and prevention of shock.

Ovarian cyst is a fluid filled sac on the ovary which can cause abdominal pain. It is not usually treated in the prehospital setting.

Appendicitis is mentioned in an earlier chapter of the text and may be a source of abdominal pain.

Cystitis or bladder infection is more prevalent in the female than the male. The female urethra is shorter, leading to a greater incidence of bladder infection. It may cause lower abdominal pain just above the symphysis pubis.

Mittleschmertz is pain associated with the release of an ovum midway through the menstrual cycle.

Other causes of abdominal pain include infections secondary to surgery, incomplete abortion, or post-partum problems.

Management of lower abdominal pain should include care directed at the signs and symptoms and patient comfort. In severe cases, oxygen should be administered and an IV started.

6. Discuss the physical and psychological implications of rape and sexual assault, and describe prehospital management.

pp. 960 to 962

Rape and sexual assault are crimes of violence which may leave the patient withdrawn or hysterical. The patient may use denial, anger or fear as defense mechanisms. Use a calming and professional approach and do not ask questions about the incident unless they are essential to emergency care. Management should ensure that no severe bleeding continues and should otherwise protect modesty. Provide a well lit environment and have the patient attended to by a female paramedic if possible.

Care should be taken to protect evidence if the victim should decided to press charges. Handle clothing as little as possible and discourage the patient from washing, bathing or douching. Place items of clothing or other blood-stained articles in paper or cloth bags and do not clean wounds unless necessary.

Do not question the victim about the incident and do not examine the genitalia.

CASE STUDY REVIEW

Reread the case study in **PARAMEDIC EMERGENCY CARE** and then read the discussion below.

This case study presents a patient with the typical signs and symptoms of a gynecological emergency. It provides the opportunity to overview the assessment and care of the female patient with lower abdominal pain and discuss the presentation and significance of ectopic pregnancy.

Chapter 31 Case Study

The paramedics of Wilmington EMS are attending a patient with a primary complaint of lower abdominal pain. The cause of that pain is very hard to differentiate in the field though some patient questioning may be helpful. The possible causes of the problem include appendicitis, pelvic inflammatory disease, ovarian cyst, bladder infection, mittleschmertz and ectopic pregnancy, to name just a few. Questioning should investigate her last menstrual period and its characteristics. Questioning should also address the pain: its onset, quality, quantity, radiation, and any alleviating or aggravating factors. The history should also address medical history including allergies, prescribed medications, recent surgery or medical conditions, and special questioning about pregnancies, children and birth control. While these elements of patient questioning might appear lengthy, they may be of great help to the emergency department staff, especially if the patient's level of consciousness drops.

The physical assessment reveals a patient who is relatively stable. The pulse rate, level of consciousness, and the negative tilt test all support a suspicion of only limited internal hemorrhage, if any. Remember that internal blood loss is a primary concern when abdominal pain is the chief complaint.

The definitive diagnosis of ectopic pregnancy reminds us of the dangers underlying abdominal pain. If the ectopic pregnancy had ruptured prior to this call, the patient might have experienced hypovolemia, shock and possibly death. It is a potentially lethal problem that can present with non-specific abdominal pain.

READING COMPREHENSION SELF-EXAM

1. The structures of the female anatomy that produce the eggs for reproduction and produce estrogen and progesterone is (are) the ....

   A. uterus.
   B. fallopian tubes.
   C. cervix.
   D. ovaries.
   E. vagina.

   Answer D

2. The patient with pelvic inflammatory disease is most likely to present with which of the following?

   A. pain around the umbilicus
   B. diffuse lower abdominal pain
   C. sharp stabbing pain along the flanks
   D. pain that is somewhat relieved during sexual intercourse
   E. painless yellow or brown vaginal discharge

   Answer B

3. Which of the following are true of the menstrual cycle?
   1. it normally begins after 16 years of age
   2. the cycle is about 28 days long
   3. an egg is released in the middle of the menstrual cycle
   4. if an egg is not fertilized, the uterine lining will slough

   Select the proper grouping.

   A. 1, 3
   B. 1, 4
   C. 2, 3, 4
   D. 1, 3, 4
   E. 1, 2, 3, 4

   Answer C

4. Which questions are important to ask of the female patient in the childbearing years with lower abdominal pain?
   1. date of the last menstrual period
   2. menstrual flow characteristics
   3. what birth control is used, if any
   4. number of pregnancies and children
   5. any chills, fever, syncope, diarrhea, constipation, etc.

   Select the proper grouping.

   A. 1, 2, 3
   B. 1, 3, 4
   C. 1, 2, 3, 5
   D. 2, 3, 4, 5
   E. 1, 2, 3, 4, 5

   Answer E

5. While somewhat similar in presentation, a good assessment can dependably differentiate PID from acute appendicitis.

   A. True
   B. False

   Answer B

6. Which of the following signs and symptoms are consistent with ectopic pregnancy?
   1. late or missed menstrual period
   2. a single day of pain midway during the menstrual cycle
   3. one-sided lower abdominal pain
   4. vaginal bleeding

   Select the proper grouping.

   A. 1, 3
   B. 2, 4
   C. 1, 2, 4
   D. 1, 3, 4
   E. 1, 2, 3, 4

   Answer D

7. Which of the following can be responsible for non-traumatic lower abdominal pain in the female?

   A. mittleschmertz
   B. cystitis
   C. ovarian cysts
   D. ectopic pregnancy
   E. all of the above

   Answer E

8. Severe and uncontrollable vaginal hemorrhage should be cared for with IV fluids and by packing the vagina with soft absorbent dressings.

A. True
B. False

Answer B

9. The patient who has been sexually assaulted or raped should not be questioned about the incident by the paramedic in the field.

A. True
B. False

Answer A

10. The articles of clothing that are blood stained after a sexual assault and need to be taken to the hospital as evidence should be ....

A. placed in separate plastic bags.
B. folded and kept together.
C. placed in separate paper or cloth bags.
D. washed with sterile cool water.
E. none of the above.

Answer C

11. List the considerations to preserve evidence in cases of sexual assault.

Handle Patients Clothing AS little AS possible
Do not examine the Peritoneal Area unless Absolutely necessary.
Do not use plastic bags to hold Blood-Stained Articles
Bag each Item seperatly, if they need to be bagged.
Do not let Patient comb her hair or Clean her fingernails.
Do not Allow Patient to douche, bathe, or Change. clothes before medical exam.
Do not Clean wounds unless Absolutely necessary.

12. List the possible causes of abdominal pain in the female.

ectopic pregnancy
Appendicittis
PID.
mittleschmertz

ovarian cysts
cystitis
endometritis
trauma.

32

OBSTETRICAL EMERGENCIES

Review of the Objectives for Chapter 32

After reading this chapter, you should be able to:

1. Identify the normal sites of fertilization and implantation of the fertilized egg.

p. 966

The fertilized ovum will implant on the interior wall of the uterus.

2. Describe fetal-maternal blood flow and the role of the placenta.

pp. 966 to 967

The placenta is the organ of exchange between the maternal and fetal circulation. The blood does not actually exchange between the mother and fetus, allowing the infant to have a different blood type. The placenta also contains an endocrine gland that produces several hormones. Circulation between the placenta and the fetus is accommodated by the umbilical cord. It has two arteries and one vein.

3. Define the following terms.

p. 970

Antepartum is the period of time immediately before the delivery of the infant.
Postpartum is the period of time immediately following the delivery of the infant.
Prenatal is the time between conception and delivery of the infant.
Natal literally means birth.
Primagravida is a woman who is pregnant for the first time.
Multigravida is a woman who has been pregnant more than once.
Primapara is a woman who has delivered a previous infant.
Multipara is a woman who has delivered more than one infant.

4. Identify the details of the history that should be obtained from an obstetrical patient.

pp. 970 to 971

In assessing the pregnant female who is about to deliver you should ask the following questions:

- How many times has the mother been pregnant?
- How many times has she delivered?
- How long since conception/when is the expected estimated date of confinement?
- Has the patient had any cesarean sections or previous gynecological or obstetrical complications?
- Has the patient had any prenatal care?
- If the patient has any pain, was its onset sudden or gradual, what is its character, and is it regular?
- Has there been any vaginal discharge or bleeding?
- Is the patient on any medications?

Does the patient have any allergies?
Does she have the urge to move her bowels or "push?"
Has the woman had a gush or dribbling of fluid?

5. Discuss the effects of pregnancy on pre-existing conditions such as diabetes, hypertension, and cardiac problems.

pp. 972

Diabetes - pregnancy often aggravates diagnosed diabetes or may induce gestational diabetes in the patient without previous diabetes. Since the oral medications for diabetes cross the placental membranes, injectable insulin is most frequently given for the pregnant patient if diet is ineffective.

Hypertension is exacerbated by pregnancy and the condition is further complicated in that the common hypertension medications cannot be given to the pregnant female. Hypertension during pregnancy may be further complicated by eclampsia and may adversely affect the placenta.

Cardiac problems - pregnancy places a great strain on the maternal heart. The cardiac output increases 30 percent and may induce congestive heart failure.

6. Define the following terms.

p. 974

Spontaneous abortion is the termination of the pregnancy before the fetus is viable, which occurs of its own accord. It is also termed a miscarriage.

Criminal abortion is the attempt to destroy a fetus by someone who is not licensed or permitted to do so.

Therapeutic abortion is a termination of the pregnancy because of a threat to the mother's life.

7. Describe the management of the patient who has suffered an abortion.

pp. 974 to 975

The patient who has experienced an abortion should be treated in the anticipation of shock including the application of PASG (inflated as needed), IVs of lactated Ringer's solution, and high-flow oxygen. Any tissue passed should be transported to the emergency department. The attending paramedic should also provide psychological support to the patient.

8. Describe the pathophysiology and management of the following conditions.

pp. 975 to 977

Ectopic pregnancy is the attachment of a fertilized egg to a location other than the uterine wall. The fetus begins to grow and will reach a size where it ruptures the blood supply of the structure supporting it. The patient will exhibit lower abdominal pain, often one sided. The patient may also display the early signs of pregnancy, including nausea, vomiting, tender breasts, and fatigue. She may also have a history of the predisposing conditions for ectopic pregnancy; PID, tubal ligation, pelvic surgery, or previous ectopic pregnancy. Management should be provided as for any patient with potential hypovolemic shock. High-flow oxygen, IVs established with crystalloid, and PASG applied (but not inflated) should all be employed. Transport the patient quickly.

Abruptio placentae is the premature, partial, or complete separation of the placenta from the uterine wall. It may be predisposed by abdominal trauma, preeclampsia, maternal hypertension or multiparity. The patient with abruptio placentae will usually complain of constant, severe abdominal pain, a very tender abdomen with a hard uterus, absent to heavy vaginal hemorrhage, and slow or absent fetal heart tones. Management includes high-flow oxygen and two large-bore IVs started with lactated Ringer's solution or normal saline. PASG may be applied, and inflated as shock develops. Transport the mother immediately.

Placenta previa occurs when the placenta develops in the proximity of the cervix. As the cervix effaces during the first stage of labor it tears the placental attachment to the uterus and bleeding begins. The patient will often experience painless vaginal bleeding following sexual intercourse, vaginal exam or at the onset of labor. Care for the patient with suspected placenta previa should include high-flow oxygen, two large-bore IVs with lactated Ringer's solution or normal saline, and the PASG (without inflating the abdominal segment).

9. Distinguish between pregnancy-induced hypertension, preeclampsia, and eclampsia.

pp. 977 to 979

Pregnancy-induced hypertension is an elevation of blood pressure that accompanies pregnancy. The blood pressure is above 140/90.

Preeclampsia is pregnancy-induced hypertension which is accompanied by abnormal weight gain, edema, headache, protein in the urine, epigastric pain and, occasionally, visual disturbances.

Eclampsia is preeclampsia with seizure activity.

10. Describe the pathophysiology and prehospital management of the hypertensive disorders of pregnancy.

pp. 977 to 979

Pregnancy-induced hypertension is a blood pressure elevated above 140/90 in a patient who was normotensive before pregnancy. Maternal and fetal vital signs should be monitored and medical control contacted if they are abnormal. Apresoline or other antihypertensive agent may be ordered.

Pre-eclampsia is the presence of hypertension and edema, abnormal weight gain, protein in the urine, headaches, or visual disturbances. Treatment includes placing the patient in the left lateral recumbent position, administered high flow oxygen, and provided with calm, quiet and rapid transport. An IV of D_5W should be started. If transport time is expected to be long, the medical control physician may order magnesium sulfate.

Eclampsia is the most serious extreme of hypertensive disorders of pregnancy. It is characterized by grand mal seizures. It can be differentiated from epilepsy in that the patient will usually be edematous, not have a history of seizure activity, will not be taking antiseizure medications, will have an elevated blood pressure, and will appear, or report, she is pregnant. Eclampsia is managed as other hypertensive conditions of pregnancy. In addition, the patient may receive valium and possibly magnesium sulfate to assist in seizure control. Calcium chloride should be available to counteract any untoward actions of magnesium sulfate.

11. Describe the stages of labor and the approximate lengths of each stage.

pp. 981 to 982

The **first stage** of labor begins with the onset of uterine contractions and ends with the complete dilatation of the cervix. It lasts about 8 hours in the first pregnancy and about 5 hours in following labors.

The **second stage** of labor begins with the complete dilatation of the cervix and concludes with the delivery of the infant. In the first birth it lasts about 50 minutes while in those following it lasts about 20 minutes.

The **third stage** of labor begins with the delivery of the infant and concludes with the expulsion of the placenta. The placenta usually delivers about 30 minutes after the delivery of the infant.

12. List and describe the steps of a normal delivery.

pp. 982 to 987

Determine if delivery is imminent - the paramedic must evaluate the expectant mother to determine the number of previous deliveries, the frequency of contractions, the urge to push, and the presence of crowning. If all elements suggest impending delivery, it should be accomplished in the field. Exceptions include earlier rupture of the membranes, fetal bradycardia, and meconium staining of the amniotic fluid.

Preparation for delivery - the paramedic should prepare an area for the delivery that is out of public view. Oxygen is administered and an IV should be established with normal saline or lactated Ringer's solution as time permits. The mother should be placed on her back and draped. The paramedic should glove, gown and open the OB kit using sterile technique. The fetal heart tones should be monitored until delivery begins.

Delivery of the head - as the delivery of the infant begins, the paramedic should place gentle pressure on the head to prevent an explosive delivery. If the head presents with the amniotic sac still intact, the sac should be ruptured. Check to see that the umbilical cord is not encircling the neck and suction the nasal and oral airway as the head delivers.

Delivery of the shoulders - support the head as the anterior and the posterior shoulders deliver. Be advised that the body will soon follow. The infant is wet and slippery; take care to keep control of it.

Cutting the umbilical cord - after the baby is delivered he or she should be kept above the level of the vagina. Do not "milk" the cord. The cord should be clamped about 10 cm from the baby and then about 5 cm from the first clamp. Cut the cord between the two clamps and be sure the cord does not continue to bleed.

Post-delivery care - the airway should be suctioned again and the infant patted dry. The infant is wrapped in a soft blanket and kept in the supine position with the head slightly lower than the body to allow for drainage of the secretions from the airway. The time of birth should be noted and an APGAR score determined.

Delivery of the placenta - the vagina will continue to ooze blood and the cord will eventually appear to lengthen as the placenta separates from the uterine wall. It should be transported, with the mother and infant, to the hospital. Do not await transport for the delivery of the placenta.

Post-partum care - the mother's abdomen should be massaged to ensure the constriction of the uterus. This will effectively control post-partum hemorrhage. The mother's vaginal opening should be inspected for tears. If any are found, they should be dressed with obstetrical pads. A second APGAR score should be taken five minutes post delivery.

13. Describe the management, during delivery, of a cord that becomes wrapped around the baby's neck.

pp. 987

As the head delivers, the neck is checked to ensure the cord is not entangled. If it is, the paramedic should try to slide it over the infant's head. Failing at this, the cord should be clamped in two places and cut between. The cord should then be untangled if more than one loop around the neck is found.

14. Describe the management of a breech presentation.

pp. 988 to 989

Transport to the hospital is recommended since the breech delivery is normally prolonged. If transport time is lengthy and the decision is made to deliver at the scene, the mother should be placed at the edge of a firm bed and asked to keep her legs flexed. Support the infant's legs or buttocks as they deliver without pulling. Insert gloved fingers along the chin to the nose and push against the vaginal wall to make an airway as the chest and neck deliver. Suction as needed and transport while maintaining the airway if the head does not deliver within three minutes.

15. Describe the pathophysiology and management of a prolapsed cord.

pp. 989

Prolapsed cord occurs as the cord precedes the infant through the birth canal. If the infant is allowed to deliver vaginally, the cord will be compressed, the fetal circulation halted, and infant death is likely. Upon seeing the umbilical cord in the vagina, the paramedic should place two fingers of a gloved hand into the vaginal canal up to the presenting part. The fingers should lift the presenting part until the cord pulsates. The pressure should be maintained while the mother is placed in the Trendelenburg or knee-chest position, given high-flow oxygen and transported rapidly to the hospital. If possible, a sterile saline soaked dressing can be applied to the exposed cord.

16. Describe the management of a multiple-birth delivery.

pp. 989 to 991

The delivery of multiple birth infants is as for single births. The first-born infant has his or her cord clamped and cut. Then, the delivery of the second infant follows. Since the infants are usually smaller than single birth babies, special care should be aimed at drying and keeping the infants warm.

17. Describe the pathophysiology and management of the following conditions.

pp. 991 to 992

Post-partum hemorrhage is the loss of more than 500 mL of fluid in the first 24 hours post delivery. Most commonly, the uterus does not maintain contraction and control hemorrhage. Other causes of post-partum hemorrhage include retained placental parts, or vaginal or cervical tears. Management of post-partum hemorrhage involves the standard shock care and gentle but firm massage of the uterus if it is found to be soft. Forced delivery of the placenta and vaginal packing are contraindicated.

Uterine inversion is a rare complication of delivery where the uterus inverts as the delivery is completed. The patient should be placed in the supine position and given high-flow oxygen. Initiate two large-bore IVs run with lactated Ringer's solution or normal saline. Make one attempt to replace the uterus using a gloved hand to push the fundus toward the vagina. If unsuccessful, cover the exposed uterus with a sterile saline soaked towel and transport the patient rapidly.

Uterine rupture is a tearing of the uterus during labor or secondary to abdominal trauma. The condition may be accompanied with a history of previous cesarean section or prolonged labor. The patient will often be in shock with labor interrupted abruptly. The abdomen will be tender and rigid, and fetal heart tones will be absent. Management includes high-flow oxygen, two large-bore IVs of lactated Ringer's solution or normal saline, and the application of the PASG without using the abdominal section. Rapid transport is indicated.

CASE STUDY REVIEW

Reread the case study in **PARAMEDIC EMERGENCY CARE** and then read the discussion below.

Childbirth is about the only circumstance in emergency medical service in which the outcome of the "emergency" is expected and natural. The paramedic plays a role, supportive of the experience and beneficial if something abnormal occurs. This case study addresses a scenario that is without complication, representing 97 percent of deliveries.

Chapter 32 Case Study

The mother presents a few bits of information that suggest an imminent delivery. The previous number of births reflect that delivery may very well move quickly. The urge to move the bowels is a sign that the cervix has fully effaced and the child is moving down the birth canal. Lastly the exam of the perineum displays the infant's head, crowning. This reflects that the cervix is fully dilated, the infant is already passing through the birth canal, and that delivery is but moments away.

Time does not permit the usual actions that would accompany a field delivery. The EMTs are not gowned, though gloves are used. Eye protection would also be advisable since body fluids may be splashed. The patient is not draped, which would protect the infant from some contamination as delivery proceeds. Lastly, there is not enough time to open the OB kit with sterile technique nor display its contents so they are easily available to the assisting EMS personnel.

The key actions of the care providers in the delivery of a newborn are those of preventing an explosive delivery, suctioning the airway, cutting the cord, monitoring post-partum hemorrhage and caring for the neonate. The EMT places a gloved hand against the delivering head to prevent the explosive delivery, and the vaginal tears and infant head trauma it might cause. The airway is suctioned as the head delivers, ensuring a clear airway and a clear respiratory track when the infant takes her first breath as the chest delivers. As the paramedics arrive, they cut the cord as the child is delivered by clamping 10 cm and then 15 cm from the infant and severing it in-between. The mother's uterus is gently massaged to keep it firm and occlude hemorrhage from its interior wall. The infant is also cared for by patting dry and covering with a soft blanket to reduce heat loss. Finally, the infant is assessed, an APGAR score is determined and the mother and child are transported to the emergency department.

READING COMPREHENSION SELF-EXAM

1. The organ of fetal/maternal exchange responsible for the production of several hormones during pregnancy is the ....

   A. uterus.
   B. vagina.
   C. placenta.
   D. fallopian tube.
   E. ovary.

   Answer C

2. The length of the normal pregnancy is about ....

   A. 280 days.
   B. 10 lunar months.
   C. 9 calendar months.
   D. 40 weeks.
   E. all of the above.

   Answer E

3. The possibility of premature infant survival begins after how many months of gestation?

   A. 5th
   B. 6th
   C. 7th
   D. 8th
   E. 9th

   Answer B

4. The fetal circulation changes to the normal circulation ....

A. with the beginning of labor.
B. with exposure to the cool environment.
C. due to the drying of the body.
D. with the first respiration.
E. with expulsion from the vaginal canal.

Answer D

5. In addition to the normal assessment and questioning of the primary and secondary assessment, the obstetrical patient should be asked ....
   1. her estimated date of confinement.
   2. her gravidity and parity.
   3. about the presence of discharge or vaginal bleeding.
   4. if she has had any cesarean sections.
   5. the character of any pain she feels.

   Select the proper grouping.

A. 1, 4
B. 2, 5
C. 1, 2, 4
D. 2, 4, 5
E. 1, 2, 3, 4, 5

Answer E

6. Which of the following might be expected in the pregnant patient who has been subjected to blunt abdominal trauma?

A. abruptio placenta
B. uterine rupture
C. premature labor
D. fetal death
E. all of the above

Answer E

7. The infant of a pregnant mother who has had trouble controlling blood sugar levels may ....

A. be of high birth weight.
B. have trouble maintaining body temperature.
C. experience hypoglycemia.
D. all of the above.
E. none of the above.

Answer D

8. Vaginal bleeding during pregnancy can be related to ....
   1. spontaneous abortion.
   2. ectopic pregnancy.
   3. menstrual period.
   4. placenta previa.
   5. abruptio placenta.

   Select the proper grouping.

A. 1, 2, 5
B. 2, 3, 5
C. 1, 2, 4, 5
D. 1, 2, 3, 4
E. 1, 2, 3, 4, 5

Answer C

9. If an abortion occurs in the second trimester and the infant is suspended from the cord the paramedic should ....

A. clamp and cut the cord.
B. leave the cord intact.
C. gently pull on the cord until placental delivery.
D. await placental delivery.
E. none of the above.

Answer A

10. Care for the patient who has just experienced an abortion should include all of the following except ....

A. high flow oxygen.
B. IV of normal saline or lactated Ringer's solution.
C. 2 mg of morphine sulfate.
D. emotional support.
E. possible PASG use.

Answer C

11. The type of pain associated with abruptio placentae is usually described as ....

A. tearing.
B. dull.
C. cramping.
D. stabbing.
E. pulsating.

Answer A

12. In the presence of any pre-partum hemorrhage the patient should receive which of the following?
   1. high-flow oxygen
   2. a vaginal exam
   3. an IV with dextrose 5% in water
   4. PASG without using the abdominal segment

Select the proper grouping.

A. 1, 2
B. 1, 4
C. 2, 3
D. 1, 2, 4
E. 1, 3, 4

Answer B

13. The cardinal signs of preeclampsia include ....
   1. seizures.
   2. excessive weight gain.
   3. edema.
   4. hypertension.
   5. protein in the urine.

Select the proper grouping.

A. 2, 3, 5
B. 1, 3, 4
C. 2, 3, 4, 5
D. 1, 2, 3, 4
E. 1, 2, 3, 4, 5

Answer C

14. The condition in which the placenta is located over or close to the cervix is called ....

A. abruptio placenta.
B. malformed placenta.
C. cervical placenta.
D. placenta previa.
E. none of the above.

Answer D

15. The drug that is indicated in preeclampsia and eclampsia and may be ordered by the medical control physician is ....

A. magnesium sulfate.
B. calcium chloride.
C. apresoline.
D. dopamine.
E. atropine.

Answer A

16. The care most often required for the late pregnancy patient with supine hypotension who does not appear to be volume depleted is ....

A. fluid infusion.
B. patient positioning.
C. PASG application.
D. dopamine administration.
E. all of the above.

Answer B

17. Which factors are taken into consideration in making the determination to stay and deliver or transport?
   1. frequency of the contractions
   2. parity
   3. urge to push
   4. crowning
   5. previous length of labor

Select the proper grouping.

A. 1, 2, 5
B. 2, 3, 4
C. 1, 2, 4, 5
D. 2, 3, 4, 5
E. 1, 2, 3, 4, 5

Answer e

18. If the cord is found protruding from the birth canal during an exam for crowning the paramedic should ....

A. clamp and cut the cord.
B. loop the cord over the infant's neck.
C. place gentle pressure against the presenting part.
D. pull the cord gently.
E. continue with the delivery in the normal and routine way.

Answer C

19. During the preparation for delivery the fetal heart rate is noted to be 120. This would necessitate ....

A. immediate transport.
B. an increase in the maternal oxygen administration.
C. the use of pitocin.
D. no unusual care steps.
E. gentle massage of the uterus until it firms.

Answer D

20. If at the conclusion of the third stage of labor, the patient experiences moderate hemorrhage the paramedic should ....

A. disregard the blood loss.
B. pack the vaginal canal.
C. massage the uterus until hard.
D. transport the mother immediately.
E. none of the above.

Answer C

21. During a breech birth the infant's head does not deliver. The infant makes chest movements as though to breath. The paramedic should ....

A. pull forcibly on the infant's legs.
B. pull gently on the infant's legs.
C. attempt to open an airway for the infant.
D. provide the mother with high-flow oxygen and transport.
E. locate the umbilical cord and clamp and cut it.

Answer C

22. If during the visual exam for crowning you notice a hand or leg protruding from the vaginal canal, you should ....
1. give high flow oxygen.
2. reassure the mother.
3. attempt to reposition the limb once.
4. provide immediate transport.
5. maintain a gentle but constant pull on the extremity.

Select the proper grouping.

A. 1, 2, 4
B. 2, 3, 4
C. 1, 3, 4, 5
D. 2, 3, 4, 5
E. 1, 2, 3, 4, 5

Answer A

23. If labor ends abruptly without the delivery of the infant, the abdomen is tender and rigid, and auscultation of the belly reveals no fetal heart tones, you should suspect ....

A. Braxton-Hicks contraction.
B. uterine inversion.
C. ectopic pregnancy rupture.
D. uterine rupture.
E. uterine exhaustion.

Answer D

24. The uterus protrudes from the vagina after the delivery of the placenta. You should ....

A. place it in dry towels.
B. attempt to replace it once.
C. attempt to replace it several times.
D. soak it in saline and transport.
E. pull firmly on the umbilical cord and let it snap.

Answer B

25. The patient you are attending develops severe dyspnea during heavy labor accompanied with a sharp chest pain, tachycardia and tachypnea. What condition would you suspect?

A. pulmonary embolism
B. aortic aneurysm
C. congestive heart failure
D. preeclampsia
E. uterine rupture or inversion

Answer A

26. List the types of abortion.

Spontaneous Abortion | threatened Abortion
inevitable Abortion | incomplete Abortion
Criminal Abortion | therapeutic Abortion
elective Abortion

27. Identify care you would provide if the umbilical cord is found wrapped around the infant's neck.

Gently loop the cord off the infants head, If they are unsuccessful, then cord should be clamped twice and cut between It should then be untangled and the delivery progress normally.

SPECIAL PROJECTS

The authoring of both the radio message to medical command and the written run report are two of the most important tasks you will perform as a paramedic. Read the following information, reread the case study in your textbook and complete the run report for this call.

The Call:

Your paramedic unit is dispatched at 3:15 p.m. to the Southside Fire Station for a possible childbirth situation. You are enroute immediately and arrive on the scene at 3:22 p.m. Upon arrival, you find EMTs Tom Johnson and Steve Lawrence in the midst of a delivery in the back seat of an auto. You step in to cut the cord (3:26), suction the airway, pat the infant dry and place the infant in a blanket.

At 3:28 the mother, Mary Kasson of 345 S. Missouri Street, has the following vitals; blood pressure of 110/88, pulse of 88, respiration of 16, and a pulse oximeter reading of 92%. She explains that her due date is in one week and that she has received pre-natal care from her obstetrician. This is her sixth child with the other births being normal deliveries after only 5 hours of labor. She is allergic to sulfa drugs and has been asked to watch her diet during the pregnancy due to a family history of diabetes.

Oxygen is applied via non-rebreather at 12 L/min and the oxygen saturation rises to 97%. A quick visual exam of the mother's vaginal canal displays moderate hemorrhage. Palpation of her abdomen reveals a soft central mass. The uterus is massaged gently and the hemorrhage slows within two or three minutes. 1,000 mL of Ringer's lactate is hung and run at 5 mL/min via a 18 ga angiocath started in the left antecubital vein. A second set of vitals are taken at 3:50: BP of 108/90, pulse of 86, respirations of 18 and regular, and a pulse oximetry of 97%. The monitor is applied with normal sinus rhythm displaying.

The infant is evaluated for APGAR scoring at one minute after birth. The score is initially 8 because the limbs are blue and the heart rate is 80. Medical control is alerted to the delivery and the ambulance is directed to Women's Hospital by the patient's request. At five minutes the score is 9 because the limbs begin to turn pink. The infant, a girl, is named Natalie by her mother and is transported with her to the hospital at 4:07. The placenta delivers enroute at 4:12. Enroute vitals (4:15) were blood pressure of 112/92, pulse of 84, respirations of 16 and regular, and a pulseox reading of 96%. The mother and child ride comfortably to the hospital and the patients arrive uneventfully at the hospital at 4:20.

The unit is reported in service at 4:45 p.m.

Using the information contained in the case study and this additional narrative, complete the run report on the following page.

Compare the radio communication and run report form which you prepared against the example in the answer key section of this workbook. As you make this comparison, realize that there are "many correct" ways to communicate this body of information. Ensure that the information you have recorded contains the major points of your assessment and care, and enough other material to describe the patient and his condition to the receiving physician and anyone else who might review the form. Remember that this document may be the only record of your assessment and care for this patient. When you are done, it should be a complete accounting of your actions.

Date 5 / 13 / 94	Emergency Medical Service Run Report		Run # 915
Patient Information	**Service Information**		**Times**
Name: MARY KASSIN	Agency: Crew 29		Rcvd 15 : 15
Address: 345 S. MISSOURI	Location: S. Side Fire Station		Enrt 15 : 15
City: Washoe St: CA Zip: 95713	Call Origin: Dispatch		Scne 15 : 22
Age: 29 Birth: 11 / 29 / 60 Sex: [M][F]	Type: Emrg[X] Non[ ] Trnsfr[ ]		LvSn 16 : 07
Nature of Call: Obstetrical			ArHsp 16 : 20
Chief Complaint: mother in Active labor/Strong & frequent contractions.			InSv 16 : 45

Description of Current Problem: A young female presented to the Fire Station in Active labor and at 16:26 gave birth to a baby girl (Natilie) The 1 min/APGAR Score was 8. The mother experienced minor Post partum hemmorrhage and a soft uterus. Uternine massage, Reduced the hemmorage and the uterus became Firm. The Five minute APGAR was 9, mother and Child arrived uneventfully at womens Hospital

Medical Problems	Past	Present
Cardiac	[ ]	[ ]
Stroke	[ ]	[ ]
Acute Abdomen	[ ]	[ ]
Diabetes	[ ]	[X]
Psychiatric	[ ]	[ ]
Epilepsy	[ ]	[ ]
Drug/Alcohol	[ ]	[ ]
Poisoning	[ ]	[ ]
Allergy/Asthma	[ ]	[ ]
Syncope	[ ]	[ ]
Obstetrical	[ ]	[X]
GYN	[ ]	[ ]

Other: none.

Trauma Scr: n/A Glascow: 15

On Scene Care: The Cord was Clamped & cut and the Infant was placed in A blanket A 18ga IV w/1000 LR @ 5ml/min Left Antecubital	First Aid: The delivery was Assisted by the Emts The patient was in the back of A Station wagon. By Whom? Johnson & Lawrence.

O2 @ 12 L 15:28 Via NRM	C-Collar n/A:	S-Immob. n/A	Stretcher 16 : 07

Allergies/Meds: Sulfa Drugs. Possible diabetes controlled by diet	Past Med Hx: 6th normal Child Birth. Previous labors were Normal

Time	Pulse	Resp.	BP S/D	LOC	EKG
15:28	R: 88 [r][i]	R: 16 [s][l]	110 / 88	[a][v][p][u]	NSR SaO2 92% NSR
Care/Comments: Immediate Post Partum, Soft uterus w/hemmorage - uterine massage.					
15:50	R: 86 [r][i]	R: 18 [s][l]	108 / 90	[a][v][p][u]	NSR SaO2 97%
Care/Comments: Hemmorage. controlled, Apgar 8, IV Started.					
16:15	R: 84 [r][i]	R: 16 [s][l]	112 / 92	[a][v][p][u]	NSR SaO2 96%
Care/Comments: Placenta delivered @ 16:12					
:	R: [r][i]	R: [s][l]	/	[a][v][p][u]	
Care/Comments:					

Destination: Womens Hospital	Personnel:	Certification
Reason: [X]pt [ ]Closest [ ]M.D[ ]Other	1. Cindy Robertson	[P][E][O]
Contacted: [X]Radio [ ]Tele[ ]Direct	2. Tom Johnson	[P][E][O]
Ar Status: [ ]Better [X]UnC[ ]Worse	3. Steve Lawrence.	[P][E][O]

33

EMERGENCY MANAGEMENT OF THE NEONATE

Review of the Objectives for Chapter 33

After reading this chapter, you should be able to:

1. Describe the routine care of the newborn.

pp. 998 to 999

Airway - the airway is of prime concern in management of the neonate. It should be suctioned as the head delivers and monitored and suctioned as needed thereafter. Both the mouth and nose should be cleared of fluids. If the infant does not spontaneously breathe or cry a few moments after delivery, stimulate the infant by patting the feet or rubbing the back.

Maintain body temperature - heat loss is an important consideration in the infant. The neonate has a large surface area to weight ratio and underdeveloped temperature regulation mechanisms. It is therefore very important to quickly pat dry the neonate and wrap him or her in a soft blanket. As necessary, place warm water bottles in the vicinity of the child.

Cut the umbilical cord - the cord should be cut after the baby is breathing and insulated from heat loss. Keep the infant at the same level as the birth canal. After 30 to 45 seconds of birth place an umbilical clamp 10 cm from the infant and another 5 cm from that. Cut between the two clamps and ensure the infant end of the cord does not continue to bleed.

Assessment - obtain the infant pulse, respiratory rate and examine the color, muscle tone and response to stimulation. Use the findings to determine the APGAR score at one minute and five minutes post-birth.

2. List four means by which heat loss occurs in neonates.

p. 998

Heat loss in the neonate occurs through the same mechanisms as it does for the adults: evaporation, conduction, convection, and radiation. Help maintain body heat by drying to reduce evaporation heat loss and place in a blanket to reduce conduction and convection losses. Keep the room temperature high to reduce radiation losses.

3. Define the parameters of APGAR scoring and the numerical values used.

pp. 999 to 1000

Signs		0	1	2
Appearance	(Color)	Blue	Pink trunk	Pink
Pulse	(Heart Rate)	None	<100	>100
Grimace	(Irritability)	Quiet	Grimace	Active Cry
Activity	(Muscle Tone)	Quiet	Motion	Active Motion
Respiration	(Breathing)	None	Slow, Irregular	Active Cry

4. Identify special considerations in the care of the premature neonate.

pp. 1000 to 1001

The premature neonate is especially susceptible to heat loss and hypothermia. Its body surface area is large compared to its weight, it does not have a fully developed temperature regulating mechanism, it has less subcutaneous fat than the normal neonate, and neonates cannot shiver to raise body temperature. Because of these considerations you must must maintain the premature infant's temperature.

5. Explain the significance of meconium staining.

p. 1001

Meconium is the first bowel movement of the newborn. If before or during the delivery process the infant is distressed, the bowels will move and stain the amniotic fluid. Not only does the meconium indicate distress, it also means that the infant may have aspirated the material. Meconium staining is a serious sign of fetal distress.

6. Describe the inverted-pyramid approach to neonatal resuscitation.

pp. 1003 to 1009

The inverted pyramid identifies the most common and significant threats to the infant. Warmth, positioning, suctioning and tactile stimulation are most important to initial resuscitation. The second level of resuscitation is supplemental oxygen followed by assisted ventilation. If the previous steps are unsuccessful, step four calls for cardiac compressions. Finally, step six involves the use of medications and fluid resuscitation. In the vast majority of pediatric patients steps one and two will successfully resuscitate the newborn.

7. Describe two methods of stimulating a distressed neonate.

p. 1005

The neonate may be stimulated by either gently slapping the soles of the feet or rubbing the back. Rigorous spanking or slapping is not recommended and will not be any more effective than gentle stimulation.

8. Describe the appropriate administration of oxygen to a neonate.

p. 1007

Oxygen should be administered to the neonate by allowing the oxygen to blow across the infant's face. Warmed oxygen is most ideal.

9. Describe the indications and procedure for endotracheal intubation of a distressed neonate.

p. 1008

Endotracheal intubation is indicated for cases when the bag-valve-mask unit is not effective, tracheal suctioning is needed, or ventilation is needed for a long time. The uncuffed tube is chosen based upon the child size and placed with the straight laryngoscope blade. Position is checked by watching for symmetrical chest wall motion and by auscultating for bilaterally equal breath sounds.

10. Describe methods and problems in ventilating the distressed infant.

p. 1008

The neonate should be ventilated via an infant bag-valve-mask. The pressure release valve should be disabled since the pressures required to ventilate the infant are relatively high. The breaths must also be administered at a rate of between 40 and 60 per minute. Endotracheal intubation is indicated if the BVM is ineffective, tracheal suctioning is needed, or prolonged ventilation will be needed. The tube should be uncuffed and the straight laryngoscope blade used for its placement.

11. Describe the technique and rates used in chest compressions in the neonate.

p. 1009

The infant's chest should be depressed 1.5 to 2.0 cm at a rate of 120 compressions per minute. The chest should be encircled or two fingers should be used to place pressure on the lower third of the chest along the sternum. If the heart rate exceeds 80, discontinue CPR.

12. List drugs and fluids used in neonatal resuscitation and give the correct dosages.

p. 1009

Epinephrine	0.1 - 0.3 mL/kg
Volume expanders	10 mL/kg
Sodium bicarbonate	2 mEq/kg
Narcan	0.5 mL/kg (0.01 mg/kg)
Dopamine	5 - 20 mcg/kg/min

CASE STUDY REVIEW

Reread the case study in **PARAMEDIC EMERGENCY CARE** and then read the discussion below.

The call to which the Bell County General Hospital paramedics respond is a typical response that addresses emergency childbirth and care of the neonate. Several elements of importance to this response are discussed below.

Chapter 33 Case Study

The paramedics determine that the delivery is imminent. They ask the patient her expected date of confinement, the number of previous deliveries, and the strength of, the length of, and time between contractions. The woman may also have had her waters break and is experiencing the urge to move her bowels. With this history, the paramedics examine the perineum only to find crowning of the infant's head with the strong contractions. There is no choice. The patient is about to deliver and the paramedics choose to do it at the scene.

The paramedics prepare for the delivery. They ready the patient by draping the thighs and abdomen so only the mother's perineum is exposed. They don gloves, open the OB kit and display the contents. As the head presents, gentle pressure is applied to prevent explosive delivery. They suction the nose and mouth as the head passes through the vaginal canal.

Once the infant has completely delivered, suctioning continues. The paramedics perform a quick APGAR score to find a baby with a blue trunk and extremities (0 points), who is breathing slowly (1 points), is limp (0 points), has a pulse of 86 (1 point), and is not responding to stimulation (0 points). They assign a score of 2 initially. The infant is ventilated via bag-valve-mask, is patted dry and wrapped in a blanket while the cord is clamped and cut. After four more minutes the infant's pulse remains at 86 though his extremities turn pink and he begins to cry vigorously and to move about. The five minute APGAR score is 9.

The mother's abdomen is soft and there is a moderate amount of vaginal bleeding. One paramedic gently massages the fundus and the hemorrhage slows. Oxygen and an IV of Lactated Ringer's solution are administered. The trip to the hospital was uneventful.

READING COMPREHENSION SELF-EXAM

1. Which of the following are true regarding the airway and breathing for the neonate?
   1. the head should be raised above the trunk
   2. both the mouth and nose need suctioning
   3. the infant is expected to breathe within one minute
   4. suctioning should begin as the delivery ends

   Select the proper grouping.

   A. 1, 4
   B. 2, 3
   C. 1, 2, 4
   D. 1, 2, 3
   E. 1, 2, 3, 4

   Answer B

2. Heat loss, normally accompanying birth, can be minimized by ....
   1. patting the infant dry.
   2. the use of heat lamps directed at the infant.
   3. placing the child in a soft receiving blanket.
   4. placing uninsulated hot water bottles next to the infant.
   5. ensuring the environment is at a temperature of 74 to 76 degrees.

   Select the proper grouping.

   A. 2, 4
   B. 1, 2, 3
   C. 2, 4, 5
   D. 1, 3, 5
   E. 1, 2, 3, 4, 5

   Answer D

3. Milking of the umbilical cord will push red blood cells into the infant's circulation. It will thereby increase the vascular volume, the blood's ability to carry oxygen and infant survival.

   A. True
   B. False

   Answer B

4. The initial respiratory rate for the newborn is normally around ....

   A. 24 to 36 breaths per minute.
   B. 40 to 60 breaths per minute.
   C. 60 to 80 breaths per minute.
   D. 80 to 100 breaths per minute.
   E. none of the above.

   Answer B

5. The infant's heart rate at birth is about 150 to 180 though it slows to 130 to 140 shortly thereafter.

   A. True
   B. False

   Answer A

6. At five minutes after birth an infant is breathing at 24 breaths per minute, responds to stimuli with vigorous crying, has a heart rate of 120, is moving all extremities briskly, and is pink. What APGAR score would you award the infant?

A. 15
B. 10
C. 9
D. 8
E. A+

Answer B

7. The premature infant loses body heat more rapidly than the full term infant because ....
   1. they have a high body surface area to weight ratio.
   2. their temperature-regulating mechanisms are immature.
   3. they have less subcutaneous fat.
   4. they cannot shiver.

Select the proper grouping.

A. 1, 3
B. 2, 4
C. 1, 4
D. 1, 2, 4
E. 1, 2, 3, 4

Answer E

8. If during delivery the amniotic fluid is stained with meconium, the attending paramedic must be sure to ....

A. not attempt any resuscitation.
B. apply high-flow oxygen early in care.
C. suction the airway thoroughly.
D. infuse an antibiotic to reduce respiratory inflammation.
E. none of the above.

Answer C

9. The infant you are caring for has a heart rate of 52 one minute after delivery. What action should you take?

A. begin CPR
B. increase the oxygen level
C. infuse 20 mL of fluid
D. stimulate the infant
E. continue normal infant care

Answer A

10. The cardiac compressions for the neonate should be delivered at which rate?

A. 60 per minute
B. 80 per minute
C. 100 per minute
D. 120 per minute
E. 140 per minute

Answer D

SPECIAL PROJECTS

Childbirth/Neonate Crossword Puzzle

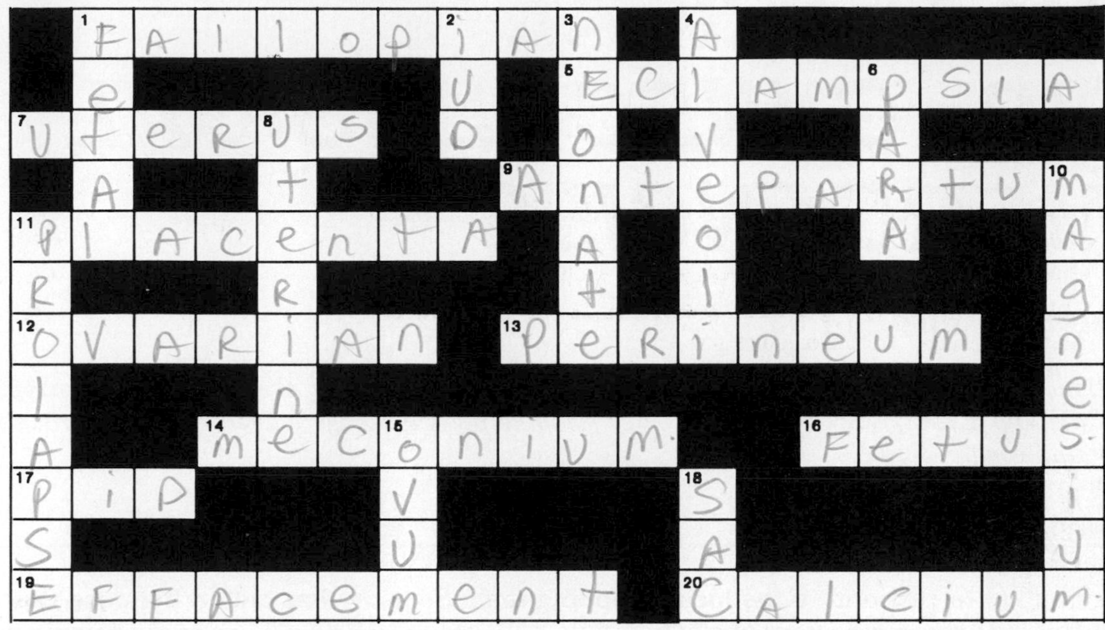

The crossword puzzle above addresses the vocabulary of chapters 32 and 33.

ACROSS

1. The tube through which the egg travels from the ovary to the uterus.
5. A hypertensive disorder of pregnancy that manifests with a grand mal seizure.
7. The muscular organ in which the fetus develops.
9. Just before the delivery of the fetus.
11. The organ of maternal and fetal circulatory exchange.
12. Having to do with or related to the ovaries.
13. The area surrounding the vagina and anus.
14. The first bowel movement of the newborn.
16. The developing infant within the uterus.
17. A lower abdominal syndrome commonly caused by a sexually transmitted disease.
19. The drawing back and thinning of the cervix in preparation for delivery.
20. The drug that is an antidote to magnesium.

DOWN

1. Refering to the developing infant while in the uterus.
2. A type of birth control in which a device is placed in the uterus to prevent fertilization.
3. The infant, immediately after birth.
4. The small air sacs where the oxygen/carbon dioxide exchange occurs.
6. A prefix meaning around or about.
8. Having to do with the organ containing the developing fetus.
10. Drug used to manage eclampsia and preeclampsia.
11. A falling or dropping down of an part.
15. The medical term for the egg.
18. The term used to describe the envelope which contains the infant and amniotic fluid.

DIVISION REVIEW

OBSTETRICAL AND GYNECOLOGICAL EMERGENCIES

Chapters 3l through 33

The following scenario based questions are designed to help you review the previous three chapters of **PARAMEDIC EMERGENCY CARE.** *They combine the knowledge gained thus far through your reading and course work.*

Scenario I

You are called to respond to the local shopping mall. Security has called because there is a lady in the bathroom who says she is in labor. You arrive to find a 24-year-old female who is clearly in the later stages of her pregnancy. The history reveals this is her second full term pregnancy, she is two days beyond her expected date of confinement, she just experienced a gush of fluid, and her pains are less than 2 minutes apart.

1. This patient is probably in which stage of labor?

A. first
B. second
C. third
D. post partum
E. none of the above

Answer B

You lay the woman on your stretcher and check for crowning. The presenting part is the babies head, which bulges the vaginal opening with each contraction. You drape the mother and prepare for delivery. It progresses uneventfully and ends with the infant's birth. You cut the cord and place the infant on the mother's chest.

2. This delivery would be referred to as ....

A. breech.
B. brow.
C. vertex.
D. occiput posterior position.
E. transverse.

Answer C

3. When cutting the umbilical cord you should do which of the following?
   1. keep the baby lower than the vagina
   2. milk the cord
   3. place one clamp 10 cm from the infant
   4. place another clamp 15 cm from the infant
   5. cut between the clamps

   Select the proper grouping.

   A. 1, 3, 4
   B. 3, 4, 5
   C. 1, 3, 4, 5
   D. 2, 3, 4, 5
   E. 1, 2, 3, 4, 5

   Answer B

4. The mother seems to be doing fine but you notice that she is still hemorrhaging moderately. What action should you take?

   A. pull gently on the umbilical cord
   B. pack the vaginal opening
   C. gently massage the uterus
   D. have the mother flex her legs over a pad
   E. B and C

   Answer C

5. The actions you employ in question number 4 are unsuccessful. You should employ which of the following?
   1. PASG
   2. oxygen
   3. force placenta delivery
   4. IV fluids
   5. magnesium sulfate IV

   Select the proper grouping.

   A. 1, 3
   B. 2, 4
   C. 3, 5
   D. 1, 2, 4
   E. 1, 3, 4, 5

   Answer D

The infant is assessed at one minute and found to have a pulse of 90, blue limbs and a pink trunk, slow and irregular respirations, a weak cry, and limited flexing of the extremities.

6. The infant described above should receive an APGAR score of ....

   A. 3
   B. 5
   C. 10
   D. 12
   E. 15

   Answer B

7. The infant described above is in need of ....

   A. no special care.
   B. routine care.
   C. oxygen and stimulation.
   D. ventilation.
   E. cardiac compression.

   Answer C

At five minutes the infant is pink in both the limbs and trunk, has a pulse of 120, cries loudly, and is writhing about.

8. What APGAR score would you give this infant?

A. 3
B. 6
C. 10
D. 12
E. 15

Answer C

Scenario II

An early morning call has you attending an 18-year-old female with lower abdominal pain. The patient has left sided abdominal pain, minor vaginal spotting, and feels very weak. She reports a history of a missed period and intermittent spotting for the past four or five weeks. She thinks she might be pregnant and reports a severe abdominal infection about a year ago.

9. Which medical situation should you anticipate?

A. abruptio placenta
B. placenta previa
C. pelvic inflammatory disease
D. eclampsia
E. ectopic pregnancy

Answer e

10. Which of the following conditions would predispose the patient to this problem?

A. pelvic inflammatory disease
B. previous ectopic pregnancy
C. previous tubal ligation
D. an IUD
E. all of the above

Answer e

11. This patient requires which of the following care approaches?

A. immediate transport with care en route
B. immediate on scene care
C. stabilizing scene care and expeditious transport
D. supportive care and gentle transport
E. routine scene care

Answer A

12. Care steps should include which of the following?
1. rapid transport
2. vaginal packing
3. high-flow oxygen
4. IV lines with lactated Ringer's or normal saline
5. PASG, ready to inflate

Select the proper grouping.

A. 1, 4, 5
B. 1, 3, 5
C. 1, 3, 4, 5
D. 2, 3, 4, 5
E. 1, 2, 3, 4, 5

Answer C

34

BEHAVIORAL AND PSYCHIATRIC EMERGENCIES

Review of the Objectives for Chapter 34

After reading this chapter, you should be able to:

1. Define the term behavioral emergency.

p. 1014

A behavioral emergency is an intrapsychic, environmental, situational or organic alteration that results in a behavior that is unacceptable to the patient or society. It requires immediate attention and entry into the mental health system.

2. Discuss the role of drugs and alcohol in behavioral emergencies.

p. 1015

Drugs and alcohol are common causes of behavioral emergencies. Alcohol is a depressant, which alone can cause the unacceptable behavior or can worsen underlying psychological problems. Abuse of prescription or street drugs can cause a wide variety of problems due to the great variation of the expected action of the pharmacologic agent.

3. List physical problems that can be manifested as psychiatric problems.

pp. 1015 to 1016

Diabetes and electrolyte disturbances can manifest as behavioral emergencies. The diabetic can display alcohol intoxication-like signs and symptoms including slurred speech, confusion and unsteady gait. Electrolyte imbalances may present with confusion, violence or anxiety. Dementia, referred to as organic brain syndrome, and Alzheimer's disease will also present with confusion, anxiety and impaired behavior. These medical problems are associated with aging.

4. Describe verbal communication techniques useful in managing the emotionally disturbed patient.

pp. 1017 to 1018

The communication between the paramedic and the patient should be unrushed, make use of open-ended questions, lead by the patient, unthreatening, and nonjudgmental. It should be quiet and relaxed. The paramedic should be concerned, empathetic, honest, self-confident, and supportive.

5. Describe the use of open-ended versus closed-ended questions.

p. 1017

Open-ended questions permit the patient to answer in sentences and phrases rather than yes, no or some other very short answer. Open-ended questioning allows the paramedic to analyze the patient's thought process, logic, and feelings, more so than close-ended questions.

6. List factors associated with increased risk of suicide.

p. 1020

Ages 15 to 24 and above 40 years
Homosexuality
A plan, mechanism to accomplish it
Previous attempts
Depression or alcohol or drug abuse
Living alone
Major separation (divorce, personal independence, death, job, etc.)
Major physical stress (surgery, childbirth, sleep deprivation)
Lack of future goals
Suicide of same sexed parent

7. Define and briefly describe the management of the following conditions:

pp. 1019 to 1029

Depression is a common disorder affecting 20% of the population. The patient loses interest and pleasure in his or her usual activities and often feels hopeless and helpless. Care is emotional support, encouragement and transport.

Suicide is a frequent cause of death and is related to stress and depression. The thoughts of suicide are more significant if the individual has a plan, has the needed materials or has made previous attempts. Management is aimed at protecting the patient from the attempt while considering your own safety. Do not leave the patient alone. Use restraints and medication to subdue the patient as necessary.

Anxiety is a normal response to stress. It can, at times, be overwhelming and leave the patient unable to function normally. The patient should be supported, calmed, and reassured. Allow the patient to talk while you look for physical causes for his or her complaints even though they may be attributed to anxiety.

Mania is generally the opposite of depression. The patient appears high and intense. Care is directed at calming the patient if he or she is nonviolent. Consider restraints and medication if violent.

Schizophrenia is characterized by a regression to a previous level of functioning, hallucinations, delusions, altered thought, inappropriate emotions, and general disorganization. Management includes transport with support and reassurance if the patient is nonviolent. If the patient is violent, restraint and medication may be required.

Behavioral problems in the elderly are of the same etiology as those of younger persons, though they may be compounded by poor hearing, sight, and mental capabilities. Management should include extra effort to explain what is happening, and employ patience, empathy and reassurance. Avoid medication unless absolutely necessary.

Behavioral problems in children - children are not immune from behavioral emergencies. Their presentation may be compounded by the stage of behavioral development and by an ability to communicate, understand and conceptualize. Management includes support from the parent, soft, calm, reassuring speech, short simple explanations and allowing the child to keep a favorite blanket or toy. Invasive procedures should be done slowly and the child should not be left alone.

Domestic violence is the use of force by one family member with the intent to cause emotional or physical injury on another. It is best to await police control of the situation and then assist the injured. Be supportive and not judgemental.

8. Describe the indications and procedure for restraining a violent patient.

pp. 1024 to 1029

The patient who presents a physical threat to either himself or others should be restrained. The patient must be disarmed before EMS personnel attempt to restrain the patient. Restraint should be attempted with police authorization and then it should be provided by at least four persons of the stature of the patient to be restrained. The patient should be approached from behind and both sides and be moved to a prone position. Restraints should be of commercial leather or other strong material, or improvised from cravats, towels, spineboard straps or kling.

CASE STUDY REVIEW

Reread the case study in **PARAMEDIC EMERGENCY CARE** and then read the discussion below.

This case study presents an interesting manifestation of a behavioral emergency. It affords us the opportunity to examine the approach to the disturbed patient and the techniques of management we should employ.

Chapter 34 Case Study

The paramedics arrive and begin to assess a patient who is obviously experiencing a psychiatric emergency. They assess the scene to ensure it is safe for themselves, the patient's mother, and the patient. They identify that the patient has no access to a weapon and is not violent at the time. They position themselves between the patient and easy exit just in case the patient's disposition changes. The police are notified in case restraint may become necessary.

As the history and the patient evaluation become more complete, it is apparent that the patient is nonviolent and cooperative. The paramedics relax a bit and approach the patient though they still maintain a safe distance and are cautious. They are supportive of the patient, appear confident in their conversation with the patient and in their body language. They do not rush the situation and take the time to establish a rapport with the patient and reduce his anxieties associated with their presence and the eventual trip to the hospital. During the conversations with the patient the paramedics listen carefully but are honest and neither support nor challenge the delusions and hallucinations.

The patient consents to transport, which simplifies the paramedic's responsibilities. Had he refused transport, the paramedics would have been unable to force the issue since the patient was no immediate threat to himself or others. The police may have consented to place him under arrest and then ordered transport or the patient's physician may have been called, made an evaluation and then requested transport via court order.

This call is typical of most behavioral emergencies in that the patient is nonviolent. Care centers around support, careful listening and a non-confrontational attitude on the part of the care providers. Transport is offered and the patient is delivered uneventfully to the emergency department. Even though the common psychological patient is nonviolent, the paramedic must be very careful to protect himself, others and the patient from harm.

READING COMPREHENSION SELF-EXAM

1. Which of the reasons listed below account for the rise in behavioral emergencies seen by prehospital personnel?
   1. the increased stress of modern society
   2. breakdown of the ozone layer
   3. drug and substance abuse
   4. the deinstitutionalization of the mentally ill

   Select the proper grouping.

   A. 1, 2
   B. 3, 4
   C. 2, 4
   D. 1, 3, 4
   E. 2, 3, 4

   Answer B

2. The patient who is acting in an intoxicated fashion and displays confusion should be suspected of alcohol abuse and ....

   A. diabetes.
   B. electrolyte imbalance.
   C. head injury.
   D. drug overdose.
   E. all of the above.

   Answer e

3. Important aspects of the patient interview include ....
   1. removing the patient from the crisis situation.
   2. avoid arguing with the patient.
   3. encouraging the patient to speak in his or her own words.
   4. being honest.
   5. discounting any delusions the patient experiences.

   Select the proper grouping.

   A. 1, 2
   B. 2, 3, 4
   C. 1, 3, 5
   D. 1, 2, 3, 4
   E. 1, 2, 3, 4, 5

   Answer D

4. The ideal type of question to use in conversation with the behavioral emergency patient are those which can be answered simply with one or two words (closed-ended questions).

   A. True
   B. False

   Answer B

5. Which of the following psychiatric disorders account for most behavioral referrals?

   A. depression
   B. anxiety
   C. paranoia
   D. schizophrenia
   E. manic disorders

   Answer A

6. Which of the following are generally true if the behavioral emergency patient is transported under police arrest?
   1. the individual must be restrained or handcuffed
   2. the paramedics act as agents of the police
   3. the patient will be transported to confinement facilities only
   4. the police officer should accompany the paramedics and the patient

   Select the proper grouping.

   A. 1, 2
   B. 2, 4
   C. 3, 4
   D. 1, 3, 4
   E. 1, 2, 3

   Answer B

7. Suicide attempts are most successful for ....

   A. females.
   B. males.
   C. persons over 45 years of age.
   D. persons under 15 years of age.
   E. those who use drugs.

   Answer B

8. Which of the following is not normally a suicide risk factor?

   A. previous attempt
   B. married persons
   C. living alone
   D. homosexuality
   E. alcohol or drug abuse

   Answer B

9. Which of the items below is commonly associated with an anxiety disorder?
   1. hyperventilation
   2. fear of losing control
   3. constipation and infrequent urination
   4. headache, palpitations and vertigo

   Select the proper grouping.

   A. 1, 3
   B. 2, 4
   C. 1, 2, 4
   D. 2, 3, 4
   E. 1, 2, 3, 4

   Answer C

10. Which behavioral disturbance may manifest with hallucinations, delusions, disorganization, inappropriate affect, and altered thought?

    A. mania
    B. anxiety
    C. depression
    D. schizophrenia
    E. dementia

    Answer D

11. Which behavioral disorder is generally considered the opposite of depression?

A. anxiety
B. schizophrenia
C. mania
D. suicide
E. dementia

Answer C

12. In the elderly patient who is experiencing a behavioral emergency the paramedic should administer drugs aggressively.

A. True
B. False

Answer B

13. Which is true regarding the handling of a child who is experiencing a behavioral emergency?
1. separate the child from the mother if possible
2. tell them what they wish to hear until at the hospital
3. encourage the child to help with care
4. discourage crying
Select the proper grouping.

A. 3
B. 1, 4
C. 1, 3, 4
D. 1, 2, 3
E. 1, 2, 3, 4

Answer A

14. When restraining a patient against his or her will it is best to ....
1. seek police authorization.
2. use at least two persons.
3. use only reasonable force.
4. offer the patient one final opportunity to cooperate.
5. place the patient prone on the stretcher, if extremely violent.
Select the proper grouping.

A. 1, 3, 4
B. 2, 4, 5
C. 1, 3, 4, 5
D. 2, 3, 4, 5
E. 1, 2, 3, 4, 5

Answer C

15. General considerations to ensure paramedic safety when presented with a violent patient should include ....
1. keeping a safe distance.
2. not letting the patient block your exit.
3. keeping furniture between you and the patient.
4. standing together with other care providers.
5. not making threatening statements.
Select the proper grouping.

A. 1, 2, 5
B. 2, 3, 4
C. 1, 2, 3, 5
D. 1, 2, 4, 5
E. 1, 3, 4, 5

Answer C

National Registry of Emergency Medical Technicians

The Authors wish to express their thanks to the National Registry of Emergency Medical Technicians for the use of these Paramedic Practical Examination Forms and their continuing efforts to improve the quality of pre-hospital emergency medical care.

Paramedic Practical Evaluation Forms

The forms contained on the next few pages are inserted to help you identify common criteria by which you will be evaluated. It may be valuable to review your practical skills by using these sheets during your class practice sessions and as a review of those skills before class, state and any national testing. Evaluation forms will often vary, however, many of the important elements of paramedic performance are common to all forms.

Please note that the skill forms are labeled advanced level, intermediate and paramedic practical examination. Advanced level skills are tested for both intermediate and paramedic candidates while skills identified either as paramedic or intermediate are used for that level alone.

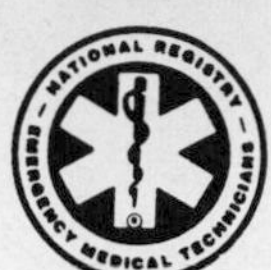

National Registry of Emergency Medical Technicians
Advanced Level Practical Examination

PATIENT ASSESSMENT/MANAGEMENT

Candidate: ____________________ Examiner: ____________________

Date: ____________________ Signature: ____________________

Scenario #________ Time Start: ____________ Time End: ____________

PRIMARY SURVEY/RESUSCITATION

		Possible Points	Points Awarded
Takes or verbalizes infection control precautions		1	
Airway with C-Spine Control	Takes or directs manual in-line immobilization of head (1 point) Opens and assesses airway (1 point) Inserts adjunct (1 point)	3	
Breathing	Assesses breathing (1 point) Initiates appropriate oxygen therapy (1 point) Assures adequate ventilation of patient (1 point) Manages any injury which may compromise breathing/ventilation (1 point)	4	
Circulation	Checks pulse (1 point) Assesses peripheral perfusion (1 point) [checks either skin color, temperature, or capillary refill] Assesses for and controls major bleeding if present (1 point) Takes vital signs (1 point) Verbalizes application of or consideration for PASG (1 point) [candidate must assess body parts to be enclosed prior to application]	5	
	Volume replacement [usually deferred until patient loaded] –Initiates first IV line (1 point) –Initiates second IV line (1 point) –Selects appropriate catheters (1 point) –Selects appropriate IV solutions and administration sets (1 point) –Infuses at appropriate rate (1 point)	5	
Disability	Performs mini-neuro assessment: AVPU (1 point) Applies cervical collar (1 point)	2	
Expose	Removes clothing	1	
Status	Calls for immediate transport of the patient when indicated	1	

PRIMARY SURVEY/RESUSCITATION SUB-TOTAL 22 ☐

SECONDARY SURVEY

NOTE: Areas denoted by "**" may be integrated within sequence of Primary Survey

		Possible Points	Points Awarded
Head	Inspects mouth**, nose**, and assesses facial area (1 point) Inspects and palpates scalp and ears (1 point) Checks eyes: PEARRL** (1 point)	3	
Neck**	Checks position of trachea (1 point) Checks jugular veins (1 point) Palpates cervical spine (1 point)	3	
Chest**	Inspects chest (1 point) Palpates chest (1 point) Auscultates chest (1 point)	3	
Abdomen/Pelvis**	Inspects and palpates abdomen (1 point) Assesses pelvis (1 point)	2	
Lower Extremities**	Inspects and palpates left leg (1 point) Inspects and palpates right leg (1 point) Checks motor, sensory, and distal circulation (1 point/arm)	4	
Upper Extremities	Inspects and palpates left arm (1 point) Inspects and palpates right arm (1 point) Checks motor, sensory, and distal circulation (1 point/arm)	4	
Posterior Thorax/Lumbar** and Buttocks	Inspects and palpates posterior thorax (1 point) Inspects and palpates lumbar and buttocks area (1 point)	2	
Identifies and treats minor wounds/fractures appropriately (1 point each)		2	

SECONDARY SURVEY SUB-TOTAL 23 ☐

CRITICAL CRITERIA

___ Failure to initiate or call for transport of the patient within 10 minute time limit
___ Failure to take or verbalize infection control precautions
___ Failure to immediately establish and maintain spinal protection
___ Failure to provide high concentration of oxygen
___ Failure to evaluate and find all presented conditions of airway, breathing, and circulation (shock)
___ Failure to appropriately manage/provide airway, breathing, hemorrhage control or treatment for shock
___ Failure to differentiate patient's needing transportation versus continued on-scene survey
___ Does other detailed physical examination before assessing & treating threats to airway, breathing & circulation

You must factually document your rationale for checking any of the above critical items on the reverse side of this form.

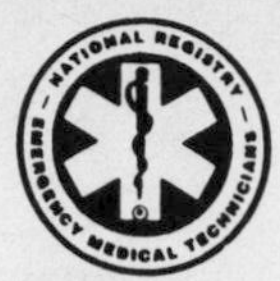

National Registry of Emergency Medical Technicians
Paramedic Practical Examination
VENTILATORY MANAGEMENT (ET)

Candidate: ______________________ Examiner: ______________________

Date: ______________________ Signature: ______________________

NOTE: If candidate elects to initially ventilate with BVM attached to reservoir and oxygen, full credit must be awarded for steps denoted by "**" so long as first ventilation is delivered within initial 30 seconds.

	Possible Points	Points Awarded
Takes or verbalizes infection control precautions	1	
Opens the airway manually	1	
Elevates tongue, inserts simple adjunct [either oropharyngeal or nasopharyngeal airway]	1	
NOTE: Examiner now informs candidate no gag reflex is present and patient accepts adjunct		
**Ventilates patient immediately with bag-valve-mask device unattached to oxygen	1	
**Hyperventilates patient with room air	1	
NOTE: Examiner now informs candidate that ventilation is being performed without difficulty		
Attaches oxygen reservoir to bag-valve-mask device and connects to high flow oxygen regulator [12-15 liters/min.]	1	
Ventilates patient at a rate of 12-20/min. and volumes of at least 800ml	1	
NOTE: After 30 seconds, examiner auscultates and reports breath sounds are present and equal bilaterally and medical control has ordered intubation. The examiner must now take over ventilation.		
Directs assistant to hyperventilate patient	1	
Identifies/selects proper equipment for intubation	1	
Checks equipment for: –Cuff leaks (1 point) –Laryngoscope operational and bulb tight (1 point)	2	
NOTE: Examiner to remove OPA and move out of way when candidate is prepared to intubate		
Positions head properly	1	
Inserts blade while displacing tongue	1	
Elevates mandible with laryngoscope	1	
Introduces ET tube and advances to proper depth	1	
Inflates cuff to proper pressure and disconnects syringe	1	
Directs ventilation of patient	1	
Confirms proper placement by auscultation bilaterally and over epigastrium	1	
NOTE: Examiner to ask "If you had proper placement, what would you expect to hear?"		
Secures ET tube [may be verbalized]	1	
TOTAL	19	

CRITICAL CRITERIA

___ Failure to initiate ventilations within 30 seconds after applying gloves or interrupts ventilations for greater than 30 seconds at any time
___ Failure to take or verbalize infection control precautions
___ Failure to voice and ultimately provide high oxygen concentrations [at least 85%]
___ Failure to ventilate patient at rate of at least 12/minute
___ Failure to provide adequate volumes per breath [maximum 2 errors/minute permissable]
___ Failure to hyperventilate patient prior to intubation
___ Failure to successfully intubate within 3 attempts
___ Using teeth as a fulcrum
___ Failure to assure proper tube placement by auscultation bilaterally **and** over the epigastrium
___ If used, stylette extends beyond end of ET tube
___ Inserts any adjunct in a manner dangerous to patient

You must factually document your rationale for checking any of the above critical items on the reverse side of this form.

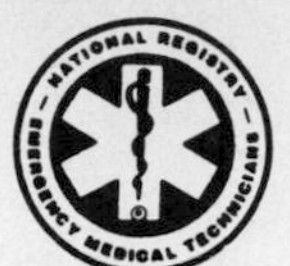

National Registry of Emergency Medical Technicians
Intermediate Practical Examination
VENTILATORY MANAGEMENT (EOA)

Candidate: ______________________ **Examiner:** ______________________

Date: ______________________ **Signature:** ______________________

NOTE: If candidate elects to initially ventilate with BVM attached to reservoir and oxygen, full credit must be awarded for steps denoted by "**" so long as first ventilation is delivered within initial 30 seconds.

	Possible Points	Points Awarded
Takes or verbalizes infection control precautions	1	
Opens the airway manually	1	
Elevates tongue, inserts simple adjunct [either oropharyngeal or nasopharyngeal airway]	1	
NOTE: Examiner now informs candidate no gag reflex is present and patient accepts adjunct		
**Ventilates patient immediately with bag-valve-mask device unattached to oxygen	1	
**Hyperventilates patient with room air	1	
NOTE: Examiner now informs candidate that ventilation is being performed without difficulty		
Attaches oxygen reservoir to bag-valve-mask device and connects to high flow oxygen regulator [12-15 liters/min.]	1	
Ventilates patient at a rate of 12-20/min. and volumes of at least 800ml	1	
NOTE: After 30 seconds, examiner auscultates and reports breath sounds are present and equal bilaterally and medical control has ordered placement of an EOA. The examiner must now take over ventilation		
Directs assistant to hyperventilate patient	1	
Identifies/selects proper equipment	1	
Assembles airway	1	
Tests cuff	1	
Inflates mask	1	
Lubricates tube [may be verbalized]	1	
NOTE: Examiner to remove OPA and move out of way when candidate is prepared to insert EOA		
Positions head properly with neck in neutral or slightly flexed position	1	
Grasps tongue and mandible and elevates	1	
Inserts tube in same direction as curvature of pharynx	1	
Advances tube until mask sealed against face	1	
Ventilates patient while maintaining tight mask seal	1	
Directs confirmation of proper placement by auscultation bilaterally and over epigastrium	1	
Inflates cuff to proper pressure and disconnects syringe	1	
Continues ventilation of patient	1	
NOTE: Examiner to ask "if you had proper placement, what would you expect to hear?"		
TOTAL	21	

CRITICAL CRITERIA

___ Failure to initiate ventilations within 30 seconds after applying gloves or interrupts ventilations for greater than 30 seconds at any time

___ Failure to take or verbalize infection control precautions

___ Failure to voice and ultimately provide high oxygen concentrations [at least 85%]

___ Failure to ventilate patient at rate of at least 12/minute

___ Failure to provide adequate volumes per breath [maximum 2 errors/minute permissable]

___ Failure to hyperventilate patient prior to placement of the EOA

___ Failure to successfully place the EOA within 3 attempts

___ Failure to assure proper tube placement by auscultation bilaterally **and** over the epigastrium

___ Inserts any adjunct in a manner dangerous to patient

You must factually document your rationale for checking any of the above critical items on the reverse side of this form.

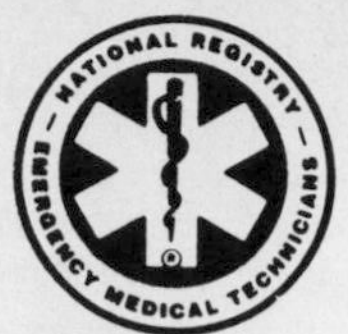

National Registry of Emergency Medical Technicians
Paramedic Practical Examination
CARDIAC ARREST SKILLS STATION
DYNAMIC CARDIOLOGY

Candidate: ______________________ Examiner: ______________________

Date: ______________________ Signature: ______________________

Set # ______________________ Time Start: __________ Time End: __________

	Possible Points	Points Awarded
Takes or verbalizes infection control precautions	1	
Checks level of responsiveness	1	
Checks ABC's	1	
Initiates CPR if appropriate [verbally]	1	
Performs "Quick Look" with paddles	1	
Correctly interprets initial rhythm	1	
Appropriately manages initial rhythm	2	
Notes change in rhythm	1	
Checks patient condition to include pulse and, if appropriate, BP	1	
Correctly interprets second rhythm	1	
Appropriately manages second rhythm	2	
Notes change in rhythm	1	
Checks patient condition to include pulse and, if appropriate, BP	1	
Correctly interprets third rhythm	1	
Appropriately manages third rhythm	2	
Notes change in rhythm	1	
Checks patient condition to include pulse and, if appropriate, BP	1	
Correctly interprets fourth rhythm	1	
Appropriately manages fourth rhythm	2	
Orders high percentages of supplemental oxygen at proper times	1	
TOTAL	24	

CRITICAL CRITERIA

___ Failure to deliver first shock in a timely manner due to operator delay in machine use or providing treatments other than CPR with simple adjuncts

___ Failure to deliver second or third shocks without delay other than the time required to reassess and recharge paddles

___ Failure to order or perform pulse checks before and after shocks

___ Failure to ensure the safety of self and others [verbalizes "All clear" and observes]

___ Inability to deliver DC shock [does not use machine properly]

___ Failure to demonstrate acceptable shock sequence

___ Failure to order initiation or resumption of CPR when appropriate

___ Failure to order correct management of airway [ET when appropriate]

___ Failure to order administration of appropriate oxygen at proper time

___ Failure to diagnose or treat 2 or more rhythms correctly

___ Orders administration of an inappropriate drug or lethal dosage

___ Failure to correctly diagnose or adequately treat v-fib, v-tach, or asystole

You must factually document your rationale for checking any of the above critical items on the reverse side of this form.

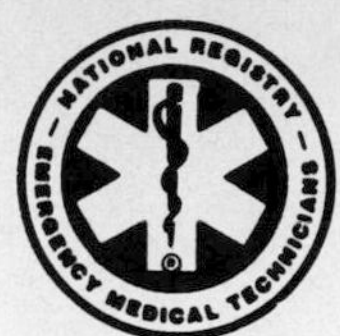

National Registry of Emergency Medical Technicians
Paramedic Practical Examination
CARDIAC ARREST SKILLS STATION
STATIC CARDIOLOGY

Candidate: ______________________ Examiner: ______________________

Date: ______________________ Signature: ______________________

Set #______________

NOTE: No points for treatment may be awarded if the diagnosis is incorrect.
Only document incorrect responses in spaces provided.

	Points Awarded	Possible Points
STRIP #1		
Diagnosis:	1	
Treatment:	2	
STRIP #2		
Diagnosis:	1	
Treatment:	2	
STRIP #3		
Diagnosis:	1	
Treatment:	2	
STRIP #4		
Diagnosis:	1	
Treatment:	2	
TOTAL	12	

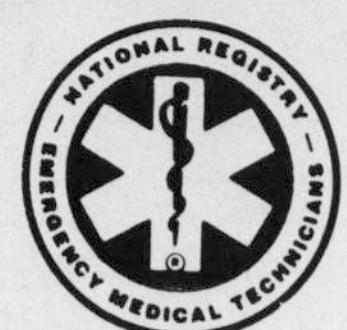

National Registry of Emergency Medical Technicians
Advanced Level Practical Examination
INTRAVENOUS THERAPY

Candidate: ______________________ Examiner: ______________________

Date: ______________________ Signature: ______________________

Time Start: __________ Time End: __________

	Possible Points	Points Awarded
Checks selected IV fluid for: –Proper fluid (1 point) –Clarity (1 point)	2	
Selects appropriate catheter	1	
Selects proper administration set	1	
Connects IV tubing to the IV bag	1	
Prepares administration set [fills drip chamber and flushes tubing]	1	
Cuts or tears tape [at any time before venipuncture]	1	
Takes/verbalizes infection control precautions [prior to venipuncture]	1	
Applies tourniquet	1	
Palpates suitable vein	1	
Cleanses site appropriately	1	
Performs venipuncture –Inserts stylette (1 point) –Notes or verbalizes flashback (1 point) –Occludes vein proximal to catheter (1 point) –Removes stylette (1 point) –Connects IV tubing to catheter (1 point)	5	
Releases tourniquet	1	
Runs IV for a brief period to assure patent line	1	
Secures catheter [tapes securely or verbalizes]	1	
Adjusts flow rate as appropriate	1	
Disposes/verbalizes disposal of needle in proper container	1	
TOTAL	21	

CRITICAL CRITERIA

___ Exceeded the 6 minute time limit in establishing a patent and properly adjusted IV
___ Failure to take or verbalize infection control precautions prior to performing venipuncture
___ Contaminates equipment or site without appropriately correcting situation
___ Any improper technique resulting in the potential for catheter shear or air embolism
___ Failure to successfully establish IV within 3 attempts during 6 minute time limit
___ Failure to dispose/verbalize disposal of needle in proper container

You must factually document your rationale for checking any of the above critical items on the reverse side of this form.

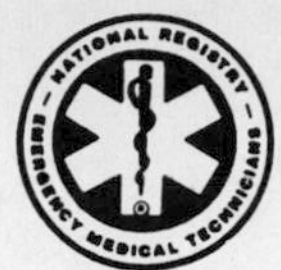

National Registry of Emergency Medical Technicians
Paramedic Practical Examination
INTRAVENOUS BOLUS MEDICATIONS

Candidate: ______________________ Examiner: ______________________

Date: ______________________ Signature: ______________________

Time Start: __________ Time End: __________

NOTE: Check here (____) if candidate did not establish a patent IV and do not evaluate these skills.

	Possible Points	Points Awarded
Asks patient for known allergies	1	
Selects correct medication	1	
Assures correct concentration of drug	1	
Assembles prefilled syringe correctly and dispels air	1	
Continues infection control precautions	1	
Cleanses injection site (Y-port or hub)	1	
Reaffirms medication	1	
Stops IV flow (pinches tubing)	1	
Administers correct dose at proper push rate	1	
Flushes tubing (runs wide open for a brief period)	1	
Adjusts drip rate to TKO (KVO)	1	
Voices proper disposal of syringe and needle	1	
Verbalizes need to observe patient for desired effect/adverse side effects	1	
IV BOLUS SUB-TOTAL	13	

CRITICAL CRITERIA

___ Failure to begin administration of medication within 3 minute time limit
___ Contaminates equipment or site without appropriately correcting situation
___ Failure to adequately dispel air resulting in potential for air embolism
___ Injects improper drug or dosage (wrong drug, incorrect amount, or pushes at inappropriate rate)
___ Failure to flush IV tubing after injecting medication
___ Recaps needle or failure to dispose/verbalize disposal of syringe and needle in proper container

INTRAVENOUS PIGGYBACK MEDICATIONS

	Possible Points	Points Awarded
Has confirmed allergies by now (award point if previously confirmed)		
Checks selected IV fluid for: –Proper fluid (1 point) –Clarity (1 point)	1 2	
Checks selected medication for: –Clarity (1 point) –Concentration of medication (1 point)	2	
Injects correct amount of medication into IV solution given scenario	1	
Connects appropriate administration set to medication solution	1	
Prepares administration set (fills drip chamber and flushes tubing)	1	
Attaches appropriate needle to administration set	1	
Continues infection control precautions	1	
Cleanses port of primary line	1	
Inserts needle into port without contamination	1	
Adjusts flow rate of secondary line as required	1	
Stops flow of primary line	1	
Securely tapes needle	1	
Verbalizes need to observe patient for desired effect/adverse side effects	1	
Labels medication/fluid bag	1	
IV PIGGYBACK SUB-TOTAL	17	

CRITICAL CRITERIA

___ Failure to begin administration of medication within 5 minute time limit
___ Contaminates equipment or site without appropriately correcting situation
___ Administers improper drug or dosage (wrong drug, incorrect amount, or infuses at inappropriate rate)
___ Failure to flush IV tubing of secondary line resulting in potential for air embolism
___ Failure to shut-off flow of primary line

You must factually document your rationale for checking any of the above critical items on the reverse side of this form.

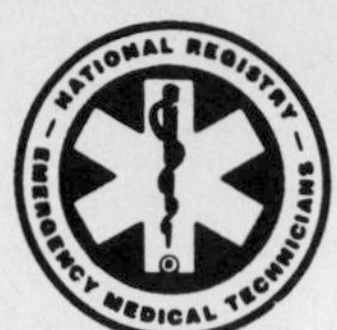

National Registry of Emergency Medical Technicians
Advanced Level Practical Examination
SPINAL IMMOBILIZATION (SEATED PATIENT)

Candidate: ______________________ **Examiner:** ______________________

Date: ______________________ **Signature:** ______________________

Time Start: __________ **Time End:** __________

	Possible Points	Points Awarded
Takes or verbalizes infection control precautions	1	
Directs assistant to place/maintain head in neutral, in-line position	1	
Directs assistant to maintain manual immobilization of head	1	
Assesses motor, sensory, and distal circulation in extremities	1	
Applies appropriately sized extrication collar	1	
Positions the immobilization device behind the patient	1	
Secures device to the patient's torso	1	
Evaluates torso fixation and adjusts as necessary	1	
Evaluates and pads behind the patient's head as necessary	1	
Secures patient's head to the device	1	
Reassesses motor, sensory, and distal circulation in extremities	1	
Verbalizes moving the patient to a long board properly	1	
TOTAL	12	

CRITICAL CRITERIA

___ Did not immediately direct or take manual immobilization of head
___ Releases or orders release of manual immobilization before it was maintained mechanically
___ Patient manipulated or moved excessively causing potential spinal compromise
___ Did not complete immobilization of the torso prior to immobilizing the head
___ Device moves excessively up, down, left, or right on patient's torso
___ Torso fixation inhibits chest rise resulting in respiratory compromise
___ Head immobilization allows for excessive movement
___ Upon completion of immobilization, head is not in neutral, in-line position

You must factually document your rationale for checking any of the above critical items on the reverse side of this form.

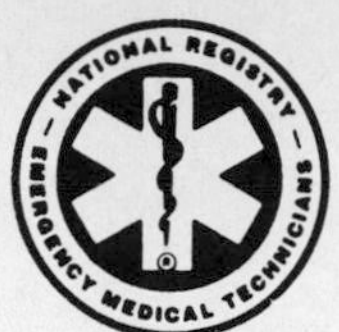

National Registry of Emergency Medical Technicians
Advanced Level Practical Examination
RANDOM BASIC SKILLS
BLEEDING–WOUNDS–SHOCK

Candidate: ______________________ **Examiner:** ______________________

Date: ______________________ **Signature:** ______________________

Time Start: __________ **Time End:** __________

	Possible Points	Points Awarded
Takes or verbalizes infection control precautions	1	
Applies direct pressure to the wound	1	
Elevates the extremity	1	
Applies pressure dressing to the wound	1	
Bandages wound	1	
NOTE: The examiner must now inform the candidate that the wound is still continuing to bleed. The second dressing does not control the bleeding.		
Locates and applies pressure to appropriate arterial pressure point	1	
NOTE: The examiner must indicate that the victim is in compensatory shock.		
Applies high concentration oxygen	1	
Properly positions patient (supine with legs elevated)	1	
Prevents heat loss (covers patient as appropriate)	1	
NOTE: The examiner must indicate that the victim is in profound shock. Medical control has ordered application and inflation of the Pneumatic Anti-shock Garment.		
Removes clothing or checks for sharp objects	1	
Quickly assesses areas that will be under the PASG	1	
Positions PASG with top of abdominal section at or below last set of ribs	1	
Secures PASG around patient	1	
Attaches hoses	1	
Begins inflation sequence (examiner to stop inflation at 15mm Hg)	1	
Checks blood pressure	1	
Verbalizes when to stop inflation sequence	1	
Operates PASG to maintain air pressure in device	1	
Reassesses vital signs	1	
TOTAL	19	

CRITICAL CRITERIA

___ Failure to take or verbalize infection control precautions
___ Did not apply high concentration of oxygen
___ Applies tourniquet before attempting other methods of hemorrhage control
___ Did not control hemorrhage or attempt to control hemorrhage in a timely manner
___ Inflates abdominal section of PASG before the legs
___ Did not reassess patient's vital signs after PASG inflation
___ Places PASG on inside-out
___ Allows deflation of PASG after inflation
___ Positions PASG above level of lowest rib

You must factually document your rationale for checking any of the above critical items on the reverse side of this form.

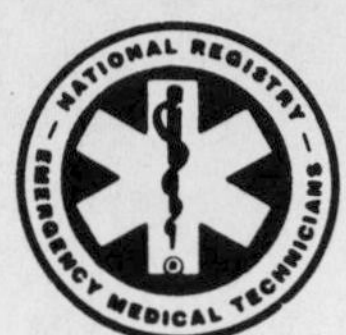

National Registry of Emergency Medical Technicians
Advanced Level Practical Examination
RANDOM BASIC SKILLS
LONG BONE IMMOBILIZATION

Candidate: ______________________ **Examiner:** ______________________

Date: ______________________ **Signature:** ______________________

Time Start: __________ **Time End:** __________

	Possible Points	Points Awarded
Takes or verbalizes infection control precautions	1	
Directs application of manual stabilization	1	
Assesses motor, sensory, and distal circulation	1	
NOTE: Examiner acknowledges present and normal		
Measures splint	1	
Applies splint	1	
Immobilizes joint above fracture	1	
Immobilizes joint below fracture	1	
Secures entire injured extremity	1	
Immobilizes hand/foot in position of function	1	
Reassesses motor, sensory, and distal circulation	1	
NOTE: Examiner acknowledged present and normal		
TOTAL	10	

CRITICAL CRITERIA

___ Grossly moves injured extremity
___ Did not immobilize adjacent joints, injury, or limb
___ Did not reassess motor, sensory, and distal circulation **after** splinting

You must factually document your rationale for checking any of the above critical items on the reverse side of this form.

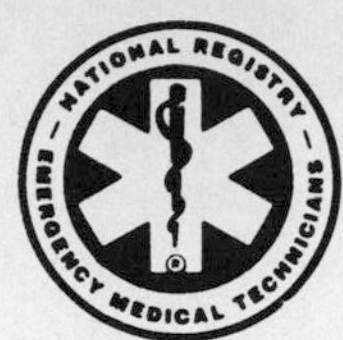

National Registry of Emergency Medical Technicians
Advanced Level Practical Examination
RANDOM BASIC SKILLS
TRACTION SPLINTING

Candidate: ______________________ **Examiner:** ______________________

Date: ______________________ **Signature:** ______________________

Time Start: ____________ **Time End:** ____________

	Possible Points	Points Awarded
Takes or verbalizes infection control precautions	1	
Directs manual stabilization of injured leg	1	
Directs application of manual traction	1	
Assesses motor, sensory, and distal circulation	1	
NOTE: Examiner acknowledges present and normal		
Prepares/adjusts splint to proper length	1	
Positions splint at injured leg	1	
Applies proximal securing device (e.g. ischial strap)	1	
Applies distal securing device (e.g. ankle hitch)	1	
Applies mechanical traction	1	
Positions/secures support straps	1	
Re-evaluates proximal/distal securing devices	1	
Reassesses motor, sensory, and distal circulation	1	
NOTE: Examiner acknowledges present and normal		
NOTE: Examiner must ask candidate how he/she would prepare for transport		
Verbalizes securing torso to long board to immobilize hip	1	
Verbalizes securing splint to long board to prevent movement of splint	1	
TOTAL	14	

CRITICAL CRITERIA

___ Loss of traction at any point after it is assumed
___ Did not reassess motor, sensory, and distal circulation **after** splinting
___ The foot is excessively rotated or extended after splinting
___ Did not secure ischial strap **before** taking traction
___ Final immobilization failed to support femur or prevent rotation of injured leg

NOTE: If Sagar is used without elevating the leg, application of manual traction is not necessary. Candidate will be awarded 1 point as if manual traction were applied.

NOTE: If the leg is elevated at all, manual traction must be applied before elevating the leg. The ankle hitch may be applied before elevating the leg and used to pull manual traction.

You must factually document your rationale for checking any of the above critical items on the reverse side of this form.

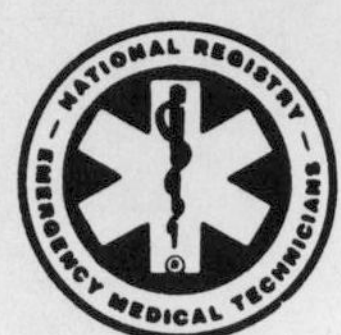

National Registry of Emergency Medical Technicians
Advanced Level Practical Examination
RANDOM BASIC SKILLS
SPINAL IMMOBILIZATION
(LYING PATIENT)

Candidate: ____________________ **Examiner:** ____________________

Date: ____________________ **Signature:** ____________________

Time Start: __________ **Time End:** __________

	Possible Points	Points Awarded
Takes or verbalizes infection control procedures	1	
Directs assistant to move patient's head to the neutral in-line position	1	
Directs assistant to maintain manual immobilization of head	1	
Evaluates motor, sensory, and distal circulation in extremities	1	
Applies cervical collar	1	
Positions immobilization device appropriately	1	
Moves victim onto device without compromising the integrity of the spine	1	
Applies padding to voids between the torso and the board as necessary	1	
Immobilizes torso to the device	1	
Evaluates and pads under the patient's head as necessary	1	
Immobilizes the patient's head to the device	1	
Secures legs to the device	1	
Secures victims arms to the board	1	
Reassesses motor, sensory, and distal circulation	1	
TOTAL	14	

CRITICAL CRITERIA

___ Did not immediately direct manual immobilization of head

___ Orders release of manual immobilization before it was maintained mechanically

___ Did not complete immobilization of the torso prior to immobilizing the head

___ Device excessively moves up, down, left or right on patient's torso

___ Head immobilization allows for excessive movement

___ Head is not immobilized in the neutral in-line position

___ Patient was moved excessively causing potential spinal compromise

___ Did not reassess motor, sensory, and distal circulation after immobilization

You must factually document your rationale for checking any of the above critical items on the reverse side of this form.

EMERGENCY DRUG CARDS

The following pages contain prepared three-by-five index cards. Each card represents one of the drugs commonly used by the paramedic. They identify the name and class of the drug, a short description, its indications, contraindications, precautions and common dosages, and routes of administration.

Detach the cards and review each one in detail. Be sure that your instructor identifies which are used in your system and which need to be modified to indicate your system's indications, contra-indications, precautions, doses, and methods of administration. You may also wish to prepare cards for the drugs used in your system yet not included with the cards contained herein.

Once your cards are prepared, begin to memorize all the information contained on the card when presented with the drug name. You will notice that the drug name appears on the back of each card. Working on just a few cards each week and then reviewing them as your course progresses will help you commit to memory the essential information you must know about each drug.

Name/Class:	**OXYGEN**
Description:	An odorless, colorless, tasteless gas that is essential for life. It is one of the most important emergency drugs.
Indications:	Hypoxia or anticipated hypoxia, cardiac arrest, chest pain, dyspnea, shock or anticipated shock.
Contra-indications:	Chronic CO_2 retention (COPD) unless respiratory failure is imminent. (Use a low-flow device.)
Precautions:	Chronic pulmonary disease and prolonged administration of high concentrations in the newborn.
Dosage/Route:	Arrest 100%, Hypoxia - 10 to 15 LPM, Chest Pain - 6 to 8 LPM, COPD - 0 to 2 LPM.

Name/Class:	**EPINEPHRINE (Adrenalin) / Sympathomimetic**
Description:	A potent alpha & beta stimulant that is diluted 1 mg in 1 mL (1:1,000) or 1 mg in 10 mL (1:10,000) of saline. It increases the electrical activity of the heart through its beta activities.
Indications:	Fine ventricular fibrillation, asystole, EMD, asthma and anaphylaxis.
Contra-indications:	None in the patient who needs aggressive resuscitation.
Precautions:	It should be protected from light and should not be infused with alkaline solutions, such as sodium bicarbonate, since they will deactivate epinephrine. The drug's actions are of short duration.
Dosage/Route:	1:10,000 - 0.5 to 1.0 mg IV repeated every 5 minutes as needed followed by a 20 mL flush. (ET - 2.0 to 2.5 mg) 1:1,000 - 0.3 to 0.5 mg SQ.

OXYGEN

EPINEPHRINE

Name/Class:	**NOREPINEPHRINE (Levophed) / Sympathomimetic**
Description:	It is a strong alpha agent that causes peripheral vasoconstriction. It is very effective in raising blood pressure in normo-volemic states.
Indications:	Cardiogenic shock and neurogenic shock.
Contra-indications:	Hypotension due to hypovolemia.
Precautions:	Blood pressure must be frequently monitored and the drug infused through the largest vein available. It may cause tissue necrosis. It may be deactivated by alkaline agents like sodium bicarbonate.
Dosage/Route:	4 mg in 250 mL or 8 mg in 500 mL of D_5W (16mcg/mL). 2 to 12 mcg/min - run IV piggyback and titrated to blood pressure.

Name/Class:	**ISOPROTERENOL (Isuprel) / Sympathomimetic**
Description:	A potent beta agent with virtually no alpha properties. It primarily affects the heart by increasing rate and strength of contraction. It increases myocardial oxygen consumption.
Indications:	Bradydysrhythmias refractory to atropine and high degree heart blocks (2nd degree Mobitz II & 3rd degree) which are symptomatic.
Contra-indications:	It should not be used to increase blood pressure in cardiogenic shock or for non-cardiogenic bradydysrhythmias.
Precautions:	Monitor for ventricular irritability (e.g.: PVCs, V-tach, etc.). Lidocaine should be readily available. May be deactivated by alkaline solutions. Isuprel may increase infarct size.
Dosage/Route:	1 mg in 500 mL of D_5W (2 mcg/mL) IV piggyback. 2 to 10 mcg/min - titrated to desired heart rate.

Name/Class:	**DOPAMINE (Intropin) / Sympathomimetic**
Description:	A beta agonist that does not appreciably increase myocardial oxygen consumption. It maintains renal and mesenteric blood flow while inducing vasoconstriction and increasing blood pressure.
Indications:	Cardiogenic shock and hypovolemic shock after fluid resuscitation.
Contra-indications:	Hypotension due to hypovolemia without aggressive fluid resuscitation.
Precautions:	Tachydysrhythmias and ventricular fibrillation or irritability. May be deactivated by alkaline solutions. Reduce the dosage if the patient is on monoamine oxidase inhibitors (antidepressant). The blood pressure should be constantly monitored.
Dosage/Route:	800 mg/500 mL or 400 mg/250 mL of D_5W (1600 mcg/mL) 2 to 5 mcg/kg/min - titrated to blood pressure IV piggyback.

NOREPINEPHRINE

ISOPROTERENOL

DOPAMINE

Name/Class:	**DOBUTAMINE (Dobutrex) / Sympathomimetic**
Description:	It is a beta agent similar to Isuprel with less inotropic effect. It increases the strength of contraction without appreciably increasing rate.
Indications:	The short term treatment of congestive heart failure.
Contra-indications:	Hypovolemic shock without aggressive fluid resuscitation.
Precautions:	Monitor for tachydysrhythmias, ventricular ectopy or irritability and elevated blood pressure. Lidocaine should be available and the blood pressure frequently monitored.
Dosage/Route:	250 mg/500 mL of D_5W (500 mcg/mL) IV. 2.5 to 20 mcg/kg/min - titrated to patient response.

Name/Class:	**LABETALOL (Trandate) (Normodyne) / Sympathetic Blocker**
Description:	It is a nonselective beta blocker that also has alpha blocker characteristics. It will reduce cardiac output, induce vasodilatation, and lower blood pressure.
Indications:	Acute management of hypertensive crisis.
Contra-indications:	Bronchial asthma, CHF, heart block, bradycardia or cardiogenic shock.
Precautions:	Monitor the vital signs and the ECG for signs of cardiovascular collapse or the development of CHF, bradycardia, heart block, or bronchospasm. The patient should be kept supine during administration of the drug.
Dosage/Route:	20 mg via slow (2 minute) IV, then 40 mg every 10 minutes until 300 mg. - or - a continuous drip of 200 mg in 250 mL of D_5W (0.8 mg/mL) - 2 mg (2.5 mL)/min.

Name/Class:	**LIDOCAINE (Xylocaine) / Antidysrhythmic**
Description:	Lidocaine is an agent that increases the fibrillation threshold thereby reducing the development of ectopy and ventricular fibrillation.
Indications:	More than 6 unifocal PVCs per minute, multifocal PVCs, couplets, runs of PVCs, ventricular tachycardia, and in ventricular fibrillation after defibrillation in the acute MI.
Contra-indications:	2nd degree Mobitz II and 3rd degree heart blocks and bradycardias.
Precautions:	Side effects include: lowering LOC, confusion, irritability, muscle spasm, seizures, coma and possibly death.
Dosage/Route:	1 to 1.5 mg/kg then 0.5 mg/kg followed by 0.5 tp0.75 mg/kg every 5 to 10 min to effect or 3mg/kg. 2 gm/500 mL D_5W(4 mg/mL) - 2 to 4 mg/min, titrated to effect.

DOBUTAMINE

LABETALOL

LIDOCAINE

Name/Class: **BRETYLIUM TOSYLATE (Bretylol) / Antidysrhythmic**

Description: Like lidocaine, bretylium raises the fibrillation threshold and thereby reduces ectopy and the potential for fibrillation. In some isolated cases bretylium has converted ventricular fibrillation.

Indications: Ventricular fibrillation, ventricular tachycardia, or ventricular ectopy which is refractory to lidocaine.

Contra-indications: None in the presence of life threatening dysrhythmias.

Precautions: Its effects are evident only after 3 to 5 minutes. It may induce postural hypotension so the patient should be kept supine. The blood pressure should be frequently monitored.

Dosage/Route: 5 mg/kg IV bolus followed by 10 mg/kg every 15 to 30 minutes. IV bolus, maximum 30 mg/kg.

Name/Class: **PROCAINAMIDE (Pronestyl) / Antidysrhythmic**

Description: It is a second line drug used in the treatment of ventricular dysrhythmias after lidocaine.

Indications: Ventricular fibrillation, ventricular tachycardia, or ventricular ectopy which are refractory to lidocaine.

Contra-indications: It should not be administered in the presence of severe conduction disturbances, especially 2nd degree Mobitz II and 3rd degree heart block.

Precautions: It may induce postural hypotension so the patient should be kept supine with the blood pressure frequently monitored. If the QRS complex is widened by more than 50% stop the administration.

Dosage/Route: 100 mg IV over 5 minutes. No more than 1 gm total.
1 gm / 500 mL D_5W (2 mg/mL) - 1 to 4 mL/min, titrated to effect.

Name/Class: **VERAPAMIL (Isoptin) (Calan) / Antidysrhythmic**

Description: It is a calcium channel blocker that suppresses dysrhythmias caused by re-entry, such as paroxysmal supraventricular tachycardia. It slows rapid ventricular responses to atrial tachydysrhythmias and reduces myocardial oxygen demand.

Indications: Paroxysmal supraventricular tachycardia, atrial flutter, and atrial fibrillation with rapid ventricular response.

Contra-indications: Hypotension, cardiogenic shock, ventricular tachycardia, and Wolff-Parkinson-White syndrome. It should not be administered to persons taking beta blockers

Precautions: Potential systemic hypotension requires constant monitoring of blood pressure.

Dosage/Route: 3 to 5 mg IV bolus over 2 to 3 minutes followed by 5 to 10 mg after 10 to 15 minutes. No more than 15 mg in a 30 minute period.

BRETYLIUM TOSYLATE

PROCAINAMIDE

VERAPAMIL

Name/Class:	**ATROPINE SULFATE / Parasympatholytic**
Description:	It blocks the parasympathetic nervous system and its inhibiting effects on heart rate. It does not increase the strength of cardiac contraction.
Indications:	Bradycardia with hypotension or escape beats, asystole, and organophosphate poisoning.
Contra-indications:	None in the emergency setting.
Precautions:	Give no more than 2.0 mg for cardiac-related problems.
Dosage/Route:	Bradycardia: 0.5 mg IV quickly every 5 minutes up to 2.0 mg. Asystole: 1.0 mg IV or ET Organophosphate: 1.0 mg, if effective give 2 to 5 mg

Name/Class:	**SODIUM BICARBONATE ($NaHCO_3$) / Alkalizing agent**
Description:	It provides bicarbonate to assist the buffer system in reducing the effects of acidosis.
Indications:	Severe acidosis, prolonged cardiac arrest (after ventilation and other problems have been taken care of), and for tricyclic anti-depressant overdose.
Contra-indications:	None when used in severe hypoxia or late cardiac arrest.
Precautions:	May cause alkalosis if given too aggressively. It may also deactivate vasopressors, and may precipitate with calcium chloride.
Dosage/Route:	1 mEq/kg initially and may be followed by 0.5 mEq/kg. It is administered IV only.

Name/Class:	**MORPHINE SULFATE / Analgesic**
Description:	It is a potent analgesic which also causes some vasodilatation. It reduces myocardial oxygen demand.
Indications:	Severe pain associated with myocardial infarction, kidney stones, etc. It may also be given for pulmonary edema with or without chest pain.
Contra-indications:	It is not given in patients with head trauma or abdominal pain, hypersensitivity to the drug, hypotension, or volume depletion.
Precautions:	It may cause respiratory depression. Naloxone should be readily available to counteract the effects of morphine.
Dosage/Route:	2 to 5 mg IV push followed by 2 mg every few minutes as needed. 5 to 15 mg may be given IM.

ATROPINE SULFATE

SODIUM BICARBONATE

MORPHINE SULFATE

Name/Class: **NITROUS OXIDE (Nitronox) / Analgesic**

Description: It is a self-administered gas composed of 50% oxygen and 50% nitrous oxide. It has strong analgesic properties which last only 2 to 5 minutes after administration ceases.

Indications: Moderate to severe pain and anxiety.

Contra-indications: It should not be administered to patients with possible bowel obstruction, pneumothorax, COPD, or severe head injury.

Precautions: It may cause nausea and vomiting.

Dosage/Route: It is self administered until the pain is relieved or the patient discontinues the administration.

Name/Class: **FUROSEMIDE (Lasix) / Diuretic**

Description: It is a potent diuretic that inhibits sodium reabsorption by the kidney. Water is eliminated with the sodium. Its effects are noted within 5 minutes.

Indications: Congestive heart failure and pulmonary edema.

Contra-indications: Pregnancy (except in life-threatening circumstances).

Precautions: Severe dehydration and electrolyte depletion may result from excessive doses of Lasix. It must be protected from light.

Dosage/Route: 20 mg (and 40 mg for those already on the medication) IV slowly. Dosages as high as 80 mg may be required.

Name/Class: **NITROGLYCERIN (Nitro Stat) / Antianginal agent**

Description: It is a rapid smooth muscle relaxant that reduces cardiac workload and, to a lesser degree, dilates the coronary arteries.

Indications: Chest pain associated with angina and myocardial infarction, and acute pulmonary edema.

Contra-indications: Increased intracranial hemorrhage.

Precautions: It may induce headache which is sometimes severe. Patients may develop tolerance. Nitroglycerin is light sensitive and will lose potency when exposed to the air.

Dosage/Route: 1 or 2 tablets (0.4 mg) sublingually.

NITROUS OXIDE

FUROSEMIDE

NITROGLYCERIN

Name/Class:	**NITROGLYCERIN SPRAY (Nitrolingual Spray) / Antianginal**
Description:	It is an aerosol preparation that delivers exactly 0.4 mg with each spray. Peak effect in four minutes.
Indications:	Chest pain associated with angina and the myocardial infarction.
Contra-indications:	Increased intracranial hemorrhage.
Precautions:	It may induce headache which is sometimes severe. Patients may develop tolerance.
Dosage/Route:	1 spray (0.4 mg) under the tongue. No more than 3 sprays in 25 minutes. The spray should not be inhaled.

Name/Class:	**NIFEDIPINE (Procardia) / Anti-hypertensive**
Description:	It is a calcium channel blocker that reduces coronary artery spasm in angina. It also decreases peripheral vascular resistance and blood pressure.
Indications:	Severe hypertension and angina.
Contra-indications:	Hypersensitivity to the drug. It should not be given to patients receiving IV beta blockers.
Precautions:	Blood pressure should be constantly watched since it can drop significantly with nifedipine use. It should be used with caution in the heart failure patient.
Dosage/Route:	One 10 mg capsule is punctured and placed under the patient's tongue. The patient may also bite and swallow the capsule.

Name/Class:	**DIAZOXIDE (Hyperstat) / Antihypertensive**
Description:	It reduces both systolic and diastolic blood pressure by causing vasodilatation of the peripheral arterioles.
Indications:	Malignant hypertension if rapid reduction in blood pressure is required.
Contra-indications:	None.
Precautions:	Blood pressure should be constantly monitored because diazoxide may cause hypotension rapidly. Hypotension should be treated with sympathomimetics.
Dosage/Route:	1 to 3 mg/kg (up to 150 mg) rapidly IV, may be repeated every 5 to 15 minutes. The drug should be given in a large vein only.

NITROGLYCERIN SPRAY

NIFEDIPINE

DIAZOXIDE

Name/Class: CALCIUM CHLORIDE

Description: It increases myocardial contractile force and may increase ventricular automaticity.

Indications: Hyperkalemia and hypocalcemia. It may also be used to counteract magnesium sulfate used in eclampsia.

Contra-indications: It may precipitate toxicity in patients taking digitalis.

Precautions: Ensure the IV line is flushed before using calcium, especially if bicarbonate is being used.

Dosage/Route: 250 to 500 mg IV repeated every 10 minutes.

Name/Class: AMINOPHYLLINE

Description: It is a dilute theophylline preparation that induces broncho-dilatation. It also is a mild diuretic and causes increased heart rate and cardiac output.

Indications: Bronchial asthma, bronchospasm in emphysema and chronic bronchitis, congestive heart failure, and pulmonary edema.

Contra-indications: Hypersensitivity to the drug.

Precautions: Caution should be exercised with any history of cardiovascular disease or hypertension. ECG monitoring is indicated to observe for PVCs or tachycardia. May cause hypotension.

Dosage/Route: 250 in 90 mL or 500 mg in 80 mL of D_5W, infused over 20 to 30 minutes. If CHF or pulmonary edema, place 250 or 500 mg in 20 mL of D_5W then infuse over 20 to 30 minutes.

Name/Class: RACEMIC EPINEPHRINE (microNEFRIN) (Vaponefrin)

Description: It is a variation of epinephrine used only for inhalation.

Indications: Croup (laryngotracheobronchitis)

Contra-indications: Epiglottitis.

Precautions: May result in tachycardia and other dysrhythmias. Patient vital signs and ECG should be monitored.

Dosage/Route: 0.5 mL of a 2.5% solution in 4 mL NS and given once by nebulizer.

CALCIUM CHLORIDE

AMINOPHYLLINE

RACEMIC EPINEPHRINE

Name/Class: **TERBUTALINE (Brethine) / Sympathomimetic**

Description: It is a synthetic sympathomimetic that causes bronchodilatation with less cardiac effect than epinephrine.

Indications: Bronchial asthma, and bronchospasm in emphysema and chronic bronchitis.

Contra-indications: Hypersensitivity to the drug.

Precautions: The patient may experience palpitations, anxiety, nausea, and/or dizziness. Vital signs must be monitored; use caution with cardiac or hypertensive patients.

Dosage/Route: 0.25 mg SQ with a second dose at 15 minutes if ineffective.

Name/Class: **ALBUTEROL (Proventil) (Ventolin) / Sympathomimetic**

Description: It is a synthetic sympathomimetic that causes bronchodilatation with less cardiac effect than epinephrine. The duration of effect is about four hours.

Indications: Bronchial asthma, and bronchospasm in emphysema and chronic bronchitis.

Contra-indications: Hypersensitivity to the drug.

Precautions: The patient may experience palpitations, anxiety, nausea, and/or dizziness. Vital signs must be monitored; use caution with cardiac or hypertensive patients.

Dosage/Route: 2.5 mg in 2 to 3 mL NS, administered by updraft nebulizer.
2 inhalations repeated every 4 to 6 hours.

Name/Class: **50% DEXTROSE IN WATER ($D_{50}W$)**

Description: Dextrose is a simple sugar that the body can rapidly metabolize while in hypoglycemic states.

Indications: Hypoglycemia, acute alcoholism with coma, and altered level of consciousness.

Contra-indications: None.

Precautions: Draw sample blood and determine glucose level before administration. Ensure good venous access.

Dosage/Route: 50 ml of $D_{50}W$ (25 gm) IV, may be repeated.

TERBUTALINE

ALBUTEROL

50% DEXTROSE IN WATER

Name/Class: **THIAMINE / Vitamin**

Description: Thiamine is vitamin B_1 which is required to convert glucose into energy. It is not manufactured by the body and must be constantly provided from ingested foods.

Indications: Coma of unknown origin, chronic alcoholism with associated coma, and delirium tremens.

Contra-indications: None.

Precautions: Known hypersensitivity to the drug.

Dosage/Route: 100 mg either IV (preferred) or IM.

Name/Class: **METHYLPREDNISOLONE (Solu-Medrol) / Steroid**

Description: It is a synthetic steroid that is often administered to patients with spinal cord injury. It is thought to minimize swelling of the cord and enhance neurological recovery.

Indications: Spinal cord injury, asthma, severe anaphylaxis.

Contra-indications: No major contraindications.

Precautions: Only a single dose should be given in the prehospital setting.

Dosage/Route: Asthma/anaphylaxis: 60 to 125 mg IV.

Spinal cord injury: An initial bolus of 30 mg/kg over 15 min., after 45 min. an infusion of 5.4 mg/kg/hr.

Name/Class: **DIAZEPAM (Valium) / Anticonvulsant**

Description: It is a smooth muscle relaxant that reduces tremors, induces amnesia, and reduces the incidence and recurrence of seizures.

Indications: Major motor seizures, status epilepticus, premedication prior to cardioversion, muscle tremors due to injury, and acute anxiety states.

Contra-indications: Hypersensitivity.

Precautions: Due to a short half-life of the drug, seizure activity may recur.

Dosage/Route: 2 to 5 mg IV (sometimes as much as 15 mg).

THIAMINE

METHYL-PREDNISOLONE

DIAZEPAM

Name/Class: **OXYTOCIN (Pitocin) / Synthetic hormone**

Description: It is a natural occurring hormone that causes the uterus to contract. It helps induce labor, encourages delivery of the placenta, and controls post-partum hemorrhage.

Indications: Severe post-partum hemorrhage.

Contra-indications: Administration prior to delivery of the infant or infants.

Precautions: May induce uterine rupture, dysrhythmias, hypertension, or anaphylaxis. Uterine tone, ECG and vital signs should be monitored during administration.

Dosage/Route: 3 to 10 units IM after delivery of the placenta.
10 to 20 units in 500 to 1000 mL D_5W IV - titrated to effect.

Name/Class: **MAGNESIUM SULFATE / Anticonvulsant**

Description: It is an anticonvulsant, especially effective in the control of seizures associated with eclampsia.

Indications: Seizures due to eclampsia (toxemia of pregnancy).

Contra-indications: Patients with heart block or recent myocardial infarction.

Precautions: May cause hypotension, circulatory collapse, or cardiac and respiratory depression. Calcium chloride should be available to counteract the untoward effects of magnesium.

Dosage/Route: 1 gm IV.

Name/Class: **DIPHENHYDRAMINE (Benadryl) / Antihistamine**

Description: It inhibits the release of histamine, thereby reducing broncho-constriction and vasodilation.

Indications: Anaphylaxis, allergic reactions, and uticaria.

Contra-indications: Asthma and other lower respiratory diseases.

Precautions: May induce hypotension, headache, palpitations, tachycardia, sedation, drowsiness, and/or disturbed coordination.

Dosage/Route: 25 to 50 mg IV or IM.

OXYTOCIN

MAGNESIUM
SULFATE

DIPHENHYDRAMINE

Name/Class:	**SYRUP OF IPECAC / Emetic**
Description:	It acts on the emetic centers of the brain and on the stomach to induce vomiting. Emesis usually occurs within 10 minutes.
Indications:	Poisoning and overdose.
Contra-indications:	Reduced level of consciousness, corrosive ingestion, petroleum distillate ingestion, alkali ingestion, or antiemetic ingestion (especially phenothiazine).
Precautions:	Monitor the airway and have suction ready. Do not administer activated charcoal until emesis has occurred.
Dosage/Route:	15 to 30 mL orally followed by 2 to 3 glasses of warm water or carbonated beverage.

Name/Class:	**ACTIVATED CHARCOAL (Actidose) (Sorbitol)**
Description:	It is a specially prepared charcoal with a surface that will absorb and bind toxins.
Indications:	Poisoning following emesis or in cases where emesis is contraindicated.
Contra-indications:	An airway that cannot be controlled.
Precautions:	Administer only after emesis or in those cases where emesis is contraindicated.
Dosage/Route:	50 gm (2 tablespoons) mixed with a glass of water, then given orally or through a nasal gastric tube.

Name/Class:	**NALOXONE (Narcan) / Narcotic antagonist**
Description:	It is an effective agent that blocks the effects of both natural and synthetic narcotics. It may be helpful in coma due to alcohol ingestion.
Indications:	Narcotic and synthetic narcotic overdose, alcohol induced coma, and coma of unknown origin.
Contra-indications:	Hypersensitivity.
Precautions:	May induce withdrawal. It also has a half-life that is shorter than most narcotics, hence the patient may return to the overdose state.
Dosage/Route:	1 to 2 mg IV, a second dose at 5 minutes if unsuccessful. 2 to 5 mg for Darvon overdoses and alcohol coma. Infusion: 2 mg / 500 mL D_5W (4 mcg/mL) - 100 mL per hour.

SYRUP OF IPECAC

ACTIVATED CHARCOAL

NALOXONE

Name/Class:	**HALOPERIDOL (Haldol) / Tranquilizer**
Description:	It is believed to block dopamine receptors in the brain associated with mood and behavior.
Indications:	Acute psychotic episodes.
Contra-indications:	Should not be given in the presence of other sedatives nor in dysphoria induced by Talwin.
Precautions:	It may impair mental and physical ability and cause orthostatic hypertension. It should be used with caution for those on anticoagulants and for patients with hypertension. The dosage should be reduced for the elderly. May cause extrapyramidal reactions.
Dosage/Route:	2 to 5 mg IM.

Name/Class:	**PROMETHAZINE (Phenergan) / Antihistamine**
Description:	It is an anticholinergic agent that enhances the effects of analgesics and is a potent antiemetic.
Indications:	Nausea and vomiting, motion sickness, and to enhance the effects of analgesics.
Contra-indications:	Comatose patients, hypersensitivity, and those who have received large amounts of depressants.
Precautions:	It may impair mental and physical ability. Avoid intra-arterial injection and do not administer subcutaneously.
Dosage/Route:	12.5 to 25 mg IV or deep IM for nausea and vomiting. 25 mg for use with analgesics.

Name/Class:	**ADENOSINE (Adenocard) / Antiarrhythmic**
Description:	It a naturally occuring agent that can "chemically cardiovert" PSVT to a normal sinus rhythm. It has a half life of 5 seconds and does not cause hypotension like verapamil.
Indications:	Narrow complex paroxysmal supraventricular tachycardia refractory to vagal maneuvers.
Contra - Indications:	Second and third degree heart block, sick sinus syndrome, or known hypersensitivity to the drug.
Precautions:	It may cause transient dysrhythmias. It may cause bronchospasm in asthma patients.
Dosage/Route:	6 mg rapidly (over 1 to 3 seconds) given near the vein. Then flush the line with saline. If ineffective, rebolus with 12 mg. in one to two minutes. Dose may be repeated.

HALOPERIDOL

PROMETHAZINE

ADENOSINE